# ACSM's Resources for the Group Exercise Instructor

**EDITOR**
**GRACE DeSIMONE, BA, ACSM-CPT, ACSM-GEI**
National Group Fitness Director
Plus One Health Management
New York, New York

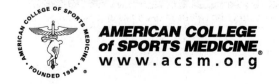

**AMERICAN COLLEGE of SPORTS MEDICINE**®
FOUNDED 1954
w w w . a c s m . o r g

Wolters Kluwer | Lippincott Williams & Wilkins
Health
Philadelphia · Baltimore · New York · London
Buenos Aires · Hong Kong · Sydney · Tokyo

*Acquisitions Editor:* Emily Lupash
*Product Manager:* Andrea Klingler
*Marketing Manager:* Christen Murphy
*Designer:* Doug Smock
*Compositor:* SPi Global

© 2012 American College of Sports Medicine

351 West Camden Street
Baltimore, MD 21201

Two Commerce Square
2001 Market Street
Philadelphia, PA 19103

Printed in China

**Library of Congress Cataloging-in-Publication Data**
DeSimone, Grace.
  ACSM's resources for the group exercise instructor / Grace DeSimone. – 1st ed.
    p. ; cm.
  Resources for the group exercise instructor
  Includes bibliographical references.
  ISBN 978-1-60831-196-5 (pbk.)
 1. Physical education and training. 2. Exercise. I. DeSimone, Grace. II. American College of Sports Medicine.
III. Title. IV. Title: Resources for the group exercise instructor.
  [DNLM: 1. Physical Education and Training. 2. Exercise—physiology. 3. Teaching—methods. 4. Vocational
Guidance. QT 255]
  GV341.D385   2012
  613.7—dc23

                                                            2011026334

To purchase additional copies of this book, call our customer service department at **(800) 638-3030** or fax orders to **(301) 223-2320**. International customers should call **(301) 223-2300**.

*Visit Lippincott Williams & Wilkins on the Internet: http://www.lww.com.* Lippincott Williams & Wilkins customer service representatives are available from 8:30 am to 6:00 pm, EST.

9 8 7 6 5 4 3 2 1

*To Jim, Lauren, and Brian for their love and support*
*and for reminding me of what is really important.*
*And to my Mom, for always being there*

# Contributors

**Ken Alan, BS, ACSM-GEL**
California State University
Fullerton, California

**Mary Ann Rumplasch, MA, ACSM-HFS, ACE-CPT, GFI**
Plus One Health Management
New York, New York

**Shirley Archer, JD, MA, ACSM-HFS**
Shirley S Archer Associates, LLC
Singer Island, Florida
Zurich, Switzerland

**Nancy J. Belli, MA, ACSM-HFS, ACE-CPT**
Asphalt Green
New York, New York

**Teri L. Bladen, MS, ACSM HFS, ACE-CPT, NIRSA-RCRSP**
Weber State University
Ogden, UT

**Grace DeSimone, BA, ACSM-CPT, ACSM-GEI**
Plus One Health Management
New York, New York

**Shannon Fable, BA**
Sunshine Fitness Resources, LLC
Boulder, Colorado

**Liza Forster, RYT**
Plus One Health Management
New York, New York

**Karen A. Kent, MS, ACSM-HFS**
Amgen BioFit Wellness Center
Narragansett, Rhode Island

**Jerry J. Mayo, PhD, RD**
Arkansas Tech University
Russellville, Arkansas

**Caroline Milani, BA, Master's Certification**
Gold's Gym
Lawrenceville, New Jersey
SuperGym
Jackson, New Jersey

**David Milani, MSHRM, SPHR, CEBS**
Plus One Health Management
New York, New York

**Gavin Moir, PhD, USAW**
East Stroudsburg University of Pennsylvania
East Stroudsburg, Pennsylvania

**Leslie Stenger, PhD, ACSM-HFS**
Indiana University of Pennsylvania
Indiana, Pennsylvania

**Felicia D. Stoler, DCN, MS, RD, FACSM**
Registered Dietitian and Exercise Physiologist
Holmdel, New Jersey

Mary Ann Rumplasch, MA, ACSM-HFS ACE-CPT, GFI
Plus One Health Management
New York, New York

Sherry Barkley, PhD, ACSM-CES, RCEP
Augustana College
Sioux Falls, South Dakota

Nancy J. Belli, MA, ACSM-HFS, ACE-CPT
Asphalt Green
New York, New York

Teri L. Bladen, MS, ACSM HFS, ACE-CPT, NIRSA-RCRSP
Weber State University
Ogden, Utah

Nikki Carosone, MS, ACSM-CPT
Plus One Health Management
New York, New York

Kim DeLeo, BS, PTA, ACSM-CPT
Health and Exercise Connections, LLC
People First Rehabilitation
Mattapoisett, Massachusetts

Julie Downing, PhD, ACSM-CPT, HFD, FACSM
Central Oregon Community College
Bend, Oregon

Gregory B. Dwyer, PhD, FACSM ACSM- CES, RCEP, PD
East Stroudsburg University of Pennsylvania
East Stroudsburg, Pennsylvania

Yuri Feito, PhD, MPH
Barry University
Miami Shores, Florida

Amanda Harris, MEd, ACSM-HFS, MES
ACAC Fitness & Wellness Center
Midlothian, Virginia

Lisa Helfrich, BS
FM Global Total Health Fitness Center
Johnston, Rhode Island

Madeline Paternostro Bayles, PhD, ACSM-CES, PD, FACSM
Indiana University of PA
Indiana, Pennsylvania

Wendy Petulla, ACE-GFI
Community Boot Camp
San Jose, California

Neal Pire, MA, ACSM-HFS, CSCS, FACSM
Inspire Training Systems
Ridgewood, New Jersey

Alicia Racela, BS, CSCS, ACSM-HFS, CWC
Phase 4, LLC
Kapolei, Hawaii

Paul Sorace, MS, ACSM-RCEP
Hackensack University Medical Center
Hackensack, New Jersey

Tom Spring, MS, FAACVPR ACSM-CES, HFS
Beaumont Health System
Royal Oak, Michiga

Leslie Stenger, PhD, ACSM-HFS
Indiana University of Pennsylvania
Indiana, Pennsylvania
New York, New York

# Foreword

Moving to music isn't a new concept. Neither is gathering a group to share the exhilarating experience of exercise. However, back in 1980, choreographing moves to music in front of people wearing athletic shoes and leotards was a new and unique idea. "Aerobics"—a word coined by Kenneth H. Cooper, MD, MPH, founder and chairman of the Cooper Aerobics Center—grapevined its way into mainstream America and then quickly spread globally. Thus began a revolution that catapulted cardiovascular health into the collective consciousness.

I taught aerobics, also known as dance exercise, in the early days and remember hauling my tapes and boom box to class so that I could lead a room full of eager participants through a routine. At the time, we knew this form of group exercise was special, but we had no idea it was going to grow as much as it has, or that it would touch so many people's lives in so many different ways. However, as this fever for creative movement grew, so too did the need for education about safety. Not only were participants getting hurt and doing exercises that were not always based on sound exercise science precepts, instructors were also getting injured. If this craze had any hope of transforming into a cause, those who were passionate about "dance exercise" had to team up and learn ways to share information about safe instruction, anatomy, and exercise physiology.

This book is a culmination of years of education, experience, and inspiration. You hold in your hands the legacy left by fitness industry experts who literally learned through sweat (and sometimes tears) how to motivate groups of people to connect and stretch their bodies and minds to new levels of health and fitness. As evolved as our industry is, it is still relatively young, and it continues to shift and change as exercise research reveals new and better ways to lead people through a wide variety of fitness classes. Expectations and standards for education are higher than ever, and the group exercise instructor is an increasingly valued member of fitness facilities.

If you're new to group exercise, welcome! You will find this book user-friendly as well as informative and timely. You will learn many new and practical methods to teach exercise and you will become an expert on the myriad ways the body moves. If you are already teaching group exercise, this manual will be an important ally as you continue to inspire the world to fitness.

The American College of Sports Medicine has carefully considered the needs of all populations when developing this book. One product of this research is the ACSM Quick Screen, which will help you quickly determine the needs of new participants when they arrive to class. You will also learn new safety protocols, the importance of biomechanics, how to handle legal issues, hospitality and conflict resolution, and, of course, you will be immersed in the world of choreography—its history and future.

Congratulations on making a commitment to help others on their path to health, fitness, and wellness. After reading the *ACSM's Resources for the Group Exercise Instructor* and absorbing the quality information, you will be more confident in your abilities to stand in front of a room full of people and lead many different styles of exercise. Keep this book as a reference, and continue your education throughout your career by making connections with other fitness professionals and organizations who share your passion.

*Kathie Davis*
*Cofounder and Executive Director*
*IDEA Health and Fitness Association*

When most people hear the term "group exercise," their thoughts immediately turn to visions of bodies clad in tight clothing sweating to the beat of loud pulsating music and moving in synchronized step to a choreographed routine. Many of today's classes still reflect this style, once called "aerobic dance," but the field has evolved to be more inclusive and less exclusive. In many ways, group exercise is the original "fusion" workout. Our roots are nestled between traditional dance (jazz and ballet), calisthenics, and cardiovascular fitness. From 1951 to 1985, Jack LaLanne hosted his television exercise show featuring timeless activities from calisthenics to balance and posture training. In 1968, Dr. Kenneth H. Cooper authored his book *Aerobics* and introduced a new word and new concept to the world. Judy Sheppard Missitt founded Jazzercise in 1969 and led a series of choreographed fitness routines still popular today. Jacki Sorensen took the next step in our evolution with "aerobic dance." Her fun, choreographed fitness routines evolved in the field as instructors experimented and churned out derivations of dance steps designed to increase and sustain heart rate. High-impact aerobics evolved to low impact and finally multi-impact. We moved from choreographed routines to "freestyle," which was less choreographed and included more repetitions and athletic moves. Gin Miller took the fitness industry by storm when her knee injury, a consequence of high-impact aerobics and poor flooring, landed her in physical therapy. Her rehabilitative exercise program included stepping up and down on a step, and in 1989, step aerobics and "equipment-based classes" were born.

As instructors, we have been the test subjects for many group exercise trends by bearing the brunt of pushing the limit—teaching repetitively week after week to realize that "more is not always better." We have helped the industry realize that better flooring, better footwear, better education, better safety recommendations, and more qualified fitness professionals will yield the most effective enjoyable product: a great fitness experience for our participants and ourselves.

Today's classes feature a buffet of choices to suit every fitness palate. For a new instructor, it can feel overwhelming, but each of us is attracted to a style of movement that we find exciting. Just as a new student needs to try different classes and instructors, the up and coming instructor needs to embark on the same journey. Once you find a style that you connect with, you can apply the basic exercise science principles in this manual to design your class. Then add practice, leadership techniques, communication skills, and hospitality and you will find yourself in front of the room leading the way for others.

In every group exercise class, there is a handful of participants who bravely attend exercise classes with the hope they will not be seen. They stand as close to the back wall or exit door as they possibly can. May the expertise shared in this text serve you, to learn to "see," reach, and bring the back row to the front of the class.

This first edition of *ACSM's Resources for the Group Exercise Instructor* recognizes the fitness professionals who touch more lives in a single hour than any other fitness pro—YOU—the group exercise instructor. Whether you teach boot camp, lead a walking club, or teach a dance-based cardio salsa class, *you* have the future of the world in your hands.

*ACSM's Resources for the Group Exercise Instructor* is intended to serve as a guide for individuals wishing to embark on a career as a fitness professional, as a resource in the university setting for those pursuing careers in health and fitness, and as a resource in the fitness industry for those seeking to add group exercise teaching skills to their toolbox. Chapter contributors have had experience teaching group fitness or were paired with an experienced instructor to ensure we provided the most up-to-date and relevant information.

## ORGANIZATION

*ACSM's Resources for the Group Exercise Instructor* is divided into three sections. Part I, Introduction to Group Exercise Instruction, covers the considerations for both the instructor and the student. Chapter 1, Profile of a Group Exercise Instructor: Education, Credentials, Scope, and Objectives, describes the role of a group exercise instructor and outlines career-based requirements and opportunities. Chapter 2, Profile of a Group Exercise Participant: Health Screening Tools, offers health screening guidelines to assist in providing the safest, most optimal experience for both the student and the teacher. Part II, Leadership and Design, balances theoretical and practical applications offering sample class outlines with communication tactics and a unique chapter on hospitality and conflict resolution for instructors. Chapter 3, Class Design and Programming, outlines the components of a class including warm-up, stimulus, and cool-down. This chapter explains the different types of classes and describes how to outline a class. Chapter 4, Communication Skills: Adherence and Motivation, is a unique chapter bridging the gap between the art and science of communication and the effect of motivation of adherence. Verbal and nonverbal skills and strategies inherent to exercise leadership are reviewed. Chapter 5, Choreography, Music, and Cueing in Class Design and Delivery, describes how to create choreography, how to cue, and how to find the beat of the music. It is a pivotal chapter of study for the group exercise instructor. Chapter 6, Teaching Your Class: A Quick Guide, outlines "day-of" class preparation and includes the "I'm Ok" policy, a unique risk management tool. Chapter 7, Hospitality and Conflict Resolution for Group Exercises Instructors, offers strategies specific to teaching in a group setting complete with tips for avoiding and handling conflicts. Chapter 8, Guidelines for Special Conditions, explains how to modify in exercise leadership, class design, and exercise selection based on a class participant's physical condition. Chapter 9, Specialty Classes, provides an overview of some common group fitness specialties—indoor cycling, Pilates, yoga, and aquatic exercise. Chapter 10, Legal Issues and Responsibilities for Group Exercise Instructor, wraps up the legalities of teaching group fitness classes.

Part III, Exercise Science for the Group Exercise Instructor, provides the foundation for all exercise selection and knowledge required for skill and leadership in the field. Chapter 11, Exercise Physiology for the Group Exercise Instructors, focuses on key biological systems such as the cardiovascular system, respiratory system, energy system, musculoskeletal system, and neurological system and their function during exercise. Chapter 12, Kinesiology, Anatomy, and Biomechanics, demonstrates why a solid knowledge of kinesiology, anatomy, and biomechanics is fundamental to the success and safety of teaching group exercise. Chapter 13, Introduction to Nutrition for Group Exercise Instructors, reviews basic nutrition and provides sound advice about weight management.

Because instructors often learn by doing, the science-based chapters frame the book in the third section. These are the bases for all practice. The manual will debut a new screen developed by the ACSM Certified GEI subcommittee called the ACSM Quick Screen, which outlines how to quickly screen new participants when they arrive to class.

## FEATURES

Information is "chunked" as much as possible and broken up with text box features. **Ask the Pros** features industry icons offering practical advice. **Boxes** throughout the chapters provide samples of exercises and valuable information. **Take Caution!** calls attention to information relating to safety or legal concerns. These also differentiate information for instructors employed as independent contractors from those employed as employees. **Recommended Resources** provide sources of additional information relevant to that being presented. The **video icon** ▶, seen throughout the chapters, refers readers to the book's Web site for video content that will provide visuals of material being discussed and described in the text.

## ADDITIONAL RESOURCES

*ACSM's Resources for the Group Exercise Instructor* includes additional resources for both instructors and students that are available on the book's companion Web site at http://thepoint.lww.com/ACSMGroupEx.

### INSTRUCTORS

- Image Bank
- WebCT/Blackboard/Angel Cartridge

### STUDENTS

- Full Text Online
- Videos

In addition, purchasers of the text can access the searchable Full Text through the book's Web site. See the front inside cover of this text for more details and include the pass code to gain access to the Web site.

*Grace DeSimone*

# Acknowledgments

This project was a true collaboration of talent. I wish to extend a heartfelt thank you to all the contributors who donated their time and expertise to the creation of this publication. I would like to acknowledge the reviewers, especially Paul Sorace and ACSM's subpublication committee. Thank you to Greg Dwyer for his guidance.

A special thank you to members of the ACSM-certified GEI subcommittee, Ken Alan, Teri Bladen, and Leslie Stenger, who went above and beyond to lend support, insight, and energy to the direction and completion of this manual.

To Madeline Paternostro Bayles, chair of ACSM's CCRB Executive Council, for hunting and gathering resources, especially at the eleventh hour. To Neal Pire, CCRB Executive Council Member at Large, for his ability to listen and counsel accordingly, and to Richard Cotton, ACSM's National Director of Certification, whose vision helped this manual become a reality.

To the fantastic team at LWW, Andrea Klingler, Emily Lupash, Christen Murphy, and Ed Shultes Jr, for their innovative ideas and unending patience and support. I am grateful to Kerry O'Rourke, ACSM's Director of Publishing, for her leadership.

To my friends and colleagues at Plus One Health Management, past, present, and future. "In teaching we will learn and in learning we will teach." Thank you all for teaching me!

A special thank you to MaryAnn Rumplasch who served as a contributor, reviewer, and video script writer. To all of the models for their beauty and talent and for doing "whatever it took." To photographer Mark Lozier for his creativity and attention to detail. To the staff of Ethos Fitness Spa for Women for allowing us to use their delightful studios, staff, and members for the photo and video shoot, and especially to Ellen Babajko, who is a pillar of support and inspiration.

# Contents

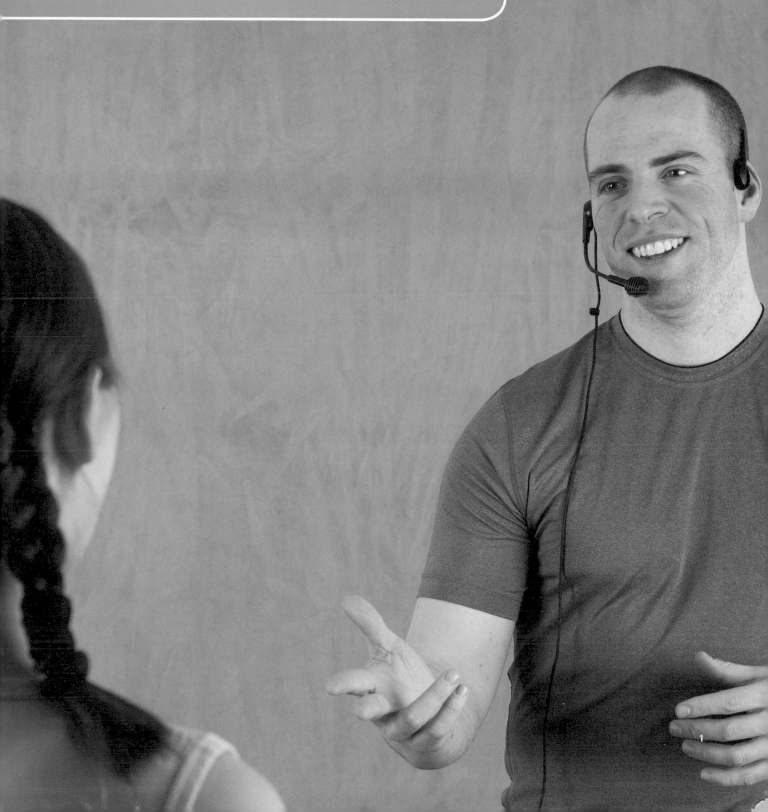

# INTRODUCTION TO GROUP EXERCISE INSTRUCTION

PART 1

# Profile of a Group Exercise Instructor: Education, Credentials, Scope, and Objectives

GRACE DeSIMONE

**At the end of this chapter you will be able to:**
- Describe the current and projected state of the fitness industry as it pertains to group exercise instructors
- Explain the minimum and suggested requirements for becoming a certified group exercise instructor
- Identify professional career paths for group exercise instructors
- Describe the difference between an employee and an independent contractor
- Identify the various styles of group exercise interviews/auditions

This chapter defines the basic responsibilities of group exercise instructors (GEIs) and outlines career opportunities that are available in the health and fitness industry.

## WHAT IS A GROUP EXERCISE INSTRUCTOR?

ACSM Certified Group Exercise Instructor$^{SM}$ works in a group exercise setting with apparently healthy individuals and those with health challenges who are able to exercise independently to enhance quality of life, improve health-related physical fitness, manage health risk, and promote lasting health behavior change. The GEI leads safe and effective exercise programs using a variety of leadership techniques to foster group camaraderie, support, and motivation to enhance muscular strength and endurance, flexibility, cardiovascular fitness, body composition, and any of the motor skills related to the domains of health-related physical fitness.

## TYPES OF WORKING ENVIRONMENTS FOR GROUP EXERCISE INSTRUCTORS

GEIs can work in a variety of settings. It is not unusual for a GEI to work in several types of environments at the same time. Generally, employment may fall into one of three general categories:

1. A GEI who works as an employee for a fitness club and teaches in addition to having other responsibilities
2. A GEI who is hired by a facility to exclusively teach classes

3. A GEI who teaches classes in a nontraditional setting such as a business, church, or school

Many GEIs teach a few classes in a commercial setting and a few classes in a community setting in the same week. This can provide the GEI with different experiences that will enhance the instructor's skill sets. GEIs may be employed in

- Commercial (for-profit) fitness centers
- Community (not-for-profit) fitness centers
- Corporate fitness/wellness centers
- University wellness/adult fitness centers
- Owner/operator (self-employed) studios, fitness centers, and in-home businesses
- Medical fitness centers (MFCs)
- Municipal/city recreation/public parks/family centers/schools
- Governmental/military fitness centers
- Activity centers/retirement centers/assisted living communities for older adults

## THE JOB MARKET FOR GROUP EXERCISE INSTRUCTORS

The United States Department of Labor Bureau of Labor Statistics predicts that fitness workers should have promising job opportunities due to job growth in health clubs, fitness facilities, community centers, hospital settings, corporate fitness centers, and other settings in which fitness workers are employed. An increasing number of people are spending time and money on fitness and more businesses are recognizing the benefits of health and fitness programs for their employees. GEIs with advanced training (at least one primary certification from a National Commission for Certifying Agencies (NCCA)-accredited provider and/or specialty certification and/or a minimum of a Bachelor's degree in a health-related field) and extensive experience are predicted to have especially good job opportunities. Many job openings will arise from the need to replace group exercise instructors who retire, transfer, or leave the field for other reasons (1).

Sedentary lifestyles, changes in the food supply, poor eating habits, and other factors contributing to the obesity epidemic will provide more opportunities for certified professionals to educate and engage the population in physical activity.

## EMPLOYMENT CHANGE

Employment of fitness workers is expected to increase 29% between 2008 and 2018, which is much faster than the average. Aging baby boomers, one group that increasingly is becoming concerned with staying healthy and physically fit, will be a primary impetus of employment growth in fitness professionals (1).

The reduction in the number of physical education programs in schools coupled with parents' growing concern about childhood obesity will increase the need for fitness professionals to work with children in nonschool settings, such as health clubs. Increasingly, parents also are hiring personal trainers for their children, and the number of weight-training gyms for children is expected to continue to grow (1).

## COMMON CATEGORIES OF EMPLOYMENT FOR THE GEI

GEIs will fall into one of the following categories of employment:

- An employee who only teaches group exercise
- An employee who has other duties such as personal trainer or floor trainer or manager who also teaches group exercise
- An independent contractor hired by a club to teach group exercise
- An independent contractor who teaches group exercise in a nontraditional setting such as a church basement and conducts their classes as a business (*e.g.*, collects fees from participants)

Each type of employment has specific benefits and responsibilities. Keep in mind that the more independent the GEI is, the more responsibility they assume. The independent contractor takes on the additional responsibility of determining the policies and procedures, ensuring the environment is safe, developing and implementing some

---

**BOX 1.1** | *Independent Contractor Versus Employee for GEIs*

Independent contractors are highlighted throughout this manual. From the member's perspective, employees and independent contractors may not appear to have different roles; however, from the business perspective, the roles are significantly different and it is extremely important that GEIs are aware of the differences. The policies and procedures concerning the separation of employees and independent contractors are governed by state and federal rules and regulations.

The courts have considered many facts in deciding whether a worker is an independent contractor or an employee. These relevant facts fall into three main categories: behavioral control, financial control, and relationship of the parties. It is very important to consider all the facts — no single fact provides the answer (2). Carefully review the following definitions:

- *Behavioral Control* covers facts that show whether the business has a right to direct or control how the work is done through instructions, training, or other means. If you receive extensive training on policies, procedures, or how your class is to be conducted, this suggests that you are an employee.

- *Financial Control* covers facts that show whether the business has a right to direct or control the financial and business aspects of the worker's job. If you have a significant investment in your work, you may be an independent contractor. If you can realize a profit or incur a loss, this suggests that you are in business for yourself and that you may be an independent contractor.

- *Type of Relationship* relates to how the workers and the business owner perceive their relationship. For example, if you receive benefits, such as insurance, pension, or paid time off, this suggests that you may be an employee.

Both employers and workers can ask the Internal Revenue Service (IRS) to make a determination on whether a specific individual is an independent contractor or an employee by filing a Form SS-8, Determination of Worker Status for Purposes of Federal Employment Taxes and Income Tax Withholding, with the IRS (3).

type of screening for participants, marketing of services, and other responsibilities often handled by employers or club management. It is critical for GEIs to understand that the situations that appear to be the least complicated (*e.g.*, teaching an exercise class to your church congregation) can often impose the most responsibility on the part of the independent contractor.

## ARE YOU A SPECIALIST OR A GENERALIST?

It is important for the GEI to understand the various opportunities within the fitness industry for their area of expertise. The GEI is often considered a specialist if they only teach classes. The GEI who only teaches certain types of classes (*e.g.*, strength training, Pilates, indoor cycling) is even more specialized and is often referred to as a **specialty instructor**. Specialty instructors often teach classes that require additional training (*e.g.*, yoga, Pilates, indoor cycling, and aquatic exercises). Being specialized or being a specialist offers the opportunity to charge a higher rate for services but can limit opportunities in the job market if the candidate is looking to teach group exercise as a career. For some, teaching a few classes per week is the perfect part-time job. For others, it can be frustrating because there are a limited number of specialty classes offered in any class program. Specialty instructors may seek work in specialty studios such as yoga studios, Pilates studios, or cycling studios. Another option is to take on a more generalized certification or consider the hybrid professional option.

The GEI can be considered a **generalist** if their only responsibility is to teach fitness classes and/or take on the more traditional roles of a fitness floor attendant or group exercise coordinator who is usually employed by the club to work with the general membership. Since club managers are tasked with the challenge of offering a variety of services while considering payroll costs, generalists satisfy a number of skill sets and can make excellent instructors.

## WHAT KIND OF TRAINING DO INSTRUCTORS NEED?

Because of the large number of certification organizations, the requirements for group exercise instructors vary greatly. Certifications such as those offered by ACSM are part of a progressive professional development pathway. The minimal requirement for an ACSM Certified Group Exercise Instructor℠ (GEI) is

- A high school diploma or General Educational Development
- 18 years of age
- Current certification in cardiopulmonary resuscitation/automated external defibrillator through the American Red Cross or American Heart Association

---

**BOX 1.2**  **GEIs' Activities and Compensation**

According to the 2010 IDEA Health & Fitness Association Fitness Industry Compensation Trends Report, group fitness instructors teach general classes set to music, such as step and mixed impact. Specialty instructors teach classes requiring specialized training (e.g., indoor cycling or martial arts). Group exercise instructors are present at 47% of the responding facilities, whereas 25% employ specialty instructors. The average number of group exercise instructors at each facility surveyed was 12.

Group fitness instructors teach an average of 6 hours per week (same as in 2008), while specialty instructors teach an average of 8 hours per week (up from 6 h/wk in 2008). Few of these individuals are salaried employees (1% of group fitness instructors, 6% of specialty instructors), though a large percentage are considered employees (64% and 61%, respectively). The number of fitness instructors who are considered employees has increased, after a dip in 2008 (58% for group fitness instructors and 41% for specialty instructors). That decline came after years of steady growth: from 2002 to 2006, the percentage increased from 49% to 59% for group fitness instructors and from 44% to 57% for specialty instructors.

Hourly rates have declined for both types of instructors, compared with past data. Instructors report earning an average of $24.50, down from $25.75 in 2008 and only slightly higher than in 2006 ($23.75). Specialty instructors are earning an average of $27.75 per hour, compared with $31.50 in 2008 and $28.50 in 2006.

Benefits (18% in 2010 and 21% in 2008) and cash incentives (17% in 2010 and 19% in 2008) have also declined over the past 2 years, while eligibility for an education fund has increased (41% in 2010 vs. 35% in 2008). Specialty instructors have seen a slight increase in benefits from 2008 (17% vs.16%), a decline in cash incentives (10% vs. 18%), and a boost in education funds (41% vs. 31%) (4).

| BOX 1.3 | Musicality Not Required |
|---------|------------------------|

Group exercise classes are rooted in dance, so many people associate dance with group exercise. This is true, but certainly not exclusive to the job. The group exercise classes we know today were born out of a term called "aerobic dance" and yes, being able to count and cue to a beat is a required skill for some but not all classes. Music should only be considered a necessary part of any group exercise class if it has purpose and adds to the class. For classes such as indoor cycling, music may actually be a necessary part of the class in that it helps the instructor and the participant stay with an intended cadence and can also help to set the mood for the type of riding performed in the class. However, group exercise has evolved to include a variety of styles; essentially, any activity that leads a group through any style of exercise qualifies. This can include aquatic exercise, boot camp or callisthenic style exercises, walking, stretching, strength training, and just about anything for any group that you can imagine. Encouraging a group of individuals to improve their health and overall well-being through physical activity is the core of this profession.

Many instructors have formal schooling in exercise science, physical education, dance, or related fields. Prospective instructors often complete courses in anatomy, kinesiology, and exercise physiology to serve as a foundation for their career. Other group instructors advance their learning through the attainment of one or more specialty certifications such as yoga, pilates, or indoor cycling.

## CONTINUING EDUCATION

Exercise professionals are constantly learning. Advancing studies and participating in continuing education credits that will assist the GEI are a key to success as exercise styles, trends, and equipment in the group setting change continuously. Staying up-to-date on the latest research and information is vital to success. Moreover, instructors who use an evidenced-based approach to understanding and vetting exercise trends will navigate the onslaught of fads. Asking the questions — Why? and Where is the research? — will separate the professionals from the garden variety enthusiasts. GEIs should take courses and attend conferences to be in a constant state of educational engagement. Current ACSM GEIs need to obtain 45 continuing education units.

## LEADERSHIP

Instructors must have excellent leadership abilities as demonstrated by very good communication and interpersonal skills. They must possess the ability to motivate and encourage a variety of exercise participants. GEIs must be able to work independently as well as be part of a team.

## GETTING STARTED

It is important to consider the impact of your choices as you embark on your career path. Group fitness instructors often get started by participating in exercise classes until they are ready to audition as instructors and, if the audition is successful, begin teaching classes. Most employers require instructors to be certified, but some will allow instructors on the job training to work toward becoming certified. Because requirements vary from employer to employer, it may be helpful to

| BOX 1.4 | Sample Class Plan |
|---------|-------------------|

### HYBRIDS: A NEW BREED OF PROFESSIONALS

There is an emerging new title called "hybrids." This term describes professionals who have chosen to work in several realms simultaneously. They have elected to combine roles, *e.g.,* group exercise instructor and personal trainer, club manager and online coach, and fitness writer.

There are many combinations. For many, they simply evolved into a hybrid out of need and for others it is a distinct choice. It is an option that will require additional training and certification but will offer a multitude of possibilities and a flexible schedule (5).

contact local fitness centers or other potential employers to find out what education, background, and training they prefer.

In the long run, earning an NCCA-accredited certification like the ACSM Certified Group Exercise Instructor℠ will provide recognition of a certification based in sound scientific principles. A recognized certification helps to raise the standards within the industry in general and may help your potential clients feel confident regarding your skills as a health fitness professional. Starting your group exercise career with a highly respected certification is an excellent first step.

## ACSM'S ROLE AND THE EDUCATIONAL CONTINUUM

ACSM is a professional member association composed of a multidisciplinary mix of more than 20,000 exercise science researchers, educators, and medical practitioners. More specifically, member categories include physicians, nurses, athletic trainers, exercise physiologists, dietitians, fitness professionals, and physical therapists, as well as many other allied health care professionals with an interest in sports medicine and the exercise sciences.

The ACSM's mission statement is:

*The ACSM promotes and integrates scientific research, education and practical applications of sports medicine and exercise science to maintain and enhance physical performance, fitness, health, and quality of life.*

Founded in 1954, ACSM was the first professional organization to begin offering health and fitness certifications (in 1975) and continues to deliver the most respected, National Commission for NCCA-accredited certifications within the health and fitness industry. Because of the multidisciplinary nature and diversity of its members, ACSM has evolved into an industry leader in the unique position of creating evidence-based best practices through the original research of its members as well as disseminating this information through its periodicals, meetings, conferences, position stands, consensus statements, and certification workshops. Respect for ACSM has earned it numerous health initiative partnerships and collaborative efforts with groups such as the American Heart Association, American Medical Association, American Cancer Society, Centers for Disease Control and Prevention, the International Health, Racquet and Sportsclub Association, National Intramural-Recreational Sports Association, National Academy of Sports Medicine, the Commission on Accreditation of Allied Health Education Programs, the National Collegiate Athletic Association, the National Center on Physical Activity and Disability, among others.

## IDENTIFICATION OF A CORE BODY OF KNOWLEDGE

Shortly after ACSM introduced professional certifications, the first edition of *ACSM's Guidelines for Exercise Testing and Prescription* was published along with its companion publication *ACSM's Resource Manual for Guidelines for Exercise Testing and Prescription*. For the first time, these publications included the consensus from subject matter experts and so provided a framework for the body of knowledge with respect to standards and guidelines for assessing fitness and prescribing exercise. Generally, all professions, regardless of the industry, have a core body of knowledge that provides guidance and clarity and also helps establish a specific ACSM-certified professional scope of practice in that profession. This initial publication proved so effective for practitioners that periodic review and revision of this book now takes place every 4 years. The year 2009 marked the publication of the eighth edition of *ACSM's Guidelines for Exercise Testing and Prescription*. Also in 2009, the sixth edition of the *ACSM's Resource Manual for Guidelines for Exercise Testing and Prescription* and the third edition of *ACSM's Certification Review Book* were published.

## ACSM CERTIFIED GROUP EXERCISE INSTRUCTOR℠ EXAM BLUEPRINT

- Domain I: Participant and Program Assessment — 10%
- Domain II: Class Design — 25%
- Domain III: Leadership and Instruction — 55%
- Domain IV: Legal and Professional Responsibilities — 10%

The percentages reflect the percentage of examination questions contained in each domain on the 100-question examination.

## THE GEI INTERVIEW/AUDITION: WHAT TO EXPECT

Once a candidate has obtained the foundational elements of leading group exercise as described in this manual and others and earned a group exercise instructor certification, he or she will need to practice his or her class. In addition to a professional resume, preparing a routine on paper (see Chapters 3 and 5) and then practicing it aloud in front of a mirror or video camera are good strategies. The candidate can find family and friends who will act as practice participants. Once the candidate has spent enough time practicing to create a class routine, he or she is ready for a job interview. Most employers will ask candidates to audition for their interview. This can be conducted in a variety of ways.

## THE GROUP AUDITION

Two or more candidates are gathered to conduct a mock class. Candidates take turns leading the class. This is sometimes conducted in a round robin style so the interviewer can observe how quickly each candidate can adapt to change. Candidates will be observed on how to give and take direction both as a leader and follower.

## THE INDIVIDUAL AUDITION

This is the most common audition. The candidate will teach the interviewer or a small group of employees. Sometimes the interviewer will participate in the class and, other times, he or she will simply observe. The GEI candidate will teach portions of a mock class. This is especially challenging since there are no actual students to direct and the GEI candidate will have to rely on any experiences they have had with actual students. See Appendix A for Sample Job Descriptions and Audition/Interview forms.

## OBSERVATION AUDITION

The GEI candidate arranges to observe or participate in an existing class the candidate may be teaching. This allows the most natural setting for the candidate and may demonstrate key aspects of leadership such class rapport. The importance of developing rapport and fine-tuning communication skills is addressed in greater detail in Chapter 4.

## VIDEO AUDITIONS

The candidate video tapes an actual or mock class and submits it to the potential employer.

## NO AUDITION

Some employers will hire candidates based on reviewing credentials, experience, and conducting a traditional interview. Sometimes the candidate will be asked to participate in a class to demonstrate movement style and how the candidate interacts with students.

### Take Caution

#### "...JUST TEACH A CLASS AS AN AUDITION..."

Some employers will ask candidates to audition by teaching a regularly scheduled class at the employer's facility. Unless the candidate is already employed at the facility, this is not recommended. If the candidate or a student is injured during the class, both the candidate and the employer are exposed for liability. The employer would be exposed for having a nonemployee teaching and the candidate is exposed for the same reason.

## INTERVIEW PREPARATION/CONDUCT RESEARCH

Candidates can request permission to attend a class or observe a program before the scheduled interview. This will provide information on student/member demographics, the teaching styles of other employees, and the variety of classes on an existing schedule. Candidates may also request to see a job description or one may be provided at the time of or prior to the interview. The job description (see Appendix A) will provide details of the employer's expectations including hours, work environment, educational requirements, and benefits if available.

## DRESS FOR SUCCESS

Candidates should not assume that an interview at a gym requires gym attire. Candidates should ask about the type of interview and dress appropriately (Fig. 1.1). It is acceptable for the candidate to inquire about attire since it varies widely from one organization to another. Many organizations will frown upon candidates who do not arrive for interviews in business attire. If the interview will be an audition, the candidate should understand what the employer's expectations are regarding attire. Interviewers will assess the candidate's awareness of their organization's culture. Jeans are never appropriate attire for any type of interview and candidates should ask clubs about their specific policy regarding body art and jewelry prior to the interview.

## HOW WILL THE CANDIDATE BE EVALUATED?

Review the Sample Instructor Interview/Audition Form (see Appendix A) for a basic understanding of the components that are observed in a typical audition.

## ETHICS AND PROFESSIONAL CONDUCT

Ethics can be described as standards of conduct that guide decisions and actions, based on duties derived from core values. Specifically, core values are principles that we use to define what is right, good, and/or just. When a professional demonstrates behavior that is consistent, or

### Take Caution

#### BE YOURSELF

It is tempting to borrow styles and classes from other instructors or to fashion a class after a popular instructor. Using concepts and best practices and making them YOURS will result in your best class and a unique product — YOU.

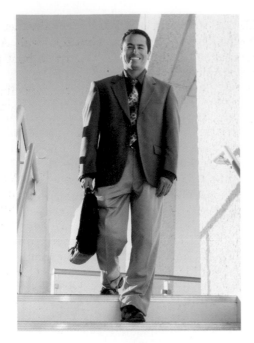

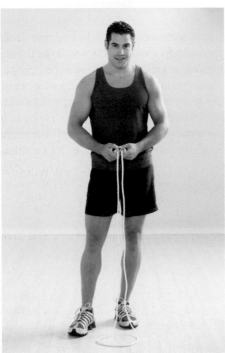

■ **FIGURE 1.1** Dress appropriately. Do not assume that an interview in a gym requires gym attire.

familiar with all aspects of the ACSM's Code of Ethics for certified and registered professionals (6).

## CODE OF ETHICS FOR ACSM CERTIFIED AND REGISTERED PROFESSIONALS

### Purpose

This Code of Ethics is intended to aid all certified and registered ACSM credentialed professionals (to establish and maintain a high level of ethical conduct, as defined by standards by which ACSM GEIs may determine the appropriateness of their conduct. Any existing professional, licensure, or certification affiliations that ACSM GEIs have with governmental, local, state, or national agencies or organizations will take precedence relative to any disciplinary matters that pertain to practice or professional conduct. This Code applies to all ACSM GEIs, regardless of ACSM membership status (to include members and nonmembers). Any cases in violation of this Code will be referred to the ACSM Committee on Certification and Registry Boards (CCRB).

### Principles and Standards

#### Responsibility to the Public

ACSM GEIs shall be dedicated to providing competent and legally permissible services within the scope of the Knowledge and Skills (KSs) of their respective credential. These services shall be provided with integrity, competence, diligence, and compassion. ACSM GEIs provide exercise information in a manner that is consistent with evidence-based practice.

- ACSM GEIs should respect the rights of clients, colleagues, and health care professionals and shall safeguard client confidences within the boundaries of the law.
- Information relating to the ACSM GEIs–client relationship is confidential and may not be communicated to a third party not involved in that client's care without the prior written consent of the client or as required by law.
- ACSM GEIs should be truthful about their qualifications and the limitations of their expertise and provide services consistent with their competencies.

#### Responsibility to the Profession

- ACSM-certified professionals (ACSMCP) maintain high professional standards. As such, an ACSM-certified professional should never represent himself or herself, either directly or indirectly, as anything other than an ACSM-certified professional unless he or she holds other license/certification that allows them to do so.

aligned, with widely accepted standards in their respective industry, that professional is said to behave "ethically." On the other hand, unethical behavior is behavior that is not consistent with industry-accepted standards. As a fitness professional, you have an obligation to stay within the bounds of the defined scope of practice for a GEI as well as to abide by all industry-accepted standards of behavior at all times. Furthermore, as a certified or registered professional through ACSM, it is your responsibility to be

- ACSM GEIs practice within the scope of their KSs and in accordance with state law.
- ACSM-certified professionals must remain in good standing relative to governmental requirements as a condition of continued credentialing.
- ACSM GEIs take credit, including authorship, only for work they have actually performed and give credit to the contributions of others as warranted. Consistent with the requirements of their certification or registration, ACSM GEIs must complete approved, additional educational course (continuing education) work aimed at maintaining and advancing their KSs.

### Principles and Standards for Candidates of ACSM Certification Examinations

Candidates applying for a credentialing examination must comply with candidacy requirements and, to the best of their abilities, accurately complete the application process.

### Public Disclosure of Affiliation

- Any ACSMCP may disclose his or her affiliation with ACSM credentialing in any context, oral or documented, provided it is currently accurate. In doing so, no ACSMCP may imply college endorsement of whatever is associated in context with the disclosure, unless expressly authorized by the college. Disclosure of affiliation in connection with a commercial venture may be made provided the disclosure is made in a professionally dignified manner; is not false, misleading, or deceptive; and does not imply licensure or the attainment of specialty or diploma status.

- ACSM GEIs may disclose their credential status.
- ACSM GEIs may list their affiliation with ACSM credentialing on their business cards without prior authorization.
- ACSM GEIs and the institutions employing an ACSMCP may inform the public of an affiliation as a matter of public discourse or presentation.

### Discipline

Any ACSMCP may be disciplined or lose his or her certification or registry for conduct that, in the opinion of the Executive Council of the CCRB goes against the principles set forth in this Code. Such cases will be reviewed by the ACSM CCRB Ethics Subcommittee, which will include a liaison from the ACSM CCRB executive council, as appointed by the CCRB chair. The ACSM CCRB Ethics Subcommittee will make an action recommendation to the executive council of the ACSM CCRB for final review and approval.

### SUMMARY

*New styles of classes and instructors are constantly emerging in today's fitness industry. The dedicated professional will have a long, satisfying career as a certified group exercise instructor working in a variety of settings including commercial clubs, not-for-profit clubs, university recreation centers, corporate fitness centers, community recreation programs, and more. Research has shown the important role of physical activity in maintaining health and preventing chronic disease. Professionally trained and certified professionals can play an integral role in leading participants to improved health and well-being.*

## References

1. Bureau of Labor Statistics. *Occupational Outlook Handbook, 2010–11 Edition*, Fitness Workers on the Internet at [cited 2011 Jan 09]. http://www.bls.gov/oco/ocos296.htm
2. Department of the Treasury Internal Revenue Service. Independent Contractor or Employee, Publication 1779 (Rev. 8-2008) Catalog Number 16134L; [cited 2011 Mar 10]. Available from: http://www.irs.gov/pub/irs-pdf/p1779.pdf
3. Internal Revenue Service. Employee vs. Independent Contractor – Seven Tips for Business Owners; [cited 2011 Mar 10]. Available from: http://www.irs.gov/newsroom/article/0,,id=173423,00.html
4. Schroeder J. 2010 IDEA fitness industry compensation trends report. *IDEA fitness Journal*. 2011;8(1):42–48.
5. Thompson W, et al. *ACSM's Resources for the Personal Trainer*, 3rd ed. Baltimore(MD) Lippincott Williams & Wilkins; 2010.
6. Williams A. Hybrid fitness professionals – The best of all worlds? *IDEA Fitness Journal* [Intenet]. 2011 [cited 2011 Jan 10];7(4). Available from: http://www.ideafit.com/fitness-library/hybrid-fitness-professionals-mdash-the-best-of-all-worlds.

# 2

# Profile of a Group Exercise Participant: Health Screening Tools

### GRACE DeSIMONE • LESLIE STENGER

## Objectives

**At the end of this chapter you will be able to:**
- Explain the importance of standardized screenings
- Identify and describe appropriate screening tools
- Deliver and describe the proper use of the ACSM Quick Screen
- Identify how to apply the various screening tools for different groups
- Describe the challenges associated with screening and teaching group exercise
- Administer basic field tests in a class setting

This chapter provides the basic tools for screening your class participants. It is common practice for group exercise instructors (GEIs) to "turn a blind eye" to the health screening area as they are under the ill-conceived notion that this responsibility lies in the hands of someone else.

The American College of Sports Medicine (ACSM) advises all GEIs to learn which screening tools are recommended for each type of teaching environment. In some cases, instructors need to administer the health screen; in other cases, instructors need to be aware that the screening occurred. GEIs should review how to properly utilize the health screening tools as they apply to their teaching.

## TYPES OF SCREENING

There is a link between physical activity, physical fitness, and overall health. By definition, physical activity is bodily movement that is produced by the contraction of skeletal muscle and that substantially increases energy expenditure, whereas physical fitness refers to a set of attributes that people have or achieve relating to their ability to perform physical activity. Health refers to a state of being associated with freedom from disease and illness that also includes a positive wellness component that is associated with a quality of life and positive well-being (3).

GEIs design their classes in order to improve participants' physical fitness and health by incorporating the most appropriate type of physical activity to achieve specific goals. Group exercise professionals must take the lead in the safety of each participant in their class. It is the GEI's responsibility to either conduct a prescreening assessment or have access to the screening results for any

participant taking a group exercise class. The extent of the screening will depend on the type of facility or program, and the role of the instructor is dependent upon the type of employment status. For example, the most common types of employment for GEI consist of:

- Full/part-time employee of a supervised fitness facility
- Independent contractor for a supervised fitness facility
- Independent contractor providing services to organizations other than supervised fitness facilities (e.g., churches, corporations, schools)

## PURPOSES OF SCREENING: SAFETY FIRST

As indicated in ACSM's Guidelines for Exercise Testing and Prescription, 8th edition (1), the rationale for screening a client is to optimize safety during exercise participation. Before students attend class, they should complete a preparticipation health screening. The purposes of this include the following:

- Identification and exclusion of participants with medical contraindications to exercise
- Identification of participants at increased risk for chronic disease due to age, symptoms, and/or risk factors. High-risk participants may need a medical evaluation and exercise testing before starting an exercise program.
- Identification of clients with clinically significant diseases who should participate in a medically supervised exercise program
- Identification of clients with other special needs

| BOX 2.1 | *Choosing Appropriate Exercise Classes* |

The type of business arrangement will dictate the most appropriate method for attaining the necessary pre-screening assessments.

The GEI can be viewed as an integral part of the health care team related to fitness programming. With this role comes the responsibility of assisting potential participants in selecting the most appropriate group exercise class for their specific health, fitness, and social needs. Conducting and/or reviewing prescreening assessments may be a critical part of the GEI's job tasks.

## THE SCREENING PROCESS

### FOR THE FULL/PART-TIME EMPLOYEE OF A SUPERVISED FITNESS FACILITY

It is recommended that a fitness facility provides a basic preactivity health screening process for every prospective member. It is during this process that the high-risk candidate, for whom medical clearance is recommended, can be identified. The GEI should be aware of how this process is structured so he or she can adapt accordingly.

### Take Caution

**KNOW YOUR EMPLOYER'S SCREENING POLICIES**

ACSM recommends that GEIs do NOT work under the employ of a facility that does not screen members. The GEI can then safely assume that participants attending class have been screened. The remaining challenge is knowing if the style of exercise and intensity are appropriate. For this reason, ACSM has created the ACSM Quick Screen.

A GEI working as a part- or full-time employee for an established fitness facility may have the opportunity to actually conduct the prescreening assessment(s) for members. This is an ideal situation since access to the information is available. It may also provide the GEI employee an opportunity to market the group exercise program.

### FOR THE INDEPENDENT CONTRACTOR

A GEI working as an independent contractor for an established fitness facility may not actually conduct the prescreening assessment(s). The screening process is typically completed by the exercise staff as discussed above in The Screening Process in a fitness facility setting.

If you are an independent GEI who is not affiliated with a supervised fitness facility, you need to be even more aware of the need for prescreening of participants since you are relying on information that you collect to determine whether your class is appropriate for each potential participant. The GEI must take the responsibility to develop, conduct, and review all prescreening assessments in order to ensure that the class is safe and effective for all potential participants.

In many instances, there is no clear definition of who has the responsibility to conduct the screening assessments. However, it is clear that all GEIs need to feel confident that they have the information necessary to protect each participant while they are in their class.

GEIs also have the unique opportunity to help participants change negative lifestyle behaviors that may influence overall health. The more information the GEI knows about the lifestyles of the participants, the more opportunity the GEI has to incorporate positive lifestyle behaviors into the class. It is not commonly the role of the GEI to determine the health status of the participants but rather to introduce the benefits of group exercise in promoting positive lifestyle behaviors. Having access to health and/or lifestyle assessment information enables the GEI to make the decision of whether their class is appropriate for each participant.

## COMMON SCREENING TOOLS

The following assessments are commonly used within the fitness industry and should be available to the GEI for review. The screening process should be followed by a discussion of the results with the client. Recommendations for each participant should be based on the results of the screening tools. Let us take a closer look at each of the screening tools.

## ACSM QUICK SCREEN

CLIP 2.1    When new participants have completed a preparticipation written questionnaire, implementing the ACSM Quick Screen (Fig. 2.1) is beneficial as it demonstrates that you are interested in the well-being of your students. It also teases out individuals who may have selected a class that is inappropriate for them.

| BOX 2.2 | Common Screening Tools (5) |

The screening process can be broken down into three distinct, yet related, phases:

Risk stratification
Health history evaluation and related assessments
Medical clearance or referral

From Thompson W. ACSM's *Resources for the Personal Trainer*. 3rd ed. Lippincott Williams & Wilkins; 2010. 257 p.

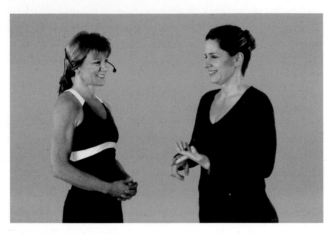

■ **FIGURE 2.1** ACSM Quick Screen.

The ACSM Quick Screen is administered verbally by the instructor to any new participant or individual returning to class after a layoff for any reason. Application of the Quick Screen will allow the instructor to know that

- The participant is in a class that is appropriate for him/her
- The participant will be able to exercise safely
- Any physical conditions that will require appropriate modifications during the class have been identified

After you introduce yourself and warmly welcome a new participant, engage the individual with the following series of fact-finding questions.

*Question: "Do you currently take any other classes? If so, which ones? When did you last attend?" OR "What other types of activities do you engage in?"*

*Purpose: You are establishing a baseline of experience and understanding the individual's exercise history, skill sets, skill levels, and likes and dislikes. Based on the response to this question, you will know if you have a neophyte who is new to classes, new to exercise, or new to your style of class.*

*Question: "Do you have any knee, shoulder, or back problems or any joint or bone issues?"*

*Purpose: This question scans the physical limitations of a participant. Does he or she have previous injuries or orthopedic concerns? You may offer modifications for exercises, suggest exercises to avoid, and, in some cases, suggest another class.*

*Question: "Do you have any medical conditions (e.g., heart/cardiovascular, blood pressure (high/low), diabetes)?"*

*Purpose: This assesses health/medical status and any acute conditions the instructor should be made aware of. Based on the responses to this question above, you may seek more information by asking some or all of the following questions:*

*Question: "When did you last have a medical checkup?"*

*Purpose: This provides the instructor with the opportunity to discuss medical conditions and suggest regular follow-up visits with a physician.*

*Question: "Are you taking any medications or getting treatment for this condition?"*

*Purpose: This question identifies that a participant is under a physician's care.*

*Question: "Has your physician ever told you that you should not exercise because of this or any other condition?"*

*Purpose: This question assesses the need for medical clearance and/or designation of specific restrictions by physician.*

| BOX 2.3 | Preactivity Screening: ACSM Quick Screen |

The ACSM Quick Screen is an abbreviated health/fitness screening tool performed verbally by the GEI. It is not intended to replace a preactivity screen, but rather to enhance it.

*Question: "Are there any physical changes you are undergoing that might affect or be affected by your exercise performance today?"*

*Purpose: The purpose of this question is to prompt the individual to share information on pregnancy, menopause, fatigue, inadequate sleep, or another condition that might indicate modification of exercises or exclusion from participation.*

In situations where it is not possible to individually converse with all new participants before class (*e.g.*, a group of new participants arrive at the same time just as you begin your class) or the class is very large and you want to make sure you have reached everyone. This is also helpful if you are new to a class and cannot recognize newcomers.

After an introduction, the GEI asks if there is anyone new taking class or anyone returning after a long vacation. The GEI offers a brief synopsis of what the class entails and offers suggested conditions that might be a concern. For example:

*"Good morning and welcome, my name is Ellen. Welcome to the Cardio Mix class. This class is aerobic in nature; we will be using step benches with a combination of low impact and high impact basic moves.*

*Is there anyone here for the first time or returning after a break?*

*Welcome! Feel free to modify any of the moves to satisfy your tolerance. Avoid 'pushing' yourself today and just get acclimated to the movement. I will offer modifications for many of the movements we are covering."*

## THE GEI AND THE SCREENING PROCESS: UNIQUE AND CHALLENGING

Remember, the general purpose of preparticipation screening is the same for all aspects of fitness training: safety. According to ACSM, it is important to provide an initial screening of participants relative to risk factors and/or symptoms for various chronic diseases in order to optimize safety during participation (5).

The screening process for GEIs can become more complicated for a variety of reasons, such as

- Not knowing all class participants on a one-to-one basis
- Working with groups rather than individuals (this limits the amount of time you can spend with each person)

- Transient population (different people participating from class to class)
- Having guests visit classes without knowing the health concerns of the guests
- Participants having various experiences with the class
- Participants exhibiting various fitness levels within the class
- Group exercise classes are often part of the membership in the fitness industry, and the GEI often assumes that participants have been prescreened to participate in his or her class.

### Take Caution

**BE SURE TO GET TO KNOW YOUR STUDENTS**

The actual role of the GEI will be dependent on the type of fitness opportunity presented to the participant. In many instances, the GEI does not have control over who participates in his or her class. It is critical that the GEI make an effort to learn as much about each participant as possible in order to assure a safe environment in which all participants can succeed.

The main purpose of prescreening for the GEI is to gather the necessary information to determine whether the class is a safe and effective training stimulus for each participant. The prescreening tool should provide information regarding the health of participants and their fitness goals. The GEI can then determine if the individual class is the appropriate method of training for the participant. According to ACSM, a prescreening assessment, or preparticipation screening, should be performed on all new participants upon entering a facility that offers exercises services (4).

### OTHER PREACTIVITY SCREENING TOOLS

**Health and Lifestyle Questionnaires**

*Definition*: Typically self-administered questionnaire to establish general health and lifestyle behaviors.

*Purpose*: Use to determine history, symptoms, and risk factors that help to direct participants to the most appropriate form of training. Also used to identify issues that should be evaluated by health care provider prior to starting program.

| BOX 2.4 | Be Sincere |
|---------|------------|

Never underestimate the value of a sincere "Welcome and tell me about you!" as the beginning to a long and successful relationship.

*Benefit*: Self-administered, valuable health information that can be used to select appropriate classes.

Self-administered questionnaires such as the Physical Activity Readiness Questionnaire (PAR-Q) (Fig. 2.2) and the AHA/ACSM Health/Fitness Facility Preparticipation Screening Questionnaire (Fig. 2.3) can be used as screening/educational tools in both health/fitness facilities and unsupervised fitness facilities. The PAR-Q focuses on symptoms of heart disease, while also identifying musculoskeletal problems that should be evaluated prior to participation in an exercise program. The one-page AHA/ACSM questionnaire is more extensive than the PAR-Q and uses history, symptoms, and risk factors to direct clients to either participate in an exercise program or contact their healthcare provider before participation.

Physical Activity Readiness
Questionnaire - PAR-Q
(revised 2002)

# PAR-Q & YOU

## (A Questionnaire for People Aged 15 to 69)

Regular physical activity is fun and healthy, and increasingly more people are starting to become more active every day. Being more active is very safe for most people. However, some people should check with their doctor before they start becoming much more physically active.

If you are planning to become much more physically active than you are now, start by answering the seven questions in the box below. If you are between the ages of 15 and 69, the PAR-Q will tell you if you should check with your doctor before you start. If you are over 69 years of age, and you are not used to being very active, check with your doctor.

Common sense is your best guide when you answer these questions. Please read the questions carefully and answer each one honestly: check YES or NO.

| YES | NO | | |
|---|---|---|---|
| ☐ | ☐ | 1. | Has your doctor ever said that you have a heart condition **and** that you should only do physical activity recommended by a doctor? |
| ☐ | ☐ | 2. | Do you feel pain in your chest when you do physical activity? |
| ☐ | ☐ | 3. | In the past month, have you had chest pain when you were not doing physical activity? |
| ☐ | ☐ | 4. | Do you lose your balance because of dizziness or do you ever lose consciousness? |
| ☐ | ☐ | 5. | Do you have a bone or joint problem (for example, back, knee or hip) that could be made worse by a change in your physical activity? |
| ☐ | ☐ | 6. | Is your doctor currently prescribing drugs (for example, water pills) for your blood pressure or heart condition? |
| ☐ | ☐ | 7. | Do you know of **any other reason** why you should not do physical activity? |

**If you answered**

## YES to one or more questions

Talk with your doctor by phone or in person BEFORE you start becoming much more physically active or BEFORE you have a fitness appraisal. Tell your doctor about the PAR-Q and which questions you answered YES.

- You may be able to do any activity you want — as long as you start slowly and build up gradually. Or, you may need to restrict your activities to those which are safe for you. Talk with your doctor about the kinds of activities you wish to participate in and follow his/her advice.
- Find out which community programs are safe and helpful for you.

## NO to all questions

If you answered NO honestly to <u>all</u> PAR-Q questions, you can be reasonably sure that you can:
- start becoming much more physically active — begin slowly and build up gradually. This is the safest and easiest way to go.
- take part in a fitness appraisal — this is an excellent way to determine your basic fitness so that you can plan the best way for you to live actively. It is also highly recommended that you have your blood pressure evaluated. If your reading is over 144/94, talk with your doctor before you start becoming much more physically active.

→ **DELAY BECOMING MUCH MORE ACTIVE:**
- if you are not feeling well because of a temporary illness such as a cold or a fever — wait until you feel better; or
- if you are or may be pregnant — talk to your doctor before you start becoming more active.

**PLEASE NOTE:** If your health changes so that you then answer YES to any of the above questions, tell your fitness or health professional. Ask whether you should change your physical activity plan.

<u>Informed Use of the PAR-Q</u>: The Canadian Society for Exercise Physiology, Health Canada, and their agents assume no liability for persons who undertake physical activity, and if in doubt after completing this questionnaire, consult your doctor prior to physical activity.

**No changes permitted. You are encouraged to photocopy the PAR-Q but only if you use the entire form.**

NOTE: If the PAR-Q is being given to a person before he or she participates in a physical activity program or a fitness appraisal, this section may be used for legal or administrative purposes.

"I have read, understood and completed this questionnaire. Any questions I had were answered to my full satisfaction."

NAME _____

SIGNATURE _____ DATE_____

SIGNATURE OF PARENT _____ WITNESS _____
or GUARDIAN (for participants under the age of majority)

**Note:** This physical activity clearance is valid for a maximum of 12 months from the date it is completed and becomes invalid if your condition changes so that you would answer YES to any of the seven questions.

 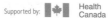
continued on other side...

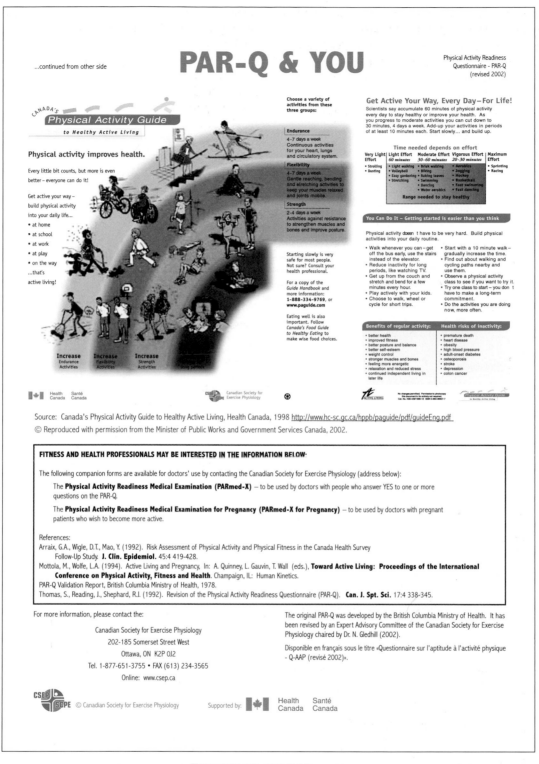

■ **FIGURE 2.2** PAR-Q & You.

**PAR-Q (Physical Activity Readiness Questionnaire)**

*Definition*: Questionnaire developed by Canadian researchers to assess general health status.

*Purpose*: Minimum screening measure for low-to-moderate intensity training.

*Benefit*: Valid, easy to administer, time-efficient.

GEIs, who work in health clubs, should not assume that because clients have been cleared for a membership based on either of these screening tools or based on more in-depth assessments collected previously, they do not require further

**AHA/ACSM   Health/Fitness Facility Preparticipation Screening Questionnaire**

### Access your health status by marking all *true* statements

**History**

You have had:

- [ ] a heart attack
- [ ] heart surgery
- [ ] cardiac catheterization
- [ ] coronary angioplasty (PTCA)
- [ ] pacemaker-implantable cardiac defibrillatory/rhythm disturbance
- [ ] heart valve disease
- [ ] heart failure
- [ ] heart transplantation
- [ ] congenital heart disease

**Symptoms**

- [ ] You experience chest discomfort with exertion
- [ ] You experience unreasonable breathlessness
- [ ] You experience dizziness, fainting, or blackouts
- [ ] You take heart medications

> If you marked any of these statements in this section, consult your physician or other appropriate health care provider before engaging in exercise. You may need to use a facility with a **m edically qualified staff.**

**Other health issues**

- [ ] You have diabetes
- [ ] You have asthma or other lung disease
- [ ] You have burning or cramping sensation in your lower legs when walking short distances
- [ ] You have musculoskeletal problems that limit your physical activity
- [ ] You have concerns about the safety of exercise
- [ ] You take prescription medications
- [ ] You are pregnant

**Cardiovascular risk factors**

- [ ] You are a man 45 years or older
- [ ] You are a woman 55 years or older
- [ ] You smoke, or quit smoking within the previous 6 months
- [ ] Your blood pressure is >140/90 mm Hg
- [ ] You do not know your blood pressure
- [ ] You take blood pressure medication
- [ ] Your blood cholesterol level is >200 mg/dL
- [ ] You do not know your cholesterol level
- [ ] You have a close blood relative who had a heart attack or heart surgery before age 55 (father or brother) or age 65 (mother or sister)
- [ ] You are physically inactive (ie, you get <30 minutes of physical activity on at least 3 days/week)
- [ ] You are >20 pounds overweight.

> If you marked two or more of the statements in this section, you should consult your physician or other appropriate healthcare provider before engaging in exercise. You might benefit from using a facility with a **professionally qualified exercise staff†** to guide your exercise program.

† Professionally qualified exercise staff refers to appropriately trained individuals who posses academic training, practical and clinical knowledge, skills and abilities commensurate with the credentials defined in Appendix D of <u>ACSM's Guidelines for Exercise Testing and Prescription 8e.</u>

- [ ] None of the above

> You should be able to exercise safely without consulting your physician or other appropriate health care provider in a self-guided program or almost any facility that meets your exercise program needs.

Modified from **American College of Sports Medicine and American Heart Association ACSM/AHA** joint position statement. Recommendations for cardiovascular screening, staffing and emergency policies at health fitness facilities. Med Sci Sports Exerc 1998:1018.

■ **FIGURE 2.3** AHA/ACSM questionnaire.

evaluation or medical clearance. Many health clubs require absolutely no health paperwork to be submitted before being accepted as a new member. GEIs should always confirm with clients that their risk stratification and health information are accurate and up-to-date before clients participate in exercise classes. Signs and symptoms suggesting cardiovascular disease can appear suddenly, medication changes are frequent, and injuries may occur without warning.

## Risk Stratification

*Definition*: Used to identify participants who should undergo a medical examination and exercise testing before beginning a moderate or vigorous exercise program. The process is based on the client's risk factors for cardiovascular, pulmonary, or metabolic disease; signs and symptoms suggestive of disease; and diagnoses of diseases (5).

*Purpose*: To identify persons with risk factors for cardiovascular, pulmonary, or metabolic disease.

*Benefit*: Helps to determine those individuals who may need a medical clearance in order to participate in exercise training.

*Special Note*: A participant at high risk should be referred to physician for clearance prior to starting classes, especially when you are working as an independent provider.

The ACSM risk stratification process has been widely used to identify clients who should undergo a medical examination and exercise testing before beginning a moderate or vigorous exercise program. The process is based on the client's risk factors for cardiovascular, pulmonary, or metabolic disease; signs and symptoms suggestive of disease; and diagnoses of diseases. This procedure provides recommendations for both medical clearance and physician involvement in submaximal or maximal cardiovascular fitness testing.

Risk stratification is the simple process of using the information provided by the preactivity screening tool (*i.e.*, ParQ) to determine whether the prospective class participant belongs in the low-risk, moderate-risk, or high-risk category. Following the checklist below will help simplify risk stratification.

- Step 1: Conduct a health history evaluation (Figs. 2.2 and 2.3).
- Step 2: Determine the number of risk factors, based on Table 2.1, "Atherosclerotic Cardiovascular Disease Risk Factor Thresholds for Use with ACSM Risk Stratification," and the number of signs and symptoms, based on Table 2.2, "Major Signs or Symptoms

| Table 2.1 | ATHEROSCLEROTIC CARDIOVASCULAR DISEASE RISK FACTOR THRESHOLDS FOR USE WITH ACSM RISK STRATIFICATION |
|---|---|
| **RISK FACTORS** | **DEFINING CRITERIA** |
| **Positive** | |
| Age | Men ≥ 45 yr; women ≥ 55 yr |
| Family history | Myocardial infarction, coronary revascularization, or sudden death before 55 yr of age in father or other male first-degree relative, or before 65 yr of age in mother or other female first-degree relative |
| Cigarette smoking | Current cigarette smoker or those who quit within the previous 6 mo or exposure to environmental tobacco smoke |
| Sedentary lifestyle | Not participating in at least 30 min of moderate-intensity (40%–60% [$\dot{V}O_2R$]) physical activity on at least 3 d of the week for at least 3 mo |
| Obesity[a] | BMI > 30 kg·m$^2$ or waist girth >102 cm (40 in) for men and >88 cm (35 in) for women |
| Hypertension | Systolic blood pressure ≥ 140 mm Hg or diastolic ≥ 90 mm Hg, confirmed by measurements on at least two separate occasions or on antihypertensive medication |
| Dyslipidemia | Low-density lipoprotein cholesterol ≥ 130 mg·dL$^{-1}$ (3.4 mmol·L$^{-1}$) or HDL-C < 40 mg·dL$^{-1}$ (1.04 mmol·L$^{-1}$) or on lipid-lowering medication; if total serum cholesterol is all that is available, use ≥200 mg·dL$^{-1}$ (5.2 mmol·L$^{-1}$) |
| Pre-diabetes | Impaired fasting glucose = fasting plasma glucose ≥ 100 mg·dL$^{-1}$ (5.50 mmol·L$^{-1}$) but <126 mg·dL$^{-1}$ (6.93 mmol·L$^{-1}$) or impaired glucose tolerance = 2-h values in oral glucose tolerance test ≥140 mg·dL$^{-1}$ (7.70 mmol·L$^{-1}$) but <200 mg·dL$^{-1}$ (11.00 mmol·L$^{-1}$) confirmed by measurements on at least two separate occasions |
| **Negative** | |
| High serum HDL-C[b] | ≥60 mg·dL$^{-1}$ (1.6 mmol·L$^{-1}$) |

BMI, body mass index; HDL-C, high-density lipoprotein cholesterol.

Hypertension threshold based on National High Blood Pressure Education Program. The Seventh Report of the Joint National Committee on Prevention, Detection, Evaluation, and Treatment of High Blood Pressure, 03-5233, 2003. Lipid thresholds based on National Cholesterol Education Program. Third Report of the National Cholesterol Education Program Expert Panel on Detection, Evaluation, and Treatment of High Blood Cholesterol in Adults (Adult Treatment Panel III). NIH Publication no. 02-5215, 2002. Impaired FG threshold based on Expert Committee on the Diagnosis and Classification of Diabetes Mellitus. Follow-up report on the diagnosis of diabetes mellitus. Diabetes Care. 2003;26:3160–7. Obesity thresholds based on Expert Panel on Detection, Evaluation, and Treatment of Overweight and Obesity in Adults. National Institutes of Health. Clinical guidelines on the identification, evaluation, and treatment of overweight and obesity in adults—the evidence report. Arch Intern Med. 1998;158:1855–67. Sedentary lifestyle thresholds based on U.S. Department of Health and Human Services. Physical activity and health: a report of the Surgeon General, 1996.

[a]Professional opinions vary regarding the most appropriate markers and thresholds for obesity, and therefore, allied health care professionals should use clinical judgment when evaluating this risk factor.

[b]It is common to sum risk factors in making clinical judgments. If HDL is high, subtract one risk factor from the sum of positive risk factors, because high HDL decreases CAD risk.

Reprinted from American College of Sports Medicine. ACSM's Guidelines for Exercise Testing and Prescription. 8th ed. Baltimore (MD): Lippincott Williams & Wilkins; 2010.

| Table 2.2 | MAJOR SIGNS OR SYMPTOMS SUGGESTIVE OF CARDIOVASCULAR, PULMONARY, OR METABOLIC DISEASES |
|---|---|
| **SIGN OR SYMPTOM**[a] | **CLARIFICATION/SIGNIFICANCE** |
| Pain, discomfort (or other anginal equivalent) in the chest, neck, jaw, arms, or other areas that may result from ischemia | One of the cardinal manifestations of cardiac disease, in particular CAD<br>Key features favoring an ischemic origin include:<br>    Character: Constricting, squeezing, burning, "heaviness" or "heavy feeling"<br>    Location: Substernal, across midthorax, anteriorly; in both arms and shoulders; in neck, cheeks, and teeth; in forearms and fingers; in interscapular region<br>    Provoking factors: Exercise or exertion, excitement, other forms of stress, cold weather, occurrence after meals<br>Key features against an ischemic origin include:<br>    Character: Dull ache; "knifelike," sharp, stabbing; "jabs" aggravated by respiration<br>    Location: In left submammary area; in left hemithorax<br>    Provoking factors: After completion of exercise, provoked by a specific body motion |
| Shortness of breath at rest or with mild exertion | Dyspnea (defined as an abnormally uncomfortable awareness of mild exertion breathing) is one of the principal symptoms of cardiac and pulmonary disease. It commonly occurs during strenuous exertion in healthy, well-trained persons and during moderate exertion in healthy, untrained persons. However, it should be regarded as abnormal when it occurs at a level of exertion that is not expected to evoke this symptom in a given individual. Abnormal exertional dyspnea suggests the presence of cardiopulmonary disorders, in particular left ventricular dysfunction or chronic obstructive pulmonary disease. |
| Dizziness or syncope | Syncope (defined as a loss of consciousness) is most commonly caused by a reduced perfusion of the brain. Dizziness and, in particular, syncope during exercise may result from cardiac disorders that prevent the normal rise (or an actual fall) in cardiac output. Such cardiac disorders are potentially life threatening and include severe CAD, hypertrophic cardiomyopathy, aortic stenosis, and malignant ventricular dysrhythmias. Although dizziness or syncope shortly after cessation of exercise should not be ignored, these symptoms may occur even in healthy persons as a result of a reduction in venous return to the heart. |
| Orthopnea or paroxysmal nocturnal dyspnea | Orthopnea refers to dyspnea occurring at rest in the recumbent dyspnea position that is relieved promptly by sitting upright or standing. Paroxysmal nocturnal dyspnea refers to dyspnea, beginning usually 2–5 h after the onset of sleep, which may be relieved by sitting on the side of the bed or getting out of bed. Both are symptoms of left ventricular dysfunction. Although nocturnal dyspnea may occur in persons with chronic obstructive pulmonary disease, it differs in that it is usually relieved after the person relieves himself or herself of secretions rather than specifically by sitting up. |
| Ankle edema | Bilateral ankle edema that is most evident at night is a characteristic sign of heart failure or bilateral chronic venous insufficiency. Unilateral edema of a limb often results from venous thrombosis or lymphatic blockage in the limb. Generalized edema (known as anasarca) occurs in persons with the nephrotic syndrome, severe heart failure, or hepatic cirrhosis. |
| Palpitations or tachycardia | Palpitations (defined as an unpleasant awareness of the forceful or rapid beating of the heart) may be induced by various disorders of cardiac rhythm. These include tachycardia, bradycardia of sudden onset, ectopic beats, compensatory pauses, and accentuated stroke volume resulting from valvular regurgitation. Palpitations also often result from anxiety states, such as anemia, fever, thyrotoxicosis, arteriovenous fistula, and the so-called idiopathic hyperkinetic heart syndrome. |
| Intermittent claudication | Intermittent claudication refers to the pain that occurs in a muscle with an inadequate blood supply (usually as a result of atherosclerosis) that is stressed by exercise. The pain does not occur with standing or sitting, is reproducible from day to day, is more severe when walking upstairs or up a hill, and is often described as a cramp, which disappears within 1 or 2 min after stopping exercise. CAD is more prevalent in persons with intermittent claudication. Patients with diabetes are at increased risk for this condition. |
| Known heart murmur | Although some may be innocent, heart murmurs may indicate valvular or other cardiovascular disease. From an exercise safety standpoint, it is especially important to exclude hypertrophic cardiomyopathy and aortic stenosis as underlying causes because these are among the more common causes of exertion-related sudden cardiac death. |
| Unusual fatigue or shortness of breath with usual activities | Although there may be benign origins for these symptoms, they with usual activities also may signal the onset of, or change in the status of, cardiovascular, pulmonary, or metabolic disease. |

CAD, coronary artery disease.

[a]These signs or symptoms must be interpreted within the clinical context in which they appear because they are not all specific for cardiovascular, pulmonary, or metabolic disease.

Reprinted from American College of Sports Medicine. ACSM's Guidelines for Exercise Testing and Prescription. 8th ed. Baltimore (MD): Lippincott Williams & Wilkins; 2010.

Suggestive of Cardiovascular, Pulmonary, or Metabolic Disease" (Tables 2.1 and 2.2).
- Step 3: Determine whether the client is at low, moderate, or high risk, based on Figure 2.4, "ACSM Preparticipation Screening Logic Model."
- Step 4: Determine whether a medical evaluation or exercise testing is necessary on the basis of Figure 2.5, "Exercise testing and test supervision recommendations based on risk stratification."

- Step 5: Obtain a medical clearance if indicated by step 3 or 4 (Figs. 2.6 and 2.7).
- Step 6: Refer the client to a physician or other health care provider if warranted.
- Step 7: Complete an informed consent (Box 2.5).
- Step 8: Conduct fitness assessments, if appropriate.

To provide some general guidance on the need for a medical examination and exercise testing prior to participation in a moderate-to-vigorous exercise program, ACSM suggests the recommendations presented in Figure 2.5 for determining when a medical examination and diagnostic exercise test are appropriate and when physician supervision is recommended during exercise testing. Although the testing guidelines are less rigorous for those clients considered to be at low risk, the information gathered from an exercise test may be useful in establishing a safe and effective exercise

prescription for these clients. The exercise-testing recommendations found in Figure 2.5 reflect the notion that the risk of cardiovascular events increases as a function of increasing physical activity intensity. GEIs should choose the most appropriate definition of their setting when making decisions about the level of screening to use prior to exercise training and whether or not it is necessary to have physician supervision during exercise testing.

**Medical Clearance**

*Definition*: Form provided to participant's physician requesting approval for exercise.

*Purpose*: Approval from physician for individuals at risk (as determined by risk stratification)

*Benefit*: Provides GEI with information regarding physical readiness of potential participant at risk.

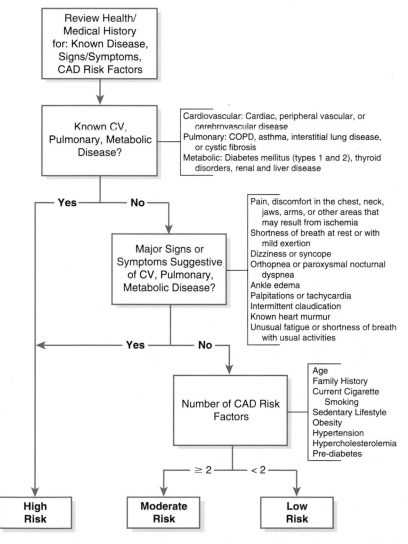

■ **FIGURE 2.4** ACSM Preparticipation Screening Logic Model.

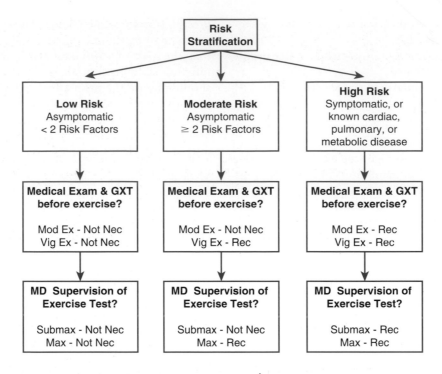

■ **FIGURE 2.5** Exercise testing and test supervision recommendations based on risk stratification. (Reprinted from American College of Sports Medicine. *ACSM's Guidelines for Exercise Testing and Prescription*. 8th ed. Baltimore (MD): Lippincott Williams & Wilkins; 2010.)

## Medical Information Release

*Definition*: Form signed by potential or existing participant that will permit physician to release medical information.

*Purpose*: Used prior to requesting any specific health information and/or medical clearance for exercise from participant's physician.

*Benefit*: Provides GEI with health information

## Informed Consent

*Definition*: Document that explains the risks and benefits of participating in physical activity (specific class) to a prospective participant. The consent should also provide the participant with an opportunity to ask questions prior to participation in the class or activity.

*Purpose*: Participant agrees that he or she knowingly understands these risks and benefits, appreciates these risks, and voluntarily assumes responsibility for taking these risks.

*Benefits*: Provides GEI and potential participant the opportunity to discuss risks associated with the class.

*Note:* It is recommended that the consent form is constructed to meet the needs of the instructor and should be reviewed by the legal staff affiliated with individual programs. The following sample informed consent has been drafted to include a release of liability waiver and a promotional waiver from XYZ Fitness (Fig. 2.8).

## Release of Liability Form

*Definition*: Document states that participant knowingly waives or releases the class instructor from liability for any acts of negligence on the part of the instructor.

*Purpose*: To protect the class instructor and/or the facility by having prospective participant waive his or her right to sue the class instructor for negligence.

*Benefit*: Helps to protect the GEI for being sued.

## Sample medical clearance form

Date: *Insert here*

Dear Dr. Rodriguez,

I am writing to you in regard to your patient, Suzanne Walker-Smith, a 40 year-old female (DOB: December 6, 1969), who indicated you are her primary physician. She would like to begin a moderate to vigorous intensity exercise program under the supervision of a certified Group Exercise Instructor. I have attached her authorization for the release of her medical information, plus her responses to our cardiovascular screening questionnaire.

Please provide your recommendation regarding her exercise participation and any restrictions and/or limitations you suggest for her program. Should you have any questions or concerns, please contact me at the number below. Thank you.

Physician recommendation:

☐ Patient may participate in unrestricted activity.

☐ Patient may participate in light to moderate activities only.

☐ Patient should not participate in activity at this time.

☐ Other: please specify: _____

_____

Please specify any restrictions or limitations you feel appropriate: _____

_____

Physician (print name):_____ Date: _____ Telephone: _____

Signature: _____

Group Exercise Instructor (name):_____ Date: _____ Telephone: _____

Send this form to:

Your first/last name, title
Company Name
Street address
City, State, Zip Code
Fax
Email address

■ **FIGURE 2.6** Sample medical clearance.

## FIELD TESTS FOR THE GROUP EXERCISE INSTRUCTOR

Physical fitness refers to the specific attributes of fitness. The five components of fitness include cardiovascular endurance, muscular fitness — consisting of muscular strength and muscular endurance, flexibility, and body composition. There are a variety of tests that can be used to determine an individual's fitness level. Having this personalized information can assist the GEI with class intensity and the types of modifications that may be necessary. The fitness testing is often referred to as field tests and should be an option for all members of a supervised fitness facility. The field tests are usually completed by the exercise staff of the supervised fitness facility. This might apply to some GEIs while others may not actually administer the tests. It

---

### Release of medical information form

Date: *Insert here*

Dear Dr. Rodriquez,

I, Suzanne Walker-Smith, a 40 year-old female, (DOB: December 6, 1969), hereby authorize the immediate release of a copy of all my medical information to the following person(s):

Your first/last name, Group Exercise Instructor
Company Name
Street address
City, Staty, Zip Code
Fax
Email address

My purpose of disclosing this information is to begin/continue an exercise program with the above Group Exercise Instructor.

Patient's signature: _____    Date: _____  Telephone: _____

■ **FIGURE 2.7**  Sample release of medical information form.

---

is critical that the GEI is familiar with the various options and, more importantly, how to interpret the results.

Field tests provide the GEI with an array of options that are appropriate in a class or group setting. The following tests may be adapted for use in a group classroom by enabling each participant to self-report and record his/her own performance.

### 3-MINUTE STEP TEST

#### Step Test Protocol/Script

▶ CLIP 2.2  During this test you will step up and down on the step (12 inches in height) always leading with the same foot at a rate of 24 steps per minute in time with the metronome (set to 96 beats per minute [bpm]) like this: (demonstrate the stepping technique to the person to be tested in a 4-count movement — right foot onto the bench on 1, left foot up on 2, right foot down to the floor on 3, and left foot down on 4) (Fig. 2.9).

The exerciser(s) should have some preliminary practice using the step before you begin, and should be well rested before you proceed to administer the test. (Prior exercise and/or not resting prior to test will affect their recovery heart rate.) If the exerciser(s) fall behind on the count, the test administrator should make them aware of that and start the 4-count out loud, so that the exerciser(s) can try to keep up. The test lasts 3 minutes. At the end of the 3 minutes, the tester instructs the participants to sit on their bench. Within 5 seconds, participants take their heart rate for 15 seconds and multiply the result by 4 to determine training heart rate for one minute. This training heart rate is the test score. Instructors can use this test score as a benchmark and retest periodically.

### PARTIAL CURL-UP

The Partial Curl-up test helps assess a client's muscular endurance. It is considered superior to the full sit-up test because it is not as sensitive to back injury or chronic

**BOX 2.5** Sample Informed Consent for Exercise Participation

**Voluntary Participation**

I desire to engage voluntarily in one or more of XYZ Fitness' exercise program(s) in order to attempt to improve my physical fitness. I understand that the activities are designed to place a gradually increasing workload on the musculoskeletal, metabolic, and/or cardio-respiratory system and thereby attempt to improve my work capacity and overall function. The reaction of the cardiorespiratory system to such activities can't be predicted with complete accuracy. There is a risk of certain changes that might occur during or following exercise. These changes might include abnormalities of blood pressure or heart rate.

**Risk and Discomforts**

There are inherent risks associated with strength training, aerobic conditioning and other forms of physical activity. Strength training may result in acute muscle and/or joint pain, pulled muscles, brief changes in blood pressure, light headedness, dizziness, delayed onset muscle soreness (DOMS), more chronic conditions such as tendonitis, and other discomforts. Training should be modified or postponed if joint injury is present or if pain or symptoms persist. Aerobic conditioning may result in fast or slow irregular heart rhythm, abnormal blood pressure changes, light-headedness, dizziness, fainting, chest pain, and other discomforts. Any type of physical activity may in rare instances lead to heart attack, stroke or death, but this is unusual, especially in participants free of known coronary heart disease (CHD), free of any signs or symptoms of CHD, and with few major risk factors of CHD. Inspire Training Systems' Coaches are trained in basic cardiac life support (CPR) and are educated to watch for any signs or symptoms associated with a poor exercise response.

**Responsibilities of the Participant**

To promote the safety and benefit of my participation in any and all XYZ Fitness' exercise programs, it is important that I fully disclose my personal health history, any medications I am taking, and any symptoms I may be experiencing during exercise. Such symptoms would include joint pain, irregular heart rhythm, tightness or pressure in my chest, unusual shortness of breath, light headedness, dizziness and the like. It is also important that I adhere to the recommendations of the XYZ Fitness' Coach(es) especially with regard to the choice and intensity of exercises I perform. I should not exceed the recommended exercise intensity (as measured by weight lifted or exercise heart rate) and I should not exercise when I am injured, sick or not otherwise feeling well.

**Benefits to be Expected**

It is expected that I will see benefits as a result of regular and consistent participation. Strength training typically results in numerous physical benefits (including improved muscle strength, increased muscle mass and increased bone density) and possibly in an improvement in physical tasks associated with work, recreation and everyday life. Aerobic conditioning typically results in health benefits (including body fat loss, reduced blood pressure and reduced risk of CHD) and possibly in changes associate with improved exercise performance (including increased aerobic capacity, improved heart and lung function and improved circulation).

**Inquiries**

An important part of the informed consent process is providing me the opportunity to inquire about any and all aspects of XYZ Fitness' exercise programs. If I have any questions or concerns about XYZ Fitness' exercise programs, I will ask a Coach on the XYZ Fitness staff.

**Use of Medical Records and Information**

Any information gathered in conjunction with XYZ Fitness exercise programs (such as health history information, signs or symptoms of disease, risk of disease, exercise risk, blood pressure, body composition, aerobic fitness, instances of joint pain, chest pain, light headedness or dizziness, etc.) will be kept confidential to the extent provided by law. I will be encouraged share or to allow XYZ Fitness to share this information with my physician or primary care provider in an attempt to diagnose or treat a current disease or reduce myrisk of developing a more serious medical condition. I may be asked to complete and sign an authorization of use and disclosure form (PF-3000) in compliance with current HIPAA laws, so that XYZ Fitness might ask my personal physician for input in developing a safe and effective exercise program for me. No identifiable information will be released or revealed to any other party without my written consent. I may be asked, however, to allow certain information (from which my identity is removed) to be used for statistical analysis or clinical research purposes.

**Freedom of Consent**

I agree to voluntarily participate in any or all XYZ Fitness' exercise programs. I understand that I am free to deny consent if I so desire now or at any point in the program.

**Please Read the Following Statements Carefully and Initial**

_____ I acknowledge that I have read this form in its entirety or it has been read to me, and I understand my responsibility in the XYZ Fitness exercise program in which I will be engaged. I accept the risks, rules, and regulations set forth. Knowing these, and having had an opportunity to ask questions which have been answered to my satisfaction, I consent to participate in all XYZ Fitness exercise programs.

_____ If I am accidentally injured during any XYZ Fitness exercise programs, the XYZ Fitness staff will offer immediate first aid (if needed) but will be unable to provide treatment. If injured, I will be responsible to seek treatment with my own physician or primary care provider.

_____ Furthermore, I, for myself and my heirs, fully release from liability and waive all legal claims against XYZ Fitness and all XYZ Fitness staff for injury or damage that I might incur during participation in the XYZ Fitness exercise programs.

_____ In additional consideration of being permitted by XYZ Fitness to participate in its training program and to use its facilities, I hereby permit XYZ Fitness to use my name, image and likeness for promotional purposes limited to its training programs and facilities. The XYZ fitness promotional mediums include but are not limited to print, radio, video, television and the Internet.

I acknowledge that I have read this release and waiver and fully understand its contents. I have been fully and completely advised of the potential dangers incidental to engaging in the activity and instruction of athlete training and conditioning, and I am fully aware of the legal consequences of signing this release. I voluntarily agree to the terms and conditions stated above.

_____     _____
Signature                                                                          Date

Please return this form when completed and signed to an XYZ Fitness Coach.

I, _____, the undersigned, wish to participate in a fitness evaluation which consists of a submaximal cardiovascular assessment (bike or treadmill), body fat analysis by skinfold, strength and flexibility assessments, muscular endurance assessment and individualized exercise program at the Fitness Center in Atlanta, Georgia, which is to be conducted on this _____ day of _____, 20_____. The evaluation will be conducted under the direction of a Personal Trainer. I understand and acknowledge that participation in the fitness evaluation activities involves an inherent risk of physical injury and I assume all such risks. I understand that I will participate in all fitness exercises in said fitness evaluation. I assume all risks of damage or injury, including death, that may be sustained by me while particpating in the fitness evaluation test.

For and in consideration of The Fitness Center allowing me to take the fitness evaluation, I hereby release and covenant not to sue The Fitness Center, the officers, agents, members and employees of each, from any and from all claims or actions, including those of negligence, which might arise as a result of any personal injury, including death, or property damage which I might suffer as a result of my participation in the fitness evaluation on the date set forth above.

By signing this document, I hereby acknowledge that I am at least 18 years of age and have read the above carefully before signing, and agree with all of its provisions this _____ day of _____, 20_____.

_____
Signature of Participant

■ **FIGURE 2.8** Sample agreement release of liability and waiver form. Note that this form is presented for information purposes only and should be not considered legal advice or used as such. The use of this form in specific situations requires substantive legal judgments, and a licensed attorney should be consulted before using the form.

back pain. This test is part of the Canadian Physical Activity, Fitness & Lifestyle Approach and has been adopted by ACSM (see Table 2.3).

### Appropriateness

Any medically cleared participant having no orthopedic limitations that would affect their ability to perform this test. Participants with significant back or neck pain or pain that is aggravated by this motion should not perform this test.

### Preparation

Before starting this test, ensure that the participant has properly prepared.

You will need to prepare that curl-up mat before administering this test. To do so, apply masking tape to a gym mat as illustrated below. Mark distances on tape as shown. Fasten strip of string or Velcro at 0 and 10 cm marks on both sides.

### Equipment

Gym mat, masking tape, metric ruler, pen, carpenter's square, metronome, and string/Velcro strip.

### Procedure

### Starting Position

The participant lies in a supine position with head resting on the mat, arms straight at sides and parallel to the trunk, palms of hands in contact with the mat, and fingertips at the "0" (zero) mark. Bend knees at an angle of 90 degrees using a square. Attach a strip of masking tape under the heels to indicate where they must maintain contact with the mat.

### Action

Set the metronome to 50 bpm. The initial phase of the curl-up must involve a "flattening-out" of the lower back region (i.e., pelvic tilt) followed by a slow "curling-up" of the upper spine, sliding the palms of the hands along the graduated tape strip until the middle fingertips of both hands touch/feel the string/Velcro at the 10-cm mark. During the curl-up, the palms of both hands must remain in contact with the mat (see "Alternatives Suggested by ACSM" below). Return to the starting position (fingertips touch/feel the string/Velcro at the 0 cm mark, shoulder blades touching the floor, head resting

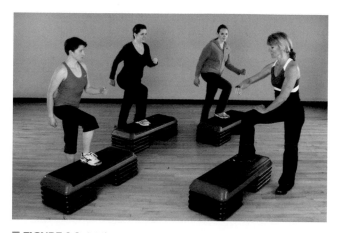

■ **FIGURE 2.9** 3-Minute step test is a tried and true cardiovascular fitness test that can be delivered and used with individuals as well as groups. This makes it an ideal field test for group exercises classes.

on the mat). The cadence is 25 curl-ups per minute. The movement is continuous and well controlled. The time to perform the raising and lowering phases is the same. Participants perform at a steady rate, counting up on one beat and down on the next, without pausing between curl-ups. The participant should continue to do curl-ups for 1 minute, or until they can no longer keep up with the metronome or they reach 25 curls-ups (the maximum).

## Alternatives Suggested by ACSM

A. To permit participants to cross their hands over their chest and to count a full rep when the trunk reaches a 30-degree position
B. Placing the hands on the thighs and curling up until the hands reach the kneecaps. Elevation of the trunk to 30 degrees is the important aspect of the movement and can be achieved by any of the three methods described here.

| Table 2.3 | FITNESS CATEGORIES BY AGE GROUPS AND GENDER FOR PARTIAL CURL-UP | | | | | | | | | |
|---|---|---|---|---|---|---|---|---|---|---|
| | **AGE** | | | | | | | | | |
| **CATEGORY** | 20–29 | | 30–39 | | 40–49 | | 50–59 | | 60–69 | |
| **GENDER** | M | F | M | F | M | F | M | F | M | F |
| Excellent | 25 | 25 | 25 | 25 | 25 | 25 | 25 | 25 | 25 | 25 |
| Very good | 24 | 24 | 24 | 24 | 24 | 24 | 24 | 24 | 24 | 24 |
| | 21 | 18 | 18 | 19 | 18 | 19 | 17 | 19 | 16 | 17 |
| Good | 20 | 17 | 17 | 18 | 17 | 18 | 16 | 18 | 15 | 16 |
| | 16 | 14 | 15 | 10 | 13 | 11 | 11 | 10 | 11 | 8 |
| Fair | 15 | 13 | 14 | 9 | 12 | 10 | 10 | 9 | 10 | 7 |
| | 11 | 5 | 11 | 6 | 6 | 4 | 8 | 6 | 6 | 3 |
| Needs improvement | 10 | 4 | 10 | 5 | 5 | 3 | 7 | 5 | 5 | 2 |

From Thompson W. *ACSM's Resources for the Personal Trainer. 3rd ed.* Lippincott Williams & Wilkins; 2010; Figure 19.4.

## PUSH-UP TEST

The push-up test is administered with male subjects starting in the standard "down" position (hands pointing forward and under the shoulder, back straight, head up, using the toes as the pivotal point) and female subjects in the modified "knee push-up" position (legs together, lower leg in contact with mat with ankles plantar-flexed, back straight, hands shoulder width apart, head up, using the knees as the pivotal point).

### Appropriateness

The test is appropriate for any medical-cleared participants having no orthopedic limitations that would affect their ability to perform this test. Participants with significant back or neck pain that is aggravated by this motion should not perform this test.

### Preparation

Before starting this test, ensure that the participant has properly prepared.

### Procedure

The subject must raise the body by straightening the elbows and return to the "down" position, until the chin touches the mat. The stomach should not touch the mat.

For both men and women, the subject's back must be straight at all times, and the subject must push up to a straight arm position.

The maximal number of push-ups performed consecutively without rest is counted as the score (Table 2.8).

## BODY COMPOSITION TESTS

Body composition can be defined as the relative proportion of fat and fat-free tissue in the body (percent body fat). The assessment of body composition is necessary for numerous reasons. There is a strong correlation (2) between obesity and increased risk of chronic diseases including coronary artery disease (CAD), diabetes, hypertension, certain cancers, and hyperlipidemia. There is a frequent need to evaluate body weight and body composition in the health and fitness field. Most often this evaluation is done to establish a target, desirable, or optimal weight for an individual. There are several ways to evaluate the composition of the human body. Body composition can be estimated with both laboratory and field techniques that vary in terms of complexity, cost, and accuracy. For the purposes of this text, the following techniques are reviewed:

- Height and weight
- Body mass index (BMI)
- Waist-to-hip ratio (WHR; waist and hip circumference measures)
- Skinfolds
- Bioelectrical impedance analysis (BIA)

- Body composition can be defined as the relative proportion of fat and fat-free tissue in the body (percent body fat).

## Height and Weight

Measure the client's height. Instruct the client with shoes removed to stand straight up; the client's heels should be together and his or her head should be level, the client should take a deep breath and hold it and look straight ahead. Record the height in centimeters or inches.

- 1 in = 2.54 cm
- 1 m = 100 cm
- For example: 6 ft = 72 in = 183 cm = 1.83 m

Measure the client's weight with his or her shoes removed and as much other clothing removed as is practical and possible. Convert weight from pounds to kilograms when necessary.

- 1 kg = 2.2 lb
- For example: 187 lb = 85 kg

With the many criticisms of the validity of the height-weight tables (including using a select group of individuals for development and the imprecise concept of "frame size"), there has been a strong trend recently to discontinue their use. Thus, this chapter discusses more advanced methods of anthropometry and body composition analysis.

## Body Mass Index

BMI, also called Quetelet's index, is used to assess weight relative to height. BMI has a similar association with body fat as the height-weight tables previously discussed. This technique compares an individual's weight (in kilograms) with his or her height (in square meters), much like a height-weight table would. The BMI gives a single number for comparison, as opposed to the weight-to-height ranges located in the tables.

$$BMI\ (kg \cdot m^{-2}) = weight\ (kg)/height\ (m^2)$$

For example, an individual who weighs 150 lb and is 5 ft, 8 in tall has a BMI of 5 ft 8 in = 173 cm = 1.73 m = 2.99 m² and 150 lb = 68.18 kg

$$BMI = 68.18/2.99 = 22.8\ kg \cdot m^{-2}$$

The major shortcoming with using BMI for body composition is that it is difficult for a client to relate to and/or interpret needed weight loss or weight gain. Also, the BMI does not differentiate fat weight from fat-free weight and has only a modest correlation with percentage body fat predicted from hydrostatic weighing. Standards and norms for BMI are presented in Table 2.4 and Figure 2.10.

## Waist-to-Hip Ratio

The WHR is a comparison between the circumference of the waist and the circumference of the hip. This ratio best represents the distribution of body weight, and perhaps body fat, in an individual. The pattern of body weight distribution is recognized as an important predictor of health risks of obesity. Individuals with more weight or circumference on the trunk are at higher risk of hypertension, type 2 diabetes, hyperlipidemia, and CAD than individuals who are of equal weight but have more of their weight distributed on the extremities. Some experts suggest that the waist circumference alone can be used as an indicator of health risk.

- Waist: The waist circumference has been frequently defined as the smallest waist circumference, typically measured 1 in (2.54 cm) above the umbilicus or navel and below the xiphoid process.
- Hip: The hip circumference has been defined as the largest circumference around the buttocks, above the gluteal fold (posterior extension).
- WHR is a ratio (thus, there are no units).
- WHR = waist circumference/hip circumference

Measure the waist and hip circumferences in either inches or centimeters (1 in = 2.54 cm). A quality tape with a spring-loaded handle (i.e., Gulick) should be used to measure circumferences. Take multiple measurements

| Table 2.4 | CLASSIFICATION OF DISEASE RISK BASED ON BMI AND WAIST CIRCUMFERENCE[a] | | |
|---|---|---|---|
| | BMI (KG·M⁻²) | DISEASE RISK RELATIVE TO NORMAL WEIGHT AND WAIST CIRCUMFERENCE: MEN < 102 CM; WOMEN < 88 CM | MEN > 102 CM; WOMEN > 88 CM |
| Underweight | <18.5 | — | — |
| Normal | 18.5–24.9 | — | — |
| Overweight | 25.0–29.9 | Increased | High |
| I | 30.0–34.9 | High | Very high |
| II | 35.0–39.9 | Very high | Very high |
| III | ≥40 | Extremely high | Extremely high |

BMI, body mass index.

[a]Disease risk for type 2 diabetes, hypertension, and cardiovascular disease. Dashes (—) indicate that no additional risk at these levels of BMI was assigned. Increased waist circumference can also be a marker for increased risk, even in persons of normal weight.

Modified from Expert Panel. Executive summary of the clinical guidelines on the identification, evaluation, and treatment of overweight and obesity in adults. Arch Intern Med. 1998;148:1855–67. Reprinted from American College of Sports Medicine. ACSM's Guidelines for Exercise Testing and Prescription. 8th ed. Baltimore (MD): Lippincott Williams & Wilkins; 2010; Table 14-2.

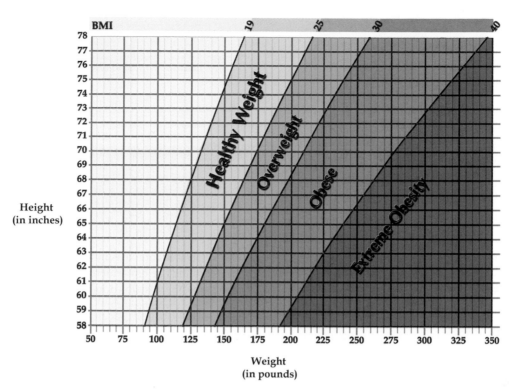

■ **FIGURE 2.10** The risks of obesity. How is body fat measured? BMI is a measure of weight in relation to a person's height. For most people, BMI has a strong relationship to weight. For adults, BMI can also be found by using this table. To use the BMI table, first find your weight at the bottom of the graph. Go straight up from that point until you reach the line that matches your height. Then look to see what weight group you fall in. BMI, body mass index. (Reprinted from Thompson W. *ACSM's Resources for the Personal Trainer*, 3rd ed. Lippincott Williams & Wilkins; 2010; Figure 14.5.)

| Table 2.5 | STANDARDIZED DESCRIPTION OF SKINFOLD SITES AND PROCEDURES |
|---|---|
| **SKINFOLD SITE** | |
| Abdominal | Vertical fold; 2 cm to the right side of the umbilicus |
| Triceps | Vertical fold; on the posterior midline of the upper arm, halfway between the acromion and olecranon processes, with the arm held freely to the side of the body |
| Biceps | Vertical fold; on the anterior aspect of the arm over the belly of the biceps muscle, 1 cm above the level used to mark the triceps site |
| Chest/pectoral | Diagonal fold; one-half the distance between the anterior axillary line and the nipple (men), or one-third of the distance between the anterior axillary line and the nipple (women) |
| Medial calf | Vertical fold; at the maximum circumference of the calf on the midline of its medial border |
| Midaxillary | Vertical fold; on the midaxillary line at the level of the xiphoid process of the sternum. An alternate method is a horizontal fold taken at the level of the xiphoid/sternal border in the midaxillary line |
| Subscapular | Diagonal fold (at a 45 degree angle); 1–2 cm below the inferior angle of the scapula |
| Suprailiac | Diagonal fold; in line with the natural angle of the iliac crest taken in the anterior axillary line immediately superior to the iliac crest |
| Thigh | Vertical fold; on the anterior midline of the thigh, midway between the proximal border of the patella and the inguinal crease (hip) |

**Procedures**

- All measurements should be made on the right side of the body with the subject standing upright
- Calipers should be placed directly on the skin surface, 1 cm away from the thumb and finger, perpendicular to the skinfold, and halfway between the crest and the base of the fold
- Pinch should be maintained while reading the calipers
- Wait 1–2 s (no longer) before reading calipers
- Take duplicate measures at each site, and retest if duplicate measurements are not within 1–2 mm
- Rotate through measurement sites or allow time for skin to regain normal texture and thickness

*Reprinted from American College of Sports Medicine. ACSM's Guidelines for Exercise Testing and Prescription. 8th ed. Baltimore (MD): Lippincott Williams & Wilkins; 2010.*

| Table 2.6 | BODY COMPOSITION (% BODY FAT) FOR MEN AND WOMEN | | | | | | |
|---|---|---|---|---|---|---|---|
| | **AGE, YR** | | | | | | |
| % | 20–29 | 30–39 | 40–49 | 50–59 | 60–69 | 70–79 | |
| **Men** | | | | | | | |
| 99 | 4.2 | 7.0 | 9.2 | 10.9 | 11.5 | 13.6 | |
| 95 | 6.3 | 9.9 | 12.8 | 14.4 | 15.5 | 15.2 | VL[a] |
| 90 | 7.9 | 11.9 | 14.9 | 16.7 | 17.6 | 17.8 | |
| 85 | 9.2 | 13.3 | 16.3 | 18.0 | 18.8 | 19.2 | |
| 80 | 10.5 | 14.5 | 17.4 | 19.1 | 19.7 | 20.4 | E |
| 75 | 11.5 | 15.5 | 18.4 | 19.9 | 20.6 | 21.1 | |
| 70 | 12.7 | 16.5 | 19.1 | 20.7 | 21.3 | 21.6 | |
| 65 | 13.9 | 17.4 | 19.9 | 21.3 | 22.0 | 22.5 | |
| 60 | 14.8 | 18.2 | 20.6 | 22.1 | 22.6 | 23.1 | G |
| 55 | 15.8 | 19.0 | 21.3 | 22.7 | 23.2 | 23.7 | |
| 50 | 16.6 | 19.7 | 21.9 | 23.2 | 23.7 | 24.1 | |
| 45 | 17.4 | 20.4 | 22.6 | 23.9 | 24.4 | 24.4 | |
| 40 | 18.6 | 21.3 | 23.4 | 24.6 | 25.2 | 24.8 | F |
| 35 | 19.6 | 22.1 | 24.1 | 25.3 | 26.0 | 25.4 | |
| 30 | 20.6 | 23.0 | 24.8 | 26.0 | 26.7 | 26.0 | |
| 25 | 21.9 | 23.9 | 25.7 | 26.8 | 27.5 | 26.7 | |
| 20 | 23.1 | 24.9 | 26.6 | 27.8 | 28.4 | 27.6 | P |
| 15 | 24.6 | 26.2 | 27.7 | 28.9 | 29.4 | 28.9 | |
| 10 | 26.3 | 27.8 | 29.2 | 30.3 | 30.9 | 30.4 | |
| 5 | 28.9 | 30.2 | 31.2 | 32.5 | 32.9 | 32.4 | |
| 1 | 33.3 | 34.3 | 35.0 | 36.4 | 36.8 | 35.5 | VP |
| n= | 1,826 | 8,373 | 10,442 | 6,079 | 1,836 | 301 | |
| Total n = 28,857 | | | | | | | |
| **Women** | | | | | | | |
| 99 | 9.8 | 11.0 | 12.6 | 14.6 | 13.9 | 14.6 | |
| 95 | 13.6 | 14.0 | 15.6 | 17.2 | 17.7 | 16.6 | VL[b] |
| 90 | 14.8 | 15.6 | 17.2 | 19.4 | 19.8 | 20.3 | |
| 85 | 15.8 | 16.6 | 18.6 | 20.9 | 21.4 | 23.0 | |
| 80 | 16.5 | 17.4 | 19.8 | 22.5 | 23.2 | 24.0 | E |
| 75 | 17.3 | 18.2 | 20.8 | 23.8 | 24.8 | 25.0 | |
| 70 | 18.0 | 19.1 | 21.9 | 25.1 | 25.9 | 26.2 | |
| 65 | 18.7 | 20.0 | 22.8 | 26.0 | 27.0 | 27.7 | |
| 60 | 19.4 | 20.8 | 23.8 | 27.0 | 27.9 | 28.6 | G |
| 55 | 20.1 | 21.7 | 24.8 | 27.9 | 28.7 | 29.7 | |
| 50 | 21.0 | 22.6 | 25.6 | 28.8 | 29.8 | 30.4 | |
| 45 | 21.9 | 23.5 | 26.5 | 29.7 | 30.6 | 31.3 | |
| 40 | 22.7 | 24.6 | 27.6 | 30.4 | 31.3 | 31.8 | F |
| 35 | 23.6 | 25.6 | 28.5 | 31.4 | 32.5 | 32.7 | |
| 30 | 24.5 | 26.7 | 29.6 | 32.5 | 33.3 | 33.9 | |
| 25 | 25.9 | 27.7 | 30.7 | 33.4 | 34.3 | 35.3 | |
| 20 | 27.1 | 29.1 | 31.9 | 34.5 | 35.4 | 36.0 | P |
| 15 | 28.9 | 30.9 | 33.5 | 35.6 | 36.2 | 37.4 | |
| 10 | 31.4 | 33.0 | 35.4 | 36.7 | 37.3 | 38.2 | |

*(Continued)*

| Table 2.6 | *(CONTINUED)* | | | | | | |
|---|---|---|---|---|---|---|---|
| | **AGE, YR** | | | | | | |
| % | 20–29 | 30–39 | 40–49 | 50–59 | 60–69 | 70–79 | |
| **Women** | | | | | | | |
| 5 | 35.2 | 35.8 | 37.4 | 38.3 | 39.0 | 39.3 | |
| 1 | 38.9 | 39.4 | 39.8, | 40.4 | 40.8 | 40.5 | VP |
| n = | 1,360 | 3,597 | 3,808 | 2,366 | 849 | 136 | |
| Total n = 12,116 | | | | | | | |

*Norms are based on Cooper Clinic patients.*
*[a]Very lean—no <3% body fat is recommended for males.*
*[b]Very lean—no <10%–13% body fat is recommended for females.*
*VL, very lean; E, excellent; G, good; F, fair; P, poor; VP, very poor.*
*From Thompson W. ACSM's Resources for the Personal Trainer. 3rd ed. Lippincott Williams & Wilkins; 2010; Table 14.3.*

until each is within 5 mm (¼ in) of each other. For example, if a male client has a waist circumference of 32 in (81.3 cm) and a hip circumference of 35 in (88.9 cm), his WHR is 32/35 = 0.91. Health risk is very high for young men when the WHR is more than 0.95 and for young women when the WHR is more than 0.86.

### Waist Circumference Alone

Some experts suggest that the waist circumference alone may be used as an indicator of health risk. For example, the health risk is high when the waist circumference is ≥35 in (88 cm) for women and 40 in (102 cm) for men. A very low risk is associated with a waist circumference <27.5 in (70 cm) for women and 31.5 in (80 cm) for men.

### Skinfolds

Skinfold determination of the percentage of body fat can be quite accurate if the technician is properly trained in the use of skinfold calipers and the caliper is of high quality (Table 2.5). It should be remembered, however, that skinfold determination of percent body fat is still an estimate or a prediction of percentage body fat, not an absolute measurement (Table 2.6). This estimate is based on the principle that the amount of subcutaneous fat is proportional to the total amount of body fat; however, the proportion of subcutaneous fat to total fat varies with gender, age, and ethnicity. Regression equations considering these factors have been developed to predict body density and percent body fat from skinfold measurements.

### Bioelectrical Impedance

BIA is a noninvasive and easy-to-administer method for assessing body composition. The basic premise behind the procedure is that the volume of fat-free tissue in the body will be proportional to the electrical conductivity of the body. Thus, the bioelectrical impedance analyzer passes a small electrical current into the body and then measures the resistance to that current. The theory

$$\text{Ideal body weight (IBW)} = \frac{\text{LBM (lean body mass)}}{1.00 - (\text{desired \% body fat}/100)}$$

For example, if a man weighs 190 lb (86.4 kg) and is determined to have 22.3% body fat, then

Fat weight = body weight × (% body fat/100)

$$= 190 \times (22.3/100)$$

$$= 42.37 \text{ lb } (19.25 \text{ kg})$$

LBW = body weight − fat weight = 190 − 42.37 = 147.63 lb (67.1 kg)

$$\text{IBW} = \frac{147.63}{1.00 - (14/100)} \text{ (15\% used for a man; as a guideline)}$$

$$= 173.68 \text{ (78.9 kg) at 15\% body fat}$$

Weight loss = body weight − IBW

In this example, 190 − 173.68 = 16.3 lb (7.4 kg) to lose to achieve ideal body weight.

■ **FIGURE 2.11** Calculation of ideal body weight.

behind BIA is that fat is a poor electrical conductor containing little water (14%–22%), whereas lean tissue contains mostly water (more than 90%) and electrolytes and is a good electrical conductor. Thus, fat tissue provides impedance to electrical current. In actuality, BIA measures total body water and uses calculations for percent body fat using some assumptions about hydration levels of individuals and the exact water content of various tissues. The following conditions must be controlled to ensure that the subject has a normal hydration level so the BIA measurement is valid.

- No eating or drinking within 4 hours of the test
- No exercise within 12 hours of the test
- Urinate (or void) completely within 30 minutes of the test
- No alcohol consumption in the previous 48 hours before test

### Densitometry

Body composition can be estimated from a measurement of whole-body density, using the ratio of body mass to body volume. In this technique, which has been used as a reference or criterion standard for assessing body composition, the body is divided into two components: the fat mass and the fat-free mass (FFM). The limiting factor in the measurement of body density is the accuracy of the body volume measurement because body mass is measured simply as bodyweight. Body volume can be measured by hydrodensitometry (underwater) weighing and by plethysmography (*e.g.*, Bod Pod).

#### Hydrodensitometry (Underwater) Weighing

This technique of measuring body composition, considered the "gold standard" is based on Archimedes principle, which states that when a body is immersed in

| Table 2.7 | FITNESS CATEGORIES BY AGE GROUPS FOR TRUNK FORWARD FLEXION USING A SIT-AND-REACH BOX (CENTIMETER)[a] | | | | | | | | | |
|---|---|---|---|---|---|---|---|---|---|---|
| | AGE, YR | | | | | | | | | |
| | 20–29 | | 30–39 | | 40–49 | | 50–59 | | 60–69 | |
| CATEGORY | M | F | M | F | M | F | M | F | M | F |
| Excellent | 40 | 41 | 38 | 41 | 35 | 38 | 35 | 39 | 33 | 35 |
| Very good | 39 | 40 | 37 | 40 | 34 | 37 | 34 | 38 | 32 | 34 |
| | 34 | 37 | 33 | 36 | 29 | 34 | 28 | 33 | 25 | 31 |
| Good | 33 | 36 | 32 | 35 | 28 | 33 | 27 | 32 | 24 | 30 |
| | 30 | 33 | 28 | 32 | 24 | 30 | 24 | 30 | 20 | 27 |
| Fair | 29 | 32 | 27 | 31 | 23 | 29 | 23 | 29 | 19 | 26 |
| | 25 | 28 | 23 | 27 | 18 | 25 | 16 | 25 | 15 | 23 |
| Needs improvement | 24 | 27 | 22 | 26 | 17 | 24 | 15 | 24 | 14 | 22 |

*The following may be used as descriptors for the percentile rankings: well above average (90), above average (70), average (50), below average (30), and well below average (10).*

[a]*These norms are based on a sit-and-reach box in which the "zero" point is set at 26 cm. When using a box in which the zero point is set at 23 cm, subtract 3 cm from each value in this table.*

*F, female; M, male.*

*From Thompson W. ACSM's Resources for the Personal Trainer. 3rd ed. Lippincott Williams & Wilkins; 2010. p. 299–304.*

## BOX 2.6 — Trunk Flexion (Sit-and-Reach) Test Procedures

**Before the test**: Participant should perform a short warm-up prior to this test and include some stretches for the targeted muscle groups (*e.g.*, modified hurdler's stretch). It is also recommended that the participant refrain from fast, jerky movements, which may increase the possibility of an injury. The participant's shoes should be removed for the assessment.

- For the Canadian Trunk Forward Flexion test, the client sits without shoes and the soles of the feet flat against the flexometer (sit-and-reach box) at the 26-cm mark. Inner edges of the soles are placed within 2 cm of the measuring scale. For the YMCA sit-and-reach test, a yardstick is placed on the floor and tape is placed across it at a right angle to the 15-in mark. The participant sits with the yardstick between the legs, with legs extended at right angles to the taped line on the floor. Heels of the feet should touch the edge of the taped line and be about 10–12 in apart. (Note the zero point at the foot/box interface and use the appropriate norms.)

- The participant should slowly reach forward (no bouncing) with both hands as far as possible (to the point of mild discomfort), holding this position approximately 2 seconds. Be sure that the participant keeps the hands parallel and does not lead with one hand. Fingertips can be overlapped and should be in contact with the measuring portion or yardstick of the sit-and-reach box. To assist with the best attempt, the participant should exhale and drop the head between the arms when reaching. Testers should ensure that the knees of the participant stay extended; however, the participant's knees should not be pressed down. The participant should breathe normally during the test and should not hold his or her breath anytime.

- The score is the most distant point (in centimeters or inches) reached with the fingertips. The better of two trials should be recorded. Norms for the Canadian test are presented in Table 2.8. Note that these norms use a sit-and-reach box in which the "zero" point is set at the 26-cm mark. If you are using a box in which the zero point is set at 23 cm (*e.g.*, Fitnessgram), subtract 3 cm from each value in this table. The norms for the YMCA test are also presented in Table 2.9.

From: Thompson W. *ACSM's Resources for the Personal Trainer*. 3rd ed. Lippincott Williams & Wilkins; 2010; Box 14.5.

water, it is buoyed by a counterforce equal to the weight of the water displaced. This loss of weight in water allows calculation of body volume. Bone and muscle tissue are denser than water, whereas fat tissue is less dense. Therefore, a person with more FFM for the same total body mass weighs more in water and has a higher body density and lower percentage of body fat. Although hydrostatic weighing is a standard method for measuring body volume and hence, body composition, it requires special equipment, the accurate measurement of residual volume, and significant cooperation by the subject. For a more detailed explanation of the technique, see Chapter 17 of ACSM's Resource Manual for Guidelines for Exercise Testing and Prescription.

### Plethysmography

Body volume also can be measured by air rather than water displacement. One commercial system uses a dual-chamber plethysmograph that measures body volume

| Table 2.8 | FITNESS CATEGORIES BY AGE GROUPS AND SEX FOR PUSH-UPS | | | | | | | | |
|-----------|-------|-------|-------|-------|-------|-------|-------|-------|-------|
| CATEGORY | AGE | | | | | | | | |
| | 20–29 | | 30–39 | | 40–49 | | 50–59 | | 60–69 | |
| GENDER | M | F | M | F | M | F | M | F | M | F |
| Excellent | 36 | 30 | 30 | 27 | 25 | 24 | 21 | 21 | 18 | 17 |
| Very good | 35 | 29 | 29 | 26 | 24 | 23 | 20 | 20 | 17 | 16 |
| | 29 | 21 | 22 | 20 | 17 | 15 | 13 | 11 | 11 | 12 |
| Good | 28 | 20 | 21 | 19 | 16 | 14 | 12 | 10 | 10 | 11 |
| | 22 | 15 | 17 | 13 | 13 | 11 | 10 | 7 | 8 | 5 |
| Fair | 21 | 14 | 16 | 12 | 12 | 10 | 9 | 6 | 7 | 4 |
| | 17 | 10 | 12 | 8 | 10 | 5 | 7 | 2 | 5 | 2 |
| Needs improvement | 16 | 9 | 11 | 7 | 9 | 4 | 6 | 1 | 4 | 1 |

Thompson W. *ACSM's Resources for the Personal Trainer*. 3rd ed. Lippincott Williams & Wilkins; 2010. 302 p; Table 14-9.

| Table 2.9 | SIT-AND-REACH NORMS PERCENTILES BY AGE GROUPS AND SEX FOR YMCA SIT-AND-REACH TEST (INCHES) | | | | | | | | | | | |
|---|---|---|---|---|---|---|---|---|---|---|---|---|
| | AGE, YR | | | | | | | | | | | |
| | 18–25 | | 26–35 | | 36–45 | | 46–55 | | 56–65 | | >65 | |
| PERCENTILE | M | F | M | F | M | F | M | F | M | F | M | F |
| 90 | 22 | 24 | 21 | 23 | 21 | 22 | 19 | 21 | 17 | 20 | 17 | 20 |
| 80 | 20 | 22 | 19 | 21 | 19 | 21 | 17 | 20 | 15 | 19 | 15 | 18 |
| 70 | 19 | 21 | 17 | 20 | 17 | 19 | 15 | 18 | 13 | 17 | 13 | 17 |
| 60 | 18 | 20 | 17 | 20 | 16 | 18 | 14 | 17 | 13 | 16 | 12 | 17 |
| 50 | 17 | 19 | 15 | 19 | 15 | 17 | 13 | 16 | 11 | 15 | 10 | 15 |
| 40 | 15 | 18 | 14 | 17 | 13 | 16 | 11 | 14 | 9 | 14 | 9 | 14 |
| 30 | 14 | 17 | 13 | 16 | 13 | 15 | 10 | 14 | 9 | 13 | 8 | 13 |
| 20 | 13 | 16 | 11 | 15 | 11 | 14 | 9 | 12 | 7 | 11 | 7 | 11 |
| 10 | 11 | 14 | 9 | 13 | 7 | 12 | 6 | 10 | 5 | 9 | 4 | 9 |

Thompson W. *ACSM's Resources for the Personal Trainer*. 3rd ed. Lippincott Williams & Wilkins; 2010; Table 14-11.

by changes in pressure in a closed chamber. This technology shows promise and generally reduces the anxiety associated with the technique of hydrodensitometry (16,23,43). For a more detailed explanation of the technique, see Chapter 17 of ACSM's Resource Manual for Guidelines for Exercise Testing and Prescription (5).

### Calculation of Ideal or Desired Body Weight

Along with the determination of percent body fat, it is often desirable to determine an ideal or desired body weight based on a desired percent of fat for the individual (Fig. 2.11). Obviously, this process can be problematic in that a desirable percent body fat for an individual must be determined. The determination of a desirable body weight is useful in weight loss and weight maintenance.

Those cardiac patients deemed low risk (e.g., persons without resting or exercise-induced evidence of myocardial ischemia, severe left ventricular dysfunction, or complex ventricular dysrrhythmias, and with normal or near-normal CRF) can perform moderate-to

high-intensity (e.g., 40%–80% 1RM) resistance testing and training safely. Additionally, research does not support the occurrence of an abnormal cardiovascular "pressure response" in cardiac patients or those with controlled hypertension, indicating that strength testing and training should be safe to include in comprehensive evaluation and training programs. However, data on the safety of muscular fitness testing in moderate- to high-risk cardiac patients, especially those with poor left ventricular function, are limited and require additional investigation.

Current guidelines suggest that the following contra-indications be recognized when considering muscular strength and endurance testing

- Unstable angina
- Uncontrolled hypertension (systolic BP ≥ 160 mm Hg and/or diastolic BP ≥ 100 mm Hg)
- Uncontrolled dysrhythmias
- Poorly managed or untreated heart failure
- Severe stenotic or regurgitant valvular disease
- Hypertrophic cardiomyopathy

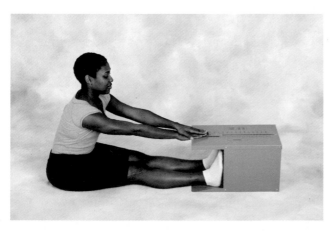
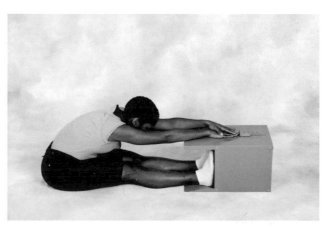

**■ FIGURE 2.12** Client performing a sit-and-reach test. From Thompson W. ACSM's Resources for the Personal Trainer. 3rd ed. Baltimore (MD): Lippincot Williams & Wilkins; 2010. Figure 14.10, p 304

Name_____ Age_____ Gender: M_____ F_____
Date_____ Resting HR_____
Ht (in)_____ Wt (lbs) _____

## BODY COMPOSITION

BMI_____ [wt (kg)/ ht2 (m)]
     Below Avg Wt_____ Avg Wt_____ Above Avg Wt_____

Circumference Measurements (in)
Neck_____ Shoulder_____ Rt Upper Arm_____ Lf Upper Arm_____ Chest _____
Waist _____ Hip_____ Rt Thigh_____ Lf Thigh_____

Waist to Hip Ratio [Waist (in)/ Hips (in)] _____ (>.80 women at risk : >.90 men at risk)

Skinfold
Chest_____ Abdominal_____ Triceps_____ Biceps _____ Midaxillary_____ Subscapular_____ Supriliac_____ Thigh_____ Medial Calf_____
% Fat_____
Rating:
Very Poor___ Poor_____ Below Avg___ Avg_____ Above Avg_____ Good_____ Excellent_____

## CARDIOVASCULAR TRAINING

3 Minute Step Test
                 Heart Rate (HR) beats/min (bpm)
Minute 1          _____
Minute 2          _____
Minute 3          _____
Rating:
Very Poor___ Poor_____ Below Avg___ Avg_____ Above Avg_____ Good_____ Excellent_____

## MUSCULAR ENDURANCE

Partial Curl-Up (metronome set at 50 rpm -25 max/min : Tape at 0-10 cm)
Curl-ups in 1 minute (#) _____
Rating:
Very Poor___ Poor_____ Below Avg___ Avg_____ Above Avg_____ Good_____ Excellent_____

Push-ups
Total # (no time limit) _____
Rating:
Very Poor___ Poor_____ Below Avg___ Avg_____ Above Avg_____ Good_____ Excellent_____

## MUSCULAR STRENGTH

YMCA Bench Press Test (metronome set at 60 rpm – 30 max/min)
Total #_____
Rating:
Very Poor___ Poor_____ Below Avg___ Avg_____ Above Avg_____ Good_____ Excellent_____

■ FIGURE 2.13 Sample fitness assessment data sheet.

In addition, it is suggested that those with cardiac disease should also have well-preserved left ventricular function and CRF (more than five or six metabolic equivalents) without anginal symptoms or ischemic ST-segment changes to participate in traditional resistance training programs. Significant care should be taken during preparticipation screening, and proper supervision should be provided in an effort to reduce the risk of a serious cardiac event during muscular strength and endurance testing.

### Flexibility Assessment: Sit-and-Reach Test

Although there exists no single best test of overall flexibility, the sit-and-reach test is the most common and most practical to use (see Fig. 2.12 ). Preceded by a proper warm-up, the sit-and-reach test can be easy to administer and interpret. The GEI should be made aware that this test measures only flexibility of the hamstrings, hip, and lower back. The practical significance of using the sit-and-reach test to measure flexibility is in the significant number of people who complain of low back pain. It is likely that this pain is caused by decreased flexibility, primarily of the hamstrings (which have their anatomical origin in the posterior hip region). For a detailed description of the procedure, see Box 2.6. Percentile rankings for men and women can be found in Table 2.7. These and other test results can be recorded on a data sheet. (see Fig. 2.13)

### SUMMARY

*This chapter describes some of the basic tools available for preactivity screening of your class participants.*

*While it is not often that a GEI actually performs preactivity screenings of class participants, it behooves him or her to be aware of any screening procedures in which participants may have participated in the supervised club environment. The ACSM advises all GEIs to learn which screening tools are recommended for each type of teaching environment. In some cases, instructors need to administer the health screen; in other cases, instructors need to be aware that the screening occurred. GEIs should review how to properly utilize the health screening tools as they apply to their teaching. Fitness assessment tools are available for use in group exercise environments, and may be utilized to set benchmarks for class participants.*

### ✔ RECOMMENDED RESOURCES:

*Kennedy-Armbruster C, Yoke MM. Methods of Group Exercise Instruction. 2nd ed., Champaign (IL): Human Kinetics; 2009.*
*The Canadian Physical Activity, Fitness & Lifestyle Approach: CSEP-Health & Fitness Program's Health-Related Appraisal & Counseling Strategy: 3rd ed. Canadian Society for Exercise Physiology; 2003.*
*Nieman DC. Exercise Testing and Prescription: A Health-Related Approach. 4th ed. Mountain View (CA): Mayfield Publishing Company; 1999.*
*Thompson W. ACSM's Guidelines for Testing and Exercise Prescription. 8th ed. Lippincot Williams & Wilkins, Baltimore (MD); 2010.*

## References

1. American College of Sports Medicine. *ACSM's Guidelines for Exercise Testing and Prescription.* 8th ed. Baltimore (MD): Lippincott Williams & Wilkins; 2010.
2. Griffin JC. *Client-Centered Exercise Prescription.* 2nd ed. Champaign (IL): Human Kinetics; 2006.
3. Pate RR, Pratt M, Blair SN, et al. Physical activity and public health. *JAMA.* 1995;5:402–7.
4. Tharrett SJ, McInnis KJ, Peterson JA. *ACSM's Health/Fitness Facility Standards and Guidelines.* 3rd ed. Champaign (IL): Human Kinetics; 2006.
5. Thompson W. *ACSM's Resources for the Personal Trainer.* 3rd ed., Baltimore (MD); Lippincott Williams & Wilkins; 2010. 267 p.

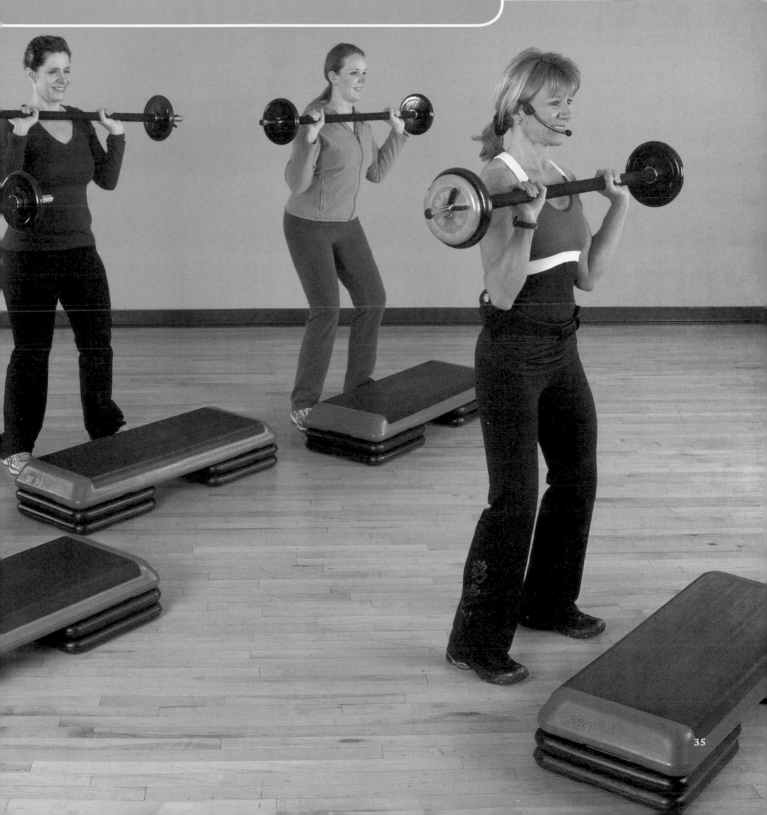

# LEADERSHIP AND DESIGN

# PART II

# Class Design and Programming

MARY ANN RUMPLASCH

**At the end of this chapter you will be able to:**
· Explain the different types of class styles
· Identify the guidelines for popular class styles
· Describe the components of class design (warm-up, stimulus, cool-down)
· Design a basic group exercise class

Group exercise program design has come a long way from the early days of aerobic dance. Today's classes offer movement options from multiple disciplines and styles. One size does not fit all when it comes to group exercise. Class participants arrive to class with varying degrees of skill, endurance, and focus. How does the group exercise instructor design a class to accommodate varying needs and skill sets while meeting the overall industry guidelines for fitness? The answer lies in the talent of the leader — you! Begin by selecting the class format that suits your style and the needs and goals of the class. Selecting the proper format and style for your class takes planning and time, but your efforts will be worthwhile as you help participants gain control of their health and improve their fitness levels.

## GROUP EXERCISE FORMATS

### CARDIOVASCULAR ENDURANCE CLASSES: HOW HARD? HOW FAST? HOW LONG?

In 2007, the American College of Sports Medicine (ACSM) and the American Heart Association (AHA) updated and clarified the 1995 Centers for Disease Control and Prevention and the ACSM recommendation on the types and amounts of physical activity needed by healthy people aged 18–65 years to improve and maintain health. The updated ACSM/AHA guidelines recommend that all healthy adults in this age category perform moderate-intensity aerobic (endurance) physical activity for a minimum of 30 minutes on 5 days each week or vigorous-intensity aerobic physical activity for a minimum of 20 minutes on 3 days each week. Also, combinations of moderate- and vigorous-intensity activity can be performed to meet the recommendation. Moderate-intensity physical activity means working hard enough to raise heart rate and break a sweat, yet still being able to carry on a conversation. Vigorous-intensity activity causes rapid breathing and a substantial increase in heart rate (19).

Group exercise offers a variety of cardio formats such as step, indoor cycling, kickboxing, and mixed impact (high/low). With so many choices, exercisers can select classes that suit their needs, goals, abilities, and sense of enjoyment. The challenge instructors face is to find ways to allow for these variations while providing a safe and effective exercise setting.

The intensity at which physical activity is performed has important implications for health and fitness benefits. To ensure that participants are reaching their cardiovascular goals without being at risk, they need to learn techniques to monitor exercise intensity. There are various field methods (requiring minimal or no equipment) to gauge cardio intensity: heart rate, talk testing, rating of perceived exertion (RPE), ventilatory threshold, and heart rate monitors, to name a few (9,37). In the group exercise setting, heart rate, RPE and heart rate monitors are most commonly used. Intensity should be checked several times during the workout so the intensity can be modified if needed. When checking heart rate, participants need to keep moving to prevent blood from pooling in the lower extremities. If heart rate is measured manually, palpation of the radial artery is preferred over the carotid pulse. However, if the measure is taken via the carotid pulse, light pressure should be used to avoid slowing the heart rate through stimulation of the carotid baroreceptors (1). Below is an overview of some popular cardiovascular endurance formats.

### STEP TRAINING

Step training was introduced in 1989. Over the years, step training has evolved to include a wide variety of workouts: dance inspired, athletic, fusion (*e.g.*, kickboxing and step). Step was developed in response to a demand for a safer, more efficient low-impact activity. The workouts can be as challenging as a rigorous jogging workout and yet produce impact forces as safe as walking (1,31). In a step class, participants step up and down on a platform. Intensity can be changed by adjusting the height of the platform. Deconditioned participants should begin on 4-in steps (platform only), while experienced and highly skilled steppers can use steps ranging from 8 to 10 in (platform plus two or three pair of risers). However, the height, injury history, and fitness level of the participants must be taken into account when selecting platform height. For safety reasons, instructors should encourage each participant to select the lowest height that will provide a training effect that meets his or her exercise goals. In addition, appropriate step cadence must be maintained to ensure proper form and stepping technique. The recommended stepping tempo is 118–128 beats per minute (bpm) (31,33).

## INDOOR CYCLING

Indoor cycling was introduced to the fitness industry in 1995 (3). It fuses elements from the sport of outdoor cycling, mind/body fitness, and traditional group exercise. Indoor cycling is performed on a specialized stationary bike. Instructors lead participants through a "virtual" road ride. The class progresses in content from bike setup, cycling terminology, and tension adjustments, to a range of hand and body positions and drills that become increasingly more challenging. Music and language are selected for motivation and to enhance the workout experience. Indoor cycling attracts a wide variety of participants due to its simple design. Because of its non–weight-bearing nature, cycling classes offer some orthopedic advantages to special populations not able to perform weight-bearing exercise. To accommodate the multiple fitness levels in class, the instructor must provide resistance or cadence options during the various class segments (36). In general, maintaining a relatively high cadence (80–100 revolutions per minute) with a low resistance produces less stress on the knees than does a low-cadence/high-resistance combination (1).

## KICKBOXING/CARDIO KICKBOXING

Kickboxing-type workouts are a hybrid of boxing, martial arts, and aerobics. These classes offer an intense and total body workout. Movements include kicks, punches, elbow strikes, hand strikes, and knee strikes. Athletic drills are mixed with recovery bouts of basic aerobic movements like rope jumping and light jogging in place. Some classes involve equipment (*e.g.*, bags, target pads, gloves). It is recommended that equipment be used only by instructors with a boxing or martial arts background who have spent many hours working with equipment in a teaching atmosphere. For safety and liability reasons, no contact should be allowed between participants. The focus should be on fitness goals, not fighters' goals. Instructors need to have proper knowledge of correct punching and kicking techniques, as well as progressive teaching skills to minimize joint-related injuries among class participants (1,3,38).

## MIXED-IMPACT

Mixed-impact classes use a combination of high-impact (*e.g.*, jumping, hopping) and low-impact (*e.g.*, step touches) moves to stimulate the cardiorespiratory system. And because the moves are weight bearing, they help to strengthen bones (3). Mixed-impact progressed from its origins of high-impact in the 1980s. The combinations, or routines, are choreographed to music and incorporate a variety of arm and leg movements, traveling steps, and directional moves. The moves range from dance based to athletic style. To modify the intensity of the exercise, participants can alter the speed of movement, modify the range of motion (ROM) of the movements, vary the amount of traveling completed with a movement, and change the vertical component of the movement. Beginner exercisers and those with certain health risks should be encouraged to use only low-impact moves. A few considerations specific to mixed-impact classes are to not hop repeatedly on one foot (*e.g.*, more than four consecutive times) to avoid excessive impact-related stress and avoid twisting hop variations that may lead to spinal stress. The recommended music tempo is 135–160 bpm (1).

## MUSCULAR ENDURANCE CLASSES

The ACSM/AHA Physical Activity guidelines (2007) recommend that all healthy adults perform muscular strength and endurance exercises for a minimum of 2 days each week (19). Like cardiovascular endurance formats, group resistance training classes offer a wide array of training options (*e.g.*, body weight, equipment based). Dumbbells, weighted bars, tubing, resistance bands, and stability and medicine balls are some examples of equipment used in class (see Box 3.1).

The success and safety of a group resistance training class depend on how well the instructor sets up the movements, provides motivation and alignment cues, and helps each participant feel challenged without going beyond his or her ability level (13). To avoid injury, instructors must teach quality of movement. For each exercise, participants need to be aware of good spinal alignment, proper starting position, individual and exercise-specific ROM, and pay equal attention to all phases of the exercise (lifting, holding, and lowering). Crews offers the following suggestions for teaching a safe and effective group resistance training class (13):

**BOX 3.1**    *Sample Class Plan*

### SAMPLE CLASS 1: ON THE BALL — CORE CONDITIONING

**Format:** Muscular endurance

**Total Time:** 45 minutes

**Equipment:** Stability ball and mat

**Music:** Music can be used as background sound

**Goal/Objective:** To develop core strength and stability utilizing the stability ball.

**Warm-up (5–10 minutes):** Basic, multijoint moves that slowly increase in intensity and raise core temperature.

**Workout (25–30 minutes)**

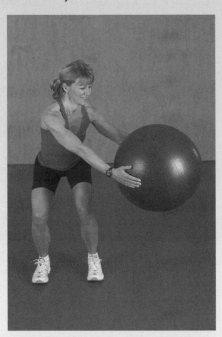

❶ **Twister Squat.** Stand with legs hip width, holding ball overhead. Squat, rotating torso to right bringing ball toward floor. Return to start position. Switch sides, rotating torso to left.

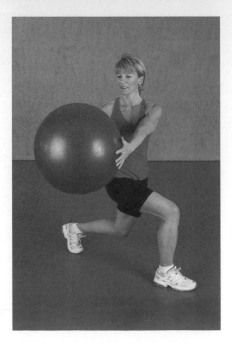

❷ **Alternating Front Lunge with Rotation.** Stand with feet together holding stability ball in front of chest, arms extended. Lunge forward with R leg while rotating torso to right. Return to start position. Switch legs; repeat.

**Modification:** Lunges can be performed in a staggered position (R leg forward/L leg back) for several repetitions. Switch legs; repeat.

**BOX 3.1, cont.**

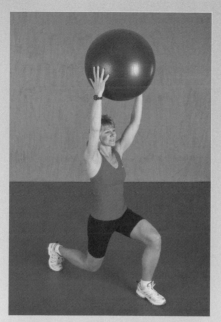

❸ **Rear Lunge with Overhead Lift**. Stand with feet together holding stability ball in front of chest, arms extended. Lunge back with R leg while lifting ball over head. Return to start position. Switch legs; repeat.

**Modification:** Lunges can be performed in a staggered position (R leg back/L leg forward) for several repetitions. Switch legs; repeat.

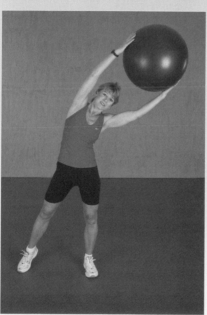

❹ **Side Pendulum with Ball.** Stand on L leg with R foot tapping floor, holding stability ball overhead. Holding ball steady, lean torso to left while R leg lifts to the side. Return to start position. Do 8–12 repetitions, then switch.

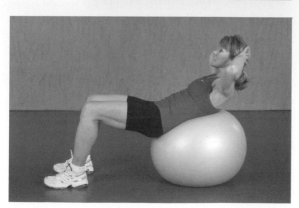

❺ **Ball Crunch**. Sit on ball, feet flat and hands behind head, elbows out. Lower upper body until back is resting on ball. Slowly crunch up. Lower to start position.

**BOX 3.1, cont.**

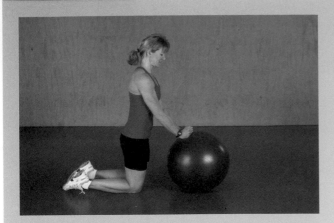

**❻ Lat Rollout.** Kneel on mat with outer edge of hands resting on ball. Keeping shoulders stacked over hips, roll out allowing ball to roll toward elbows. Return to start position.

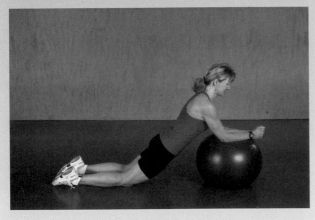

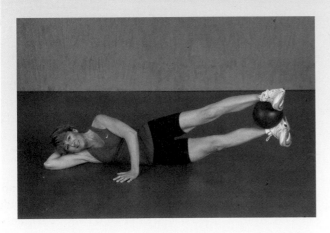

**❼ Side Leg Lifts with Ball.** Lie on right side, legs stacked holding ball between lower legs, head resting on right arm. Place left hand on floor in front of torso. Keeping hips stacked, engage abs and raise legs about 12 in off the floor. Return to start. Do 12 repetitions, then switch.

**BOX 3.1, cont.**

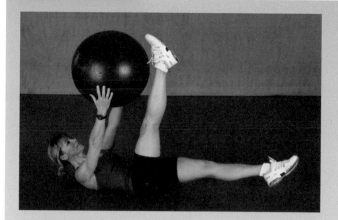

❽ **Bicycle with Ball**. Lie supine with legs elevated, ball over chest, arms extended. Lift shoulder blades, lower right 45 degrees, and rotate torso/ball toward right. Switch sides, rotating torso to left. (Photo shown without rotation.)

**Modification:** Bend knees at 90-degree angle and/or eliminate rotation.

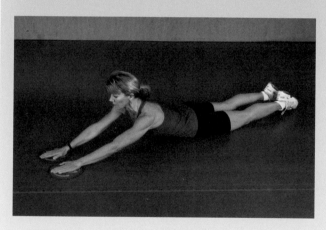

❾ **Prone Back Extension with Disks under Palms**. Lie prone with arms extended and disks under your hands. Keeping pelvis on the floor, slowly extend your spine while drawing the disks toward you.

**Stretch (5–10 minutes):** Stretches can be performed sitting and lying on the ball; include both upper- and lower-body stretches. Although this class has focused primarily on the core musculature, be sure to cover some of the other affected areas (*e.g.*, quadriceps, hamstrings, gluteals, piriformis, adductors, chest, back).

- Before class starts, tell participants to get several levels of resistance equipment so they can make adjustments during class.
- If music is used, keep the tempo in the range of 110–126 bpm.
- First teach each movement pattern without using any weight; add resistance only after correct technique and alignment have been established.
- Ensure that participants perfect their alignment before progressing loads.
- Establish the correct movement pattern before adding speed.
- Offer variations and modifications to accommodate different body types/fitness levels and to reduce the risk of overuse injuries.
- Control the number of repetitions.
- Use progressions when teaching multiple skill levels.
- For multijoint movements, offer beginner, intermediate, and advanced progressions.
- Plan exercise breaks for participants who have less strength, but make sure they don't feel unsuccessful

if they rest. For example, during a set of push-ups, let participants choose to rest on the step platform or hover over the platform during the lowering phase.

## COMBINED CONDITIONING

Combined conditioning classes blend two formats into one class (see Box 3.2). The variety these classes provide has the potential to attract a diverse base of participants. Likewise, it is a time-saving way to exercise.

## CIRCUIT TRAINING

Circuit training is another training method that can be an attractive alternative to those seeking improvement in more than one aspect of fitness (see Box 3.3). Traditional circuit training has been around for over 50 years. It was developed by R.E. Morgan and G.T. Anderson in 1953 at the University of Leeds in England (23). *Circuit* refers to a number of carefully chosen exercises arranged in a specific order. With this approach, a

BOX 3.2 · *Sample Class Plan*

### SAMPLE CLASS 2: 20/20 — STEP AND GLIDE

**Format:** Combined training

**Total Time:** 55 minutes

**Equipment:** Steps and gliding discs

**Music:** 118–128 bpm

**Goal/Objective:** To improve cardiorespiratory fitness by using basic step moves and muscular strength and endurance by using the gliding discs.

**Warm-up (10 minutes):** Use moves such as step touches and hamstring curls on the floor and then progress to moves on the bench such as basic step and knee lift. Focus on moves that will loosen hips and calves.

**Step Segment (20 minutes):** Since time is limited, keep choreography basic. Use a variety of patterns (e.g, basic step, v-step, lift steps, turn step, repeaters) and approaches (*e.g.*, front, side, top). For greater intensity, propulsion movements can be added for advanced steppers. However, do not perform propulsion steps for more than 1 minute at a time. At the end of the step segment, select a basic pattern, and slowly return to moves on the floor.

**Gliding Segment (20 minutes):** Standing patterns may include sliding squats, double sliding squats, rear lunges, and side lunges. Core work may include Hovers (weight supported on either forearms or hands with discs under toes) with hip abduction/adduction, Bridges (lying supine with discs under heels) with alternating heel slides, and Prone Lying (discs under palms) with extension press up.

**Cool-down/Stretch (5 minutes):** Stretches can be performed with the discs (*e.g.*, cat stretch with alternating lat and shoulder stretch, low lunge stretch).

person lifts a weight between 40% and 55% of the one-repetition maximum. The weight is then lifted as many times as possible for 30 seconds. After a 15-second rest, the exerciser moves to the next resistance exercise station and so on to complete the circuit. Between 8 and 15 exercises are usually used. The circuit is repeated several times to allow for 30–50 minutes of continuous exercise (27).

## INTERVAL TRAINING

Interval training classes are another way participants can increase fitness and save time on exercise. Interval training combines bouts of high-intensity exercise followed by brief periods of active recovery. Some of its benefits are enhanced utilization of fats and carbohydrates, efficient stimulation of fast- and slow-twitch muscle fibers, improved aerobic and anaerobic power and capacity, and potential reduction in injury due to variation of workout intensity (22). This method of training can be applied to a number of class formats. It works well with any cardio-based class. The issue with interval training is how long to spend in the effort phase versus the recovery phase. In deciding on the duration of each interval, the work/rest ratio comes into play. Work/rest ratio refers to how long a person

exercises at a higher-than-normal intensity compared to how long he or she recovers at or below steady-state activity (35). Instructors should plan work intervals that allow participants to sustain a solid effort (RPE of 4 or 5 on a scale of 1–10) without sacrificing proper form and technique. The recovery time (RPE of 2 or 3 on a scale of 1–10) should be proportional to the intensity and the length of the all-out phase. An interval training format will challenge athletic participants while giving a safe, fun, and effective workout to the general population. The key is to choose exercises that will get the heart pumping to increase maximal oxygen consumption. The exercises must use large muscles and be performed in a biomechanically correct manner. As always, instructors need to provide modifications and encourage participants to self-monitor and work at their own pace.

## SPECIALTY CLASSES

Specialty classes such as yoga and Pilates require specialized training. Instructor training programs vary from 10-hour workshops to significant hours of coursework and extensive practice teaching. As in traditional group exercise formats, instructors must include modifications for participants with injuries and postural issues.

| BOX 3.3 | Sample Class Plan |
| --- | --- |

## SAMPLE CLASS 3: SHORT CIRCUIT

**Format:** Circuit training (see Fig. 3.9 for sample setup)

**Total Time:** 30 minutes

**Equipment:** None

**Music:** Music can be used as background sound

**Goals/Objectives:** To improve cardiorespiratory fitness and muscular strength and endurance by alternating basic cardio moves with body weight strength moves.

To accommodate participants with limited time by offering a shorter duration class.

To provide an effective workout without the use of equipment.

**Warm-up (5 minutes):** Basic, multijoint moves that slowly increase in intensity and raise core temperature.

**Workout (20 minutes):** Alternate 3 minutes of cardio moves with 1 minute of body weight strength moves. Use both high- and low-impact cardio moves as well as movements that move forward/backward and side to side. For example:

- Heel jacks/jumping jacks/knee lifts/double knee lifts/knee crossovers
- Marches/jogs/high knee jogs/wide marches/jogs
- Walks/jogs forward/backward
- Grapevines/lateral shuffles

Body weight strength moves may include

- Squats (various stances/speeds)
- Lunges (multidirectional/multiplanar)

As a safety precaution, supine (*e.g.*, crunches) and prone (*e.g.*, push-ups) moves should be performed at the end of class.

**Cool-down/Stretch (5 minutes):** Use a combination of stretches: static (where the end ROM is held) and dynamic (where the stretches are moved through).

**Sample Circuit Setup (Fig. 3.10):** In the group exercise setting, circuit classes typically incorporate a cardio element. They also feature an extensive assortment of innovative equipment and props, including hula hoops, kickboxing equipment, balance boards, and minitrampolines. When designing a circuit class, instructors need to consider the following (26):

- There needs to be enough room to set up the different stations and to allow for traffic flow of the class.

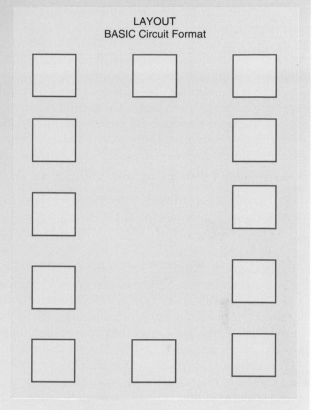

LAYOUT
BASIC Circuit Format

■ **FIGURE 3.10** Sample circuit setup.

- To accommodate various fitness levels, exercise variations and modifications need to be included.
- As a safety measure, instructors must demonstrate the exercises at each station at the beginning of class so that participants observe proper form and technique.
- Post simple instructions/diagrams at all stations to show which exercises are done where.
- During class, instructors must control the speed of reps, rest intervals, cardio elements, and transitions. They also need to constantly monitor participants' exertion and fatigue levels.
- If class size fluctuates from class to class, the design can be modified so that participants do not move from station to station. With this variation, the participants set up their own personal stations. The instructor leads each exercise, and the participants follow without moving around the room (22).

## YOGA

Yoga originated in India more than 5,000 years ago. It gained acceptance in the western world in the 1950s. The repertoire of yoga is described in Sanskrit, the language of India's classical texts and scriptures. Yoga is a philosophy that addresses the whole person and life discipline. In Sanskrit, yoga means to unite or "yoke" the mind, body, and spirit. Hatha yoga is the physical component of this discipline and includes several different styles (*e.g.*, Iyengar, Ashtanga). The repertoire of yoga consists of asanas (postures or poses) and pranayama or breathing techniques. Postures are performed while seated, standing, supine, or prone. The postures are designed to move the spine through extension, hyperextension, forward and lateral flexion, and rotation.

Yoga offers many physical and psychological benefits. It helps to build flexibility, strength, concentration, and stamina. Yoga is practiced by healthy populations, as well as by patients with cancer, heart disease, AIDs, and drug addiction (32). Some poses are contraindicated for certain health issues. Inverted postures (where the head is lower than the heart) may not be appropriate for participants with glaucoma, high blood pressure, or vertigo. Also, pregnant women should not practice breath retention and/or breath suspension. Many instructors use props such as yoga blocks, straps, and blankets to help participants modify a pose or help correct spinal alignment (12,14). Like all forms of exercise, yoga injuries do occur when participants try to perform movements they are not ready for, or don't listen to their bodies (see the Take Caution! box below).

### Take Caution

#### SOME COMMON YOGA INJURIES

- **Muscle strains involving the hip flexors (deep lunges), neck (plow), and low back (overflexing the lumbar spine in seated or forward bends).**
- **Bursitis or tendonitis in the shoulder or elbow joints (downward-facing dog or "yoga push-up").**
- **Participants who hyperextend their knees (triangle pose) or elbows (upward-facing dog) place additional stress on stabilizing ligaments and tendons, potentially causing inflammation of joint structures.**

Adapted from Crews L. Injury prevention: Yoga. *IDEA Fit J.* 2006;3(2):77–8.

## PILATES

Pilates is a method of exercise that was developed by Joseph H. Pilates in the early 20th century for physical rehabilitation. He later opened a studio in New York City to train dancers. Pilates uses many different types of apparatus, as well as exercises on a mat. The benefits of Pilates include improved body mechanics, balance, coordination, strength, and flexibility. Pilates mat workouts vary widely in energy cost depending on both the skill level and intensity of the workout and the particular exercise movement being performed (29). Although Pilates is a very challenging and effective means of building core strength and stability, its aerobic conditioning effect is limited. In a study conducted at the University of Wisconsin, LaCrosse, researchers examined whether Pilates mat training could be categorized as having an aerobic component. The results showed that the subjects' average percentage of maximal heart rate was below the ACSM-recommended guidelines for improving cardiorespiratory fitness (5).

## PRE-DESIGNING YOUR EXERCISE CLASS

### CLASS GOALS AND OBJECTIVES

When it comes to designing a safe and effective group exercise class, the first step is knowing the participants' health histories and fitness levels. The primary safety goal of a preparticipation health appraisal is to identify individuals who should receive further medical evaluation to determine whether there are contraindications to exercise training or whether referral to a medically supervised exercise program is necessary (2). The Physical Activity Readiness Questionnaire is a standardized form used in health/fitness facilities to prescreen health assessment. ACSM recommends that the form be viewed as a minimal standard for entry into a new exercise program.

The second step is setting class goals and objectives. One of the major differences between learning, as it occurs naturally, and teaching is in setting of the action goal (17). As it relates to group exercise, goals define what the instructor expects the participants to learn or gain from the class. A primary performance goal might be to complete daily tasks efficiently by improving the components of cardiorespiratory function, body composition, muscular strength and endurance, and flexibility. Once the goal is established, the instructor must then create specific objectives to meet the goal. For example, in a circuit training class, the objective would be to alternate basic cardio moves with upper- and lower-body strength moves for 25–30 minutes to improve cardiorespiratory fitness and muscular strength and endurance.

The last step in designing a well-structured class is planning the class. It is recommended that instructors map out their class designs on paper. The lesson plan needs to include the class objectives, total time, equipment, and music (if applicable to the format), class components (warm-up, workout, cool-down/stretch), time

# How do you create your class blueprint?

**MARJORIE O'CONNOR (MOC)**
*Fit International, CAN*

The methods I use for planning a class lesson varies from the type of program I teach. I structure the class by the goals the class attendees expect to achieve. Each section of the class is designed with a goal and purpose in mind. This makes the creation of a blueprint easy.

My MIND/Body class is structured differently than my cardio-focused programs. For example, in mind/body classes (yoga, pilates, Tai Chi, NIA, etc.) I focus on the progression of movements from simple to complex. In a cardio-based class (step, rebounder, hi/lo, dance style, boot drills), the class is structured with the energy systems manipulated: intervals, level of participants, length of class, and goal of class.

## SAMPLE MIND/BODY CLASS BLUEPRINT

**Preparation.** MOC MIND/Body is practiced without shoes to strengthen lower ankle mechanism, ROM, balance, and proprioception and strengthening of foot and to work on creating a solid foundation without the stabilizing factor of shoes.

**Warm-up.** The goal of any warm-up should be to prepare the body both physically and mentally for the upcoming activity. An effective warm-up increases metabolic rate, blood flow to the muscles, and lubrication of joints and elevates core body temperature. The MOC MIND/Body warm-up is a mental, emotional, and physical experience. Mentally, the MOC warm-up demonstrates all the exercise fundamentals that will be used during all the class components (*i.e.*, rib cage placement, pelvic awareness, and breath control). Also, ritualizing the pre-class warm up is an important aspect of entering a flow state for yourself and your participants.

**Upper body isolation/ROM.** Preparation for more challenging functional exercises.

**Lower body/muscle endurance and integrated strength component**. Series of functional exercises using various mobile pieces of equipment for additional challenge (*i.e.*, BOSU, rollers, suspension trainers (*e.g.*, TRX), balance disks, gliders).

**Floorwork.** Supine/prone/lateral positions. Traditional floor work exercises focusing on joint position, muscle imbalances, and breathing techniques. Fusion of Pilates and yoga inspired movements.

**Supine stretch/relaxation sequence.** Focus on key muscle groups with a blend of static and passive exercises using a stretch strap.

allocations for each component, and appropriate exercise/movement selections, variations, and modifications. The instructor also needs to plan how the exercises/choreography will transition from one move/combination to the next, as well as prepare visual and verbal cues. Exercises or movement patterns should progress from simple to complex by starting with a base move and then changing one element at a time (*e.g.*, planes, levers, direction, and rhythm).

## CLASS DURATION

For some participants, it may be difficult to fit hour-long classes into their schedules. To accommodate participants with limited time, instructors can offer 30-minute "express" classes (see Box 3.2). Half-hour formats also work well for beginner-level classes. However, regardless of the duration, it is important to start and end class on time. By starting class late, an instructor sends a message to the participants that they are not important. A class that runs beyond its allotted time is disruptive to the schedule and discourteous to other instructors and their participants.

## ENVIRONMENTAL CONCERNS/ EQUIPMENT CONSIDERATIONS

Environmental factors such as heat, humidity, altitude, and pollution can increase the heart rate response to work. A person's heart rate response is the best indicator of the relative stress being experienced due to the interaction of exercise, intensity, duration, and environmental factors (20).

The exercise facility's ambient temperature should range between 60°F–70°F (3). Other facility considerations include space and flooring. Participants need sufficient space to move comfortably and to avoid touching fellow participants. The floor needs to effectively absorb shock and offer proper foot stability. Insufficient shock absorption causes activity-related injuries to the ankle and knee joints. Inadequate surface stability has the potential to cause foot rollover. For good shock absorption and surface stability, a suspended hardwood floor is preferred. Concrete is not recommended because it absorbs little shock and can be dangerous if a participant falls. Carpeting is appropriate for classes that do not require dynamic lateral movements or pivoting. Because carpeting does not offer proper surface stability and friction, performing these moves on the carpet may result in ankle sprains or knee injuries. Since not all facilities provide ideal floors, instructors may need to adapt moves to accommodate the flooring surface. For instance, if an instructor has to teach a kickboxing class on a carpet, the moves must be kept unidirectional to eliminate the need for pivots.

## MUSIC

Music has an impact on physiology and mood. Over the past several years, researchers have studied the interactions between music and the cardiovascular, respiratory, and neural systems. The findings suggest that music can facilitate exercise performance by reducing the feeling of fatigue, increasing the levels of psychological arousal, limiting some of the uncomfortable physical sensations associated with exercise, and improving motor coordination (18). In a study conducted at Pavia University in Pavia, Italy, researchers found that music has a constant dynamic influence on cardiorespiratory responses. Music crescendos (loudness or intensity) increase systolic/diastolic blood pressures and heart rate, while decrescendos and silent pauses create a reduction in heart rate and other variables (10).

In the group exercise setting, music can be used to motivate participants and to connect them as a group. Group exercise formats like step and kickboxing are usually taught to a musical beat. Moving to a beat can help participants execute movements at the proper speed and exercise at an appropriate level of intensity. When working to a beat, music speed, or tempo, needs to be maintained within recommended limits in order to minimize risk and maximize benefits.

Other group exercise formats such as yoga and group indoor cycling often use music as background sound. Since these types of classes rely less on choreography, instructors do not have to match the movements to the beat. Instead, music serves to inspire participants and enhances the overall exercise experience.

When it comes to music selection, instructors have many options: pop, rock, hip hop, oldies, classical, and disco, to name a few. In designing a signature sound,

instructors must make sure the genre of music suits the class format, their participants' preferences, and their own personalities. Some instructors use digital technology to create custom mixes, while others prefer to purchase mixed music selections from professional music companies. Due to copyright law, there are legal issues relating to buying, selling, and playing music. An instructor may play copyrighted music in a fitness class if he or she has paid for the appropriate performing-rights license from either the American Society of Composers, Authors and Publishers (ASCAP), Broadcast Music, Inc. (BMI) or SESAC (originally the Society of European Stage Directors and Composers), or if he or she teaches at a facility that has obtained a performance license. Instructors who choose to purchase music from a reputable music company do not have to obtain performance licenses because the company pays a licensing fee to the copyright owners to sell music to instructors. From a legal and ethical standpoint, it is important that instructors do not sell or give away copies of music they've bought online, at a music store or from a fitness music company (3,6).

Group exercise instructors must be aware of music volume when playing music in class. Since participants need to hear the instructor's verbal cues, music volume has to be kept at a reasonable level. In addition, chronic exposure to loud noise can cause hearing damage such as ringing in the ears (tinnitus) or hearing loss. Hearing loss occurs when the tiny hairs in the cochlea, the snail-shaped, fluid-filled chambers in the inner ear, are damaged. The United States Occupational Safety and Health Administration (OSHA) has established safety standards for noise levels based on approximately 60 minutes of continuous exposure. Based on the OSHA guidelines, IDEA Health & Fitness Association (1997) recommends the following with regard to music volume in the fitness class (21):

- Music intensity during a group exercise class should not exceed 90 dB.
- Since an instructor's voice needs to be heard, the instructor's voice should not exceed 100 dB. Exposure at that level should last no longer than 1 hour.
- To motivate clients, fitness instructors should use creativity and enthusiasm instead of raising music volume, and they should educate clients about the risks of continuous exposure to excessive music volume.

### Take Caution

### PROJECT AND PROTECT!

Talking or shouting over loud music can cause vocal cord damage. To prevent vocal abuse, instructors are advised to use a microphone.

## EQUIPMENT

The types of equipment available to the instructor will dictate the format of the class. In addition to the portable resistance training equipment listed earlier in the chapter, some other options include steps, Gliding discs, stability balls, core boards, and the BOSU Balanced Trainer. Steps can be utilized for a variety of classes. Stability balls and BOSUs can add balance or increase functional challenge. Since risks are increased when equipment is added, instructors need to show participants how to use the equipment and where to place it when not in use. Furthermore, instructors must perform regular inspections of the equipment. Stability balls can become worn and burst. The surface matting of the step can separate from the platform, potentially causing a participant to trip as he or she steps up on the platform.

## PARTICIPANTS

Instructors must address the needs, interests and limitations of their participants. Therefore, the choice of equipment, activities, and the pace of the class must be considered when planning for young/old, less fit/very fit, and more skilled/less skilled participants. For example, children require exercise for healthy growth and development. Children's classes need to include elements of fun and play. Some kid-friendly equipment might include jump ropes, agility ladders, and colorful stability balls. Older adults need exercises to increase functional independence in activities of daily living and to reduce risk of falling. Resistance training, aerobic exercise, and balance drills will improve muscular strength and endurance, cardiovascular fitness, and balance. Also, since the fraction of leisure time that older adults spend socializing modestly declines with age, exercising in a group setting may promote social interaction and a sense of community among older adults (25).

## CLASS DESCRIPTIONS

Surveys have shown that health club member retention is higher among those members who participate in group exercise because they tend to use the club consistently (16). So, how do instructors draw a broad range of participants into their classes? How do they increase class attendance and interest? Oftentimes, participants choose classes based on the class name and description. Therefore, it is important that the name creates the correct impression and the words in the description carefully match the format. From the description, participants should be able to decide if the class will meet their needs as well as their fitness and skill levels. Typically, the majority of class participants are women. Men usually tend to shy away from classes because they perceive them as being "dancey." To attract men to the group exercise arena, class names and descriptions should use words that appeal to men's preferences for sports-specific or athletic-style movements. Words like "power," "strength," or "conditioning" fare better than "firming" or "toning."

## DESIGNING YOUR CLASS

### ANATOMY OF A WARM-UP

 **CLIP 3.1** The purpose of the warm-up is to help participants prepare both physiologically and psychologically for their workout. Commonly, warm-ups are

---

### Ask the Pro

# How do you weave the "fun factor" into your classes?

**JULZ ARNEY**
*Team Arney, Inc.*
*Fitness Consultants*
*California*

Occasionally surprising my class with a campy song or a "classic" tune is one of my favorite ways to lighten the mood and get students to laugh, relax, sometimes even sing along!

In yoga and in dance-based classes, I like to insert one pose option or one dance move where you just might surprise yourself! It's a chance to try something perceived to be beyond your reach without any assumptions that you'll be able to master it today. The results range from eye rolls, to laughter, to sheer delight at the outcome.

Whether it's a dance-off with groups battling to do their best, partner yoga where students help each other in a balance pose, or a team challenge in indoor cycling, pulling students out of their normal spaces (both physically and mentally) always raises the fun factor in class.

classified as either general or specific, but often overlap. A general warm-up includes movements that loosen up the body and are unrelated to the specific neuromuscular actions of the planned workout. A specific warm-up provides a skill rehearsal for the actual movements that will be used in the workout. An effective warm-up has the potential to improve physical performance as a result of (27)

- Increased speed of muscle action and relaxation
- Greater economy of movement because of lowered viscous resistance within active muscles
- Facilitated oxygen delivery by the muscle because hemoglobin releases oxygen more readily at higher temperatures
- Facilitated nerve transmission and muscle metabolism resulting from the direct effect temperature has on accelerating the rate of bodily processes; a specific warm-up may also facilitate the recruitment of motor units required for physical activity
- Increased blood flow through active tissue as the local vascular bed dilates with levels of metabolism and muscle temperature

Overall, the warm-up should be gradual and lead to an increase in core and muscle temperature without being too intense. ACSM recommends that the warm-up be at least 5–10 minutes.

In group exercise classes, the warm-up needs to include time-efficient, targeted, and timely movements that keep participants moving consistently and continuously. It also should consist of two phases: a rehearsal phase and a ROM phase (4). The rehearsal phase introduces new moves or movement patterns. It provides the instructor an opportunity to review proper technique and form and to assess the participants' levels and abilities. It lets participants practice the moves so they can feel confident and progress more quickly during the main workout.

The ROM phase increases joint ROM. As multiple joints flex and extend, the major muscles are pulled through an active ROM; as a result, heart rate and core temperature continue to increase. During this phase, the instructor will also want to use moves or movement sequences that challenge balance and core control. In a kickboxing class, the participants could perform a knee strike/lunge combo. The knee strike involves hip/knee flexion with ankle plantar flexion; the lung involves hip/knee extension with ankle dorsiflexion. For the upper body, they could reach the arms on a high diagonal (shoulder flexion/elbow extension/wrist pronation) while lunging and then pull the arms toward the body (shoulder extension/elbow flexion/wrist supination) while performing the knee strike.

Since movement is more limited in indoor cycling classes than choreography-based classes, the instructor would use the warm-up to introduce various hand positions, various body positions (*e.g.*, seated climb, standing climb), and real road situations (8). The instructor would use time to ensure that participants are riding in the proper position: neutral posture, the ball of the foot centered over the pedal, and focusing body weight away from the hands.

## TO STRETCH OR NOT TO STRETCH IN THE WARM-UP

Should static stretching be part of the warm-up? Based on research studies, there appears to be weakening of the muscle after static stretching. The thought is that the weakness is caused by some kind of muscle or tendon slack produced by static stretching. Since the poststretching weakness can last about 15 minutes, it is recommended that exercisers should probably not perform static stretches immediately prior to exercise (11).

## THE WORKOUT (AKA STIMULUS)

CLIP 3.2 No matter the class format, the exercises used in the main workout need to be safe, effective, and purposeful. To accommodate the varied fitness and skill levels among participants, instructors are obliged to

- Ensure that intensity increases gradually
- Provide modifications for various intensities, and when applicable, varying impact options to allow participants to make a choice
- Create movement patterns that progress from simple to complex
- Utilize a variety of muscle groups and encourage muscle balance
- Incorporate various planes of motion (front-to-back, side-to-side, and rotating movements)
- Use a variety of muscle contractions (alternating quick movements with slow and controlled motions)

Besides providing an effective workout, instructors must ensure the successful learning of skills. Group exercise leaders need to move around the room correcting inappropriate movements and paying special attention to beginners. To help participants take charge of their own workout, instructors should teach self-monitoring techniques (*e.g.*, heart rate monitoring, RPE). They should always give visual and verbal cues. They need to give visual cues by demonstrating proper posture and exercise execution for the moves. Verbal cues need to be clear and concise. When working with unskilled exercisers or when teaching a complex movement pattern, the instructor needs to use many visual and verbal cues. Once exercisers have acquired basic skills or participants have become proficient at executing the movement pattern, the instructor can limit the cues (3,15,34).

## COOL-DOWN

**CLIP 3.3** The end of class is just as important as the workout. Whether it's kickboxing, step, or indoor cycling, all cardiovascular endurance classes require an active recovery period. According to McArdle et al. (27), submaximal aerobic exercise is performed under the assumption that continued movement in some way prevents muscle cramps and stiffness. It also prevents hypotension, which may occur with sudden cessation of exercise. Light postexercise physical activity plays a role in facilitating venous return and in restoring the elevated heart rate to the preexercise level. Inadequate venous return causes blood to pool in the lower extremities. This insufficient blood flow to the brain may cause an exerciser to feel dizzy or faint.

During the cool-down, participants need to move at a slower pace. The moves must be kept simple with smaller arm and leg movements. In an indoor cycling class, the participants would go into a lower gear and pedal gradually for a few minutes. Regardless of the cardio format, a 5–10-minute cool-down should be performed.

## THE FINAL STRETCH

**CLIP 3.4** The intrinsic property of muscles and joints to go through a full or optimal ROM is referred to as flexibility (24). It is developed through the use of various stretching methods: passive, dynamic, ballistic, static, and proprioceptive neuromuscular facilitation. Flexibility is related to body type, sex, age, bone and joint structure, and other factors beyond an individual's

control (30). It is predominantly a function of habits of movement, activity, and inactivity.

Although the acute effects of stretching on exercise and sport performance have been and are currently debatable, ACSM recommends that stretching exercise be included in an exercise training environment for all adults and should be performed at least 2–3 days per week. Research suggests that stretching may elicit positive long-term performance outcomes when done at times other than *before* performance. Consequently, the appropriate time to stretch the muscle groups that were worked during the workout is after the cool-down when the muscles are warm (2,7).

In most exercise classes, static and dynamic stretches are commonly used. Static stretches gradually stretch a muscle or muscle group to the point of a mild, even tension. The position is then held for 15–30 seconds. Dynamic stretches are rhythmic in nature and involve movements around single or multiple joints. To make the transition from workout to cool-down and flexibility both functional and seamless, McCormick (28) suggests that participants perform stretches from a standing posture. If participants remain standing, they can also work on balance skills. According to McCormick, an example of a static/dynamic stretch combo that also trains for balance is the Standing Hip Flexion and Knee Extension Stretch. Participants stand with feet hip width apart and grab right leg beneath knee, using both hands. Maintain hip alignment and extend knee while performing ankle plantar flexion and dorsiflexion. Perform four to six repetitions of knee flexion and extension, continuing to move through ankle joint, and then place fingertips behind ears

## Ask the Pro

# What techniques do you use to command attention and communicate to your group of participants?

**CHRIS FREYTAG**
*Fitness Expert/Columnist, Prevention Magazine*
*American Council on Exercise Board Member*

I use lots of encouraging phrases and words; "Yes, you can!" has become kind of my trademark. I tell them they are awesome and thank them for working hard.

I use lots of helpful cues for good form. I take the time to slow down the movements and explain how, why, and which muscle group they are using. I give them modifications to make it easier if needed so

they feel they have permission. At the same time, I encourage them to work to their potential.

I use high energy beat-driving music, and I change it up from time to time to keep them interested.

I always introduce myself and offer my assistance before or after class if there are questions. I always ask who is new so I can keep my eye on them.

I encourage my participants to wear a heart rate monitor to help track progress and zones and motivate them to work to their potential.

and hold extended knee out to stretch hamstring. Hold for 6–10 seconds and focus on maintaining balance.

## SUMMARY

*Group exercise is challenging because of the great variety of physical activities employed and the wide range of fitness and skill among participants. Effective group exercise instructors understand that modifications, variations, and individualized intensity monitoring are essential to ensure safe and enjoyable participation by all. As leaders, they must be in command and communicate a positive attitude. As teachers, they must be aware that skill development is enhanced by appropriate instruction. Therefore, they must create a learning environment that meets specific requirements for effective performance.*

## References

1. American College of Sports Medicine. *ACSM's Resource Manual for Guidelines for Exercise Testing and Prescription.* 6th ed. Baltimore (MD): Lippincott Williams & Williams; 2009.
2. American College of Sports Medicine. *ACSM's Guidelines for Exercise Testing and Prescription.* 8th ed. Baltimore (MD): Lippincott Williams & Williams; 2009.
3. American Council on Exercise. *ACE Group Fitness Instructor Manual.* 2nd ed. Healthy Learning, Monterey, CA: 2007.
4. Anderson P. The active range warm-up: Getting hotter with time. *IDEA Fitness Edge.* 2000;3(2):6–10.
5. Archer S. Can Pilates do it all? *ACE FitnessMatters.* 2005;11(6):10–11.
6. Arney J. Music matters! *IDEA Fit J.* 2006;3(7):54–60.
7. Asp K. The role of stretching exercises: From warm-ups to cool-downs. *IDEA Fitness Edge.* 2001;4(5) (download).
8. Asp K. How to design hot cardio warm-ups. *IDEA Fitness Edge.* 2002;5(4) (download).
9. Benko-Livingston D, Williams-Evans K. Monitoring aerobic intensity. *IDEA Fitness Edge.* 2002;3(3):8–12.
10. Bernardi L, Porta C, Cassuci G, et al. Dynamic interactions between musical, cardiovascular, and cerebral rhythms in humans. *Circulation.* 2009;119:3171–80.
11. Bracko MR. Can stretching prior to exercise and sports improve performance and prevent injury? *ACSM's Health Fitn J.* 2002;6(5):17–22.
12. Carrico M. Yoga. *ACE FitnessMatters.* 1997;3(6):1–4.
13. Crews L. Group resistance training: Guidelines and safety suggestions. *IDEA Fitness Edge.* 2000;3(5):1–6.
14. Crews L. Sun salutations. *IDEA Fit J.* 2010;7(6):68–72.
15. Francis L. Teacher or performer? *IDEA Today.* 1989;5:30–4.
16. Freytag C. Bring on the men: How to attract more men to your group fitness programs. *ACE Certified News.* 2008;14(5):3–5.
17. Gentile AM. Skill acquisition: Action, movement and neuromotor processes. In: Carr JH, Shepherd RB, editors. *Movement Science Foundations for Physical Therapy in Rehabilitation.* Rockville (VA): Aspen Publishers Inc.; 1987. p. 93–149.
18. Harmon NM, Kravitz L. The beat goes on: The effects of music on exercise. *IDEA Fit J.* 2007;4(8):72–7.
19. Haskell WL, Lee IM, Pate RR, et al. Physical activity and public health: Updated recommendation for adults from the American College of Sports Medicine and the American Heart Association. *Med Sci Sport Exer.* 2007;39(8):1423–34.
20. Howley ET, Franks BD. *Health Fitness Instructor's Handbook.* 3rd ed. Champaign (IL): Human Kinetics; 1997.
21. IDEA. Recommendations for music volume in fitness classes. *IDEA Today.* 1997;6:50.
22. Kravitz L. The fitness professional's complete guide to circuits and intervals. *IDEA Today.* 1996;14(1):32–43.
23. Kravitz L. New insights into circuit training. *IDEA Fit J.* 2005;2(4):24–26.
24. Kravitz L. Stretching—A research retrospective. *IDEA Fit J.* 2009;6(10):30–43.
25. Kravitz L. Senior fitness research roundup. *IDEA Fit J.* 2010;7(2):30–7.
26. Lofshult D. Circuit classes come full circle. *IDEA Health & Fitness Source.* 2003;21(10):21–3.
27. McArdle WD, Katch FI, Katch VL. *Exercise Physiology.* 4th ed. Baltimore (MD): Williams & Wilkins; 1996.
28. McCormick I. Stand up for flexibility. *IDEA Fit J.* 2010;7(5):58.
29. Olson M, Williford HN, St. Martin R, et al. The energy cost of a basic, intermediate, and advanced Pilates' mat workout. *Med Sci Sport Exer.* 2004;36(5):S357 (abstract).
30. Rasch PJ. *Kinesiology and Applied Anatomy.* 7th ed. Philadelphia (PA): Lea & Febiger; 1989.
31. Reebok International Ltd. *The Step Reebok Training Manual for Fitness Professionals.* Reebok University Press, Stoughton, MA: 1994.
32. Robert-McComb JJ. Yoga: A modality in complementary therapy. *ACSM's Certified News.* 2009;19(3):1–3.
33. Smith J. Step: Guidelines & safety benchmarks. *IDEA Fitness Edge.* 2000;3(1):1–6.
34. Stevenson C. The four elements of perfect class design. *IDEA Fit J.* 2010;7(5):54–57.
35. Vogel A. Incorporating interval training into traditional group fitness classes. *ACE Certified News.* 2010;16(1):8–9.
36. Vogel AE. Indoor cycling: Guidelines & safety suggestions. *IDEA Fitness Edge.* 2000;3(2):1–5.
37. Webster AL, Aznar-Lain S. Intensity of physical activity and the "Talk Test." *ACSM's Health Fit J.* 2008;12(3):13–17.
38. Williams A. Kickboxing: Guidelines & safety suggestions. *IDEA Fitness Edge.* 2000;3(3):1–6.

# Communication Skills: Adherence and Motivation

LESLIE STENGER

*objectives*

**At the end of this chapter you will be able to:**

- Identify the importance of good communication skills for success as a group exercise instructor
- Describe how motivation of class participants is influenced by the group exercise instructor
- Define feedback and the link to adherence
- Recognize the importance of both nonverbal and verbal communication skills
- Distinguish between nonverbal and verbal communication skills as they apply to teaching group exercise
- Distinguish between client-centered versus instructor-centered instruction
- Identify three theories of human behavior as they apply to physical activity
- Apply the *Motivational Readiness to Change* model to participants in a group exercise setting
- Distinguish between behavioral and cognitive strategies as they apply to participants in a group exercise setting
- Explain how to adapt instruction to address the various learning styles of participants in a group exercise setting

Beyond exercise instruction, teaching group classes is also about establishing and maintaining relationships. The more you understand how to communicate with participants, the more effective an instructor you will be. Good communication is the foundation of successful relationships, and success in the health and fitness industry is dependent on your ability to establish relationships and create a positive rapport. Refining your communication skills will increase your opportunities for success in this dynamic field. In this case, the word dynamic means constant and unpredictable change and is the reason why many people choose the field of health and fitness.

Good communication skills may also enhance your relationship with your colleagues, management, and other professionals. The health and fitness profession is unique due to the fact that the product people pay for is our expertise and our ability to motivate, so how we communicate that knowledge is vital.

As group exercise instructors, we often place a great deal of value on the process of giving information without recognizing the importance of receiving information. The challenge for many fitness professionals is to become proficient at listening to others and sharpening our observation cues. This concept of giving and receiving information is a form of communication referred to as feedback.

There is a very close connection between the terms communication, exercise adherence, and motivation in the fitness industry and specifically when teaching group exercise. Exercise adherence in group exercise refers to retention of participants for any given group exercise activity. According to the International Health and Racquet Sports Association (IHRSA), 44% of health club users participate in group exercise and are avid health club users with over 53% attending at least 100 times per year (8). Group exercise opportunities should be designed to provide a platform for individuals to learn and grow in a supportive environment. People will be motivated to continue if they feel they have the support from the instructor and if they are successful or believe they have the capability to be successful.

While we strive to ensure that all participants enjoy the health benefits of regular exercise, it is understood that many group exercise instructors view adherence as a critical aspect of the business. Many opportunities for group exercise instructors will depend on class attendance and retention of participants. Application of the communication skills covered in this chapter will enable group exercise instructors to become valuable leaders within the health and fitness industry.

This chapter addresses the importance of good communication skills as they apply to group exercise instructors.

## Ask the Pro

# How can you evaluate your own communication skills?

**KRISTIE ABT, PHD, NASM CES, ASCM HFI, AFAA GEI, CORE CERT I & II**
*Assistant Clinical Professor*
*Department of Health and Physical Activity*
*University of Pittsburgh*

Videotape yourself teaching and how the participants respond on a semiannual basis. This allows you to critique yourself with regard to your body language, vocal tone, feedback, and cueing techniques. You should always be trying to improve your ability to establish a good rapport with your participants.

Your role as a group exercise instructor is very similar to that of an educator, mentor, or teacher. We will look at the various types and styles of learners as well as the stages of learning. It is helpful to look at the literature and research in education to help you — as a group exercise instructor — develop your own unique style. Other strategies include team-building activities, which can help to enhance the group dynamic. Think about what makes a good teacher, who was your favorite teacher, and why? What qualities did he or she possess? For many of us, our favorite teachers may not have even taught our favorite subject, but they were able to keep us interested and engaged, while learning more about that subject. Group exercise instructors have an advantage since participants elect to take the class and therefore present at least some interest in the subject matter. Motivation is the key to adherence. The ability to motivate is highly dependent on the instructor's understanding of behavior change and the application of specific strategies to promote positive physical activity behavior.

## VERBAL AND NONVERBAL COMMUNICATION SKILLS

The basis of how we communicate can be described by "what we say" (verbal communication) and "how we say it" (nonverbal communication). Understanding the importance and proper application of each can significantly impact your success as a group exercise instructor. For instance, the actual delivery of the message is more than simply what you say, as explained by the 7%–38%–55% rule (14): When delivering a message, 7% is the content of the words, 38% is tone of voice, and 55% is body language. If body language, tone of voice, and words disagree, then body language and tone of voice will carry more weight than the words (Fig. 4.1).

## NONVERBAL COMMUNICATION SKILLS

Understanding the importance of nonverbal communication skills is critical for instructors (Fig. 4.2). The body language of an instructor can have a major impact on the perception of the participants. Let us identify the body language components that will influence the perception of the participants.

CLIP 4.1

Participants will be evaluating your nonverbal communication skills from the moment you enter the room (see Table 4.1), which plays a major role in setting the tone for your class. There is a great deal of research supporting the importance of body language and effective communication. This is especially relevant for the fitness industry since motivation is often influenced by the energy of the instructor and his or her ability to establish rapport. It is also extremely important for the instructor to be able to

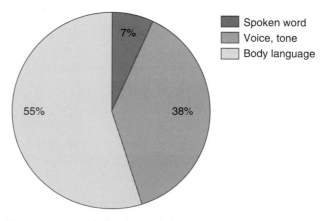

**■ FIGURE 4.1** Verbal and nonverbal communication: the 7%–38%–55% rule.

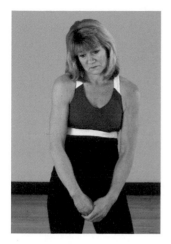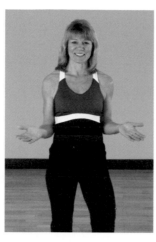

■ **FIGURE 4.2** Understanding the importance of nonverbal communication skills is critical for group exercise instructors.

recognize class participants' nonverbal cues. Responding to their body language will aid the instructor in applying the proper cue or correction.

## HOW TO REINFORCE POSITIVE BODY LANGUAGE

Check your nonverbal communication skills.

### Eye Contact and Facial Expression

- Are you able to make direct eye contact with participants?
- Are you able to engage participants with eye contact and a smile?
- Does your face express enthusiasm?

### Tone and Rhythm of Voice

- Does the tone of your voice include inflections?
- Does the tone of your voice express confidence and enthusiasm?
- Does the rhythm of your voice reinforce the rhythm of the class?

### Posture and Gestures

- Does your body posture convey enthusiasm with open body gestures?
- Does your body posture appear to be relaxed and stress free?
- Are your palms up or down when providing instruction?

### Touch

- Are you comfortable using touch as a cue?
- Can you read the body language of a participant before using touch as a cue?

## VERBAL COMMUNICATION SKILLS

Verbal communication is often referred to by group exercise instructors as "feedback" and is a critical component to success for any instructor. Feedback includes two-way communication — it implies that the instructor will be providing information in a manner that requires a response from the participants. For example, rather than an instructor saying, "you should feel it in your bicep," they could phrase it as "touch your bicep to feel it working." Participants then respond nonverbally by palpating their muscle. The instructor can then observe participants to ensure that they know where their bicep is and that they are performing the exercise correctly. Tone of voice and the rhythm of speech are also critical components of verbal communication. Both factors are directly related to the potential of motivating the class. Tone of voice refers to inflection and shows the genuine excitement of the instructor. Rhythm of speaking directly impacts the ability of participants to understand directions. Rhythm of speaking also influences motivation.

### The Key to Feedback

As previously mentioned, feedback is two-way communication and serves two main purposes. From the perspective of the instructor, appropriate feedback is a means to provide corrections that will either reinforce or improve the performance of each participant (this is stated in the beginning of the chapter). From the perspective of the participant, appropriate feedback includes following the visual and/or verbal suggestions and ensuring that the instructor knows whether or not you understand his or her directions. The key to providing appropriate feedback is to constantly watch the participants and provide information based upon their responses. Instructors should provide participants with information that will enhance their opportunities for success while maintaining a safe exercise environment. Instructors can enhance the motivation of the participants by applying a few simple skills when communicating to participants. Feedback should always be growth-oriented and positive so that participants understand the correct way to perform and not how to adapt the incorrect method of performing. Make corrections relevant to their lifestyle; use analogies that participants can relate to. For example, when describing the importance of a strong core, you might ask participants to get onto all fours and practice stabilization of the core by asking them to maintain a flat back position. For those individuals who are not able to maintain the flat back position, it is helpful to provide immediate feedback that is specific and that they can relate to. For example, the instructor would immediately point out that the back should be flat, like a tabletop where you could balance a glass of water (analogy). Be specific regarding how long to hold the position or criteria checkpoints. The instructor could emphasize that having

| Table 4.1 | COMPONENTS OF BODY LANGUAGE |
|---|---|
| **COMPONENT** | **POSSIBLE PERCEPTION/INTERPRETATION** |
| Facial expression 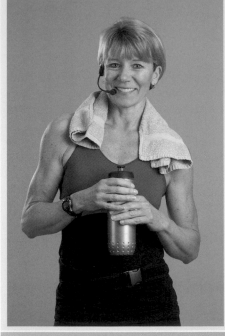 | Can express enthusiasm or disinterest. Key factor: smile |
| Eye contact 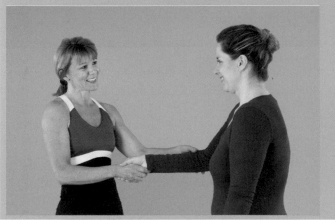 | Can express personal interest, sincerity, and trust |
| Tactile/touch 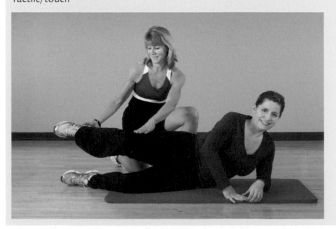 | (Always ask permission before using touch.) This type of cueing can show genuine interest in helping to successfully, and safely, perform skill |

| Respect of personal space | General rule is one arm's length in distance, unless using tactile (touch) cueing |
|---|---|
| 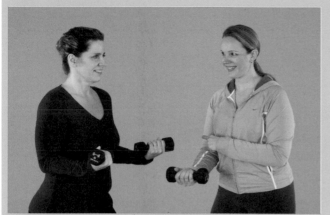 | |
| Hand gestures | Open hand invokes trust; centers on the student<br>Hand closed or facing down commands authority; centers on instructor. Gestures coordinate with verbal instructions |
| 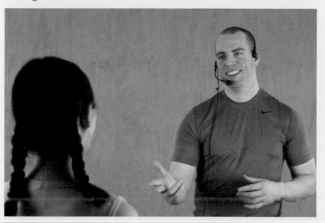 | |
| Posture | Can convey confidence or disinterest. Avoid slouching and keep body open to participants (avoid crossing arms across body) |
| 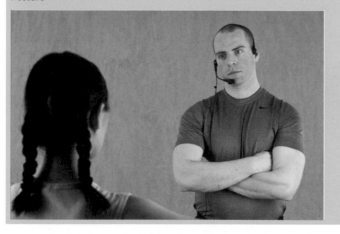 | |

a strong core may help to reduce chronic back pain and then reinforce the fact that 80% of the adult population will experience chronic low back pain. The key to feedback is to

- Provide information immediately (once the instructor observes the need for a correction)
- Be specific with comments
- Make comments growth-oriented
- Make comments relevant to their lives
- Use analogies they understand

See Figure 4.3 for a summary of verbal and nonverbal characteristics and their influence on motivation.

## INSTRUCTIONAL CONSIDERATIONS

One of the primary responsibilities for the group exercise instructor is to present the information in a safe environment that is informative, motivating, and supportive of their individual needs. In education, this is viewed as student-centered versus teacher-centered

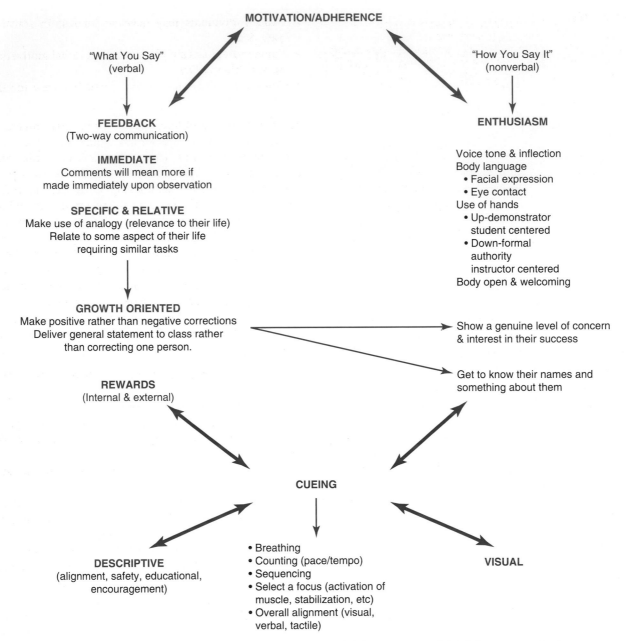

**■ FIGURE 4.3** Motivation and adherence chart summarizes verbal and nonverbal characteristics and their influence on motivation.

instruction. In the fitness industry, we might refer to this as participant/client-centered versus instructor-centered instruction. Let us look at the differences between client-centered and instructor-centered instruction. Though client-centered instruction addresses meeting the needs of each participant by keeping the focus of the class on relevant content, instructor-centered instruction focuses on the overall delivery of concepts, rather than how the participant will process the information. There is a major difference between being able to perform a skill and being able to instruct another person on how to perform the skill — a good instructor should know the difference and be able to do both.

CLIP 4.2    Think back to the question presented early in the chapter about your favorite

teacher. Was he or she more client-centered or instructor-centered? It is key to possess the attributes listed for instructor-centered instruction (see Table 4.2); however, if you do not possess the ability to apply the skills in the client-centered instruction, you may not actually be facilitating change for the participants in your class. Let us look at an example that illustrates both types of instruction. Let's say an instructor is teaching the warrior pose in a Hatha yoga class. An instructor applying instructor-centered yoga will stay in front of the class and explain and demonstrate the warrior pose and then have the participants perform the pose. The instructor may point out form errors observed in the class as a whole and state the physical purpose of the pose. A client-centered instructor will teach the warrior pose in front of the class

| Table 4.2 | CLIENT- VERSUS INSTRUCTOR-CENTERED INSTRUCTION |
|---|---|
| **PARTICIPANT/CLIENT-CENTERED INSTRUCTION** | **INSTRUCTOR-CENTERED INSTRUCTION** |
| Focus on external influences that may affect learning | Focus on internal influences that may affect learning |
| 1. Physical environment (lighting, temperature, ability to hear and see instructor)<br>2. Awareness of specific group dynamics<br>3. Ability to use a variety of teaching styles<br>4. Ability to address all learning styles<br>5. Ability to establish relationships<br>6. Interest in participant having a positive experience | 1. Knowledge of exercise specialty<br>2. Knowledge of teaching techniques<br>3. Knowledge of learning styles<br>4. Ability to perform specific exercises |

while explaining the physical purpose of the pose for a variety of health benefits. This provides multiple opportunities for each participant to relate to at least one of the benefits on a personal level. After explaining and demonstrating the pose, the instructor may walk around the class and provide individual corrections and suggestions while maintaining positive reinforcement to the group as a whole. This enables the instructor to provide personalized modifications based on individual needs. While it is critical to have the knowledge regarding specialty, learning styles, and teaching styles and ability to perform skills for demonstration purposes, what will set you apart as a "great group exercise instructor" is your ability to focus on each participant and work to ensure that each person leaves your class with a positive experience.

## GROUP DYNAMICS

Working with a group presents a unique challenge for the instructor since he or she is responsible for helping each participant reach their individual goal while nourishing the group dynamic. It is critical for group exercise instructors to be able to adapt to the dynamics provided by each and every group they work with. Each class will present their own group dynamic, and a successful group exercise instructor will know to look for cues from the group and adapt the environment in a positive fashion to enhance the dynamic, resulting in success for all participants.

Each participant has a personal reason for attending a group exercise class. Being aware of the most common reasons may aid instructors in establishing a supportive and effective environment for the group (1).

- Some individuals exercise independently and participate in group exercise to experience group success.
- Some individuals join in order to be part of a group even though they prefer to maintain their privacy.
- Some individuals feel intimidated when working out on their own and enjoy the social support from the instructor and other participants.

- Some individuals may have an interest in learning new skills.
- Some individuals simply need the external motivation to push themselves.
- Some individuals join group exercise purely for the social reasons.

The techniques used to create a positive environment in one class may not work as well in another class due to the specific class dynamics. In many instances, the participants in a group exercise program or class establish a very positive rapport with each other, similar to that experienced in team sports. Aristotle proposed the theory that the whole is greater than the sum of its parts. This is especially true when we consider the dynamics of a group exercise class. Each participant comes with a specific and individual personality and skill level. As an instructor, you have to recognize the group as a whole and will find that each class has a unique personality and combined skill level.

The group dynamic can be a motivating power for the instructor. The following team-building activities may help to improve group dynamics:

- Post information specific to benefits of exercise outside of class.
- Provide motivational handouts.
- Have class/facility procedures available in writing.
- Have survey or questionnaires available (e.g., readiness of exercise).
- Include informative dialogue during warm-up and cool-down.
- Provide written materials dealing with problem-solving techniques that address barriers to physical activity and how to overcome challenges.
- Encourage social support from within the class.
- Use class participants as role models for other participants.
- Enable participants to develop focus groups.
- Purposefully promote social support among participants and encourage exercise partnerships during class and in other forms of exercise.
- Give the class a group name or theme name and have participants provide input for class name.
- Provide class with external rewards such as T-shirts, wristbands, and headbands (participants will normally not mind paying a nominal fee for a reward).
- Combine fun and play into the class format.

## BENEFITS OF "PLAY"

"What do most Nobel laureates, innovative entrepreneurs, artists and performers, well-adjusted children, happy couples and families, and the most successfully adapted mammals have in common? They play enthusiastically throughout their lives," states Stuart Brown, Institute of Play (4). Although The Institute of Play defines play as a time when we feel most alive, we often take it for granted and may even completely forget about it.

| Table 4.3 | EXPLANATION OF THE FLOW OF PLAY |
| --- | --- |
| **COMPONENT** | **EXPLANATION** |
| Involvement | Complete focus and concentration, either due to innate curiosity or as the result of training |
| Delight | A sense of bliss and positive detachment from everyday reality |
| Clarity | A built-in understanding about the state of affairs |
| Confidence | An innate sense that the activity is doable and that your skills are adequate to the task. Additionally, you do not feel anxious or bored. |
| Serenity | A sense of peace and an absence of worries about self |
| Timeliness | Thorough focus on the present and a lack of attention to the passing of time |
| Motivation | Intrinsic understanding about what needs to be done and a desire to keep the moment of play moving |

*Reprinted with permission from Helpguide.org © 2001-2010. All rights reserved. For more information, visit www.Helpguide.org*

| Table 4.4 | MOTIVATIONAL THEORY |
| --- | --- |
| Level of concern | Individuals are more likely to succeed when they know that they are in a supportive environment. |
| Feeling/tone | Refers to the atmosphere or environment set by the instructor. It should be inviting and positive. Refrain from a competitive environment. |
| Interest | Reinforce personal improvement and encourage individual progress. |
| Success | Design class in order for all participants to see some level of success (present skills in a progressive, systematic manner). |
| Knowledge of results | Provide participants with constant feedback throughout class |
| Rewards | Intrinsic (all participants should have a positive experience) and extrinsic (tangible rewards such as snacks, T-shirts, etc.). |

The ability to play can influence our physical health as well as positively affect our sleep, nutrition, and exercise. According to the National Institute of Play, it transforms negative emotions and enhances learning, helps to relieve stress, and nurtures our connection to others. These are some of the same benefits participants can achieve in group exercise. Incorporating opportunities that will specifically address these factors will benefit the overall class environment.

Play has been described as a flow state by psychiatrist Mihaly Csikszentmihalyi (4). A flow state can be measured in any type of physical activity and includes the following factors: involvement, delight, clarity, confidence, serenity, timeliness, and motivation. Table 4.3 describes each component of a flow state.

## UNDERSTANDING MOTIVATION AND THE THEORIES OF HUMAN BEHAVIOR

Success as a group exercise instructor is dependent on two factors, what you teach and how you teach it. Both are critical to your success. Your exercise specialty and class topic may get participants into your class, but it will be your presentation of the class that will keep them returning. The ability to motivate participants for long-term behavior change is a blending of the art and science of group exercise. The application of the most appropriate motivational strategy is dependent on the setting and type of class you are teaching. Table 4.4 identifies six variables of the Motivational Theory (7) that have a direct link to motivation and can be instrumental to the group exercise instructor.

## UNDERSTANDING HOW BEHAVIOR AFFECTS PHYSICAL ACTIVITY

Research studies (6,10) indicate that programs based on various theoretical frameworks may increase physical activity behaviors among sedentary adults. Let us explore three theories focused on explaining physical activity behavior.

### SOCIAL COGNITIVE THEORY

This theory describes human behavior as actions based on individual thoughts and feelings. Individuals are seen as active agents in their own lives. The social cognitive theory denotes the thought that behavior is a function of personality traits or environmental influences. These factors are recognized as contributing influences, but the individual still has the ability to select his or her own behavior. According to the research of Bandura (2), people are proactive agents in their own lives.

### THEORY OF PLANNED BEHAVIOR

This theory focuses on attitudes and intentions, and the ability to transform intentions into behavior. Intentions and attitudes can be influenced by the social environment in either a positive or negative manner. For example, we assume that each group exercise instructor has a positive attitude toward their specialty and possesses good intentions with regard to teaching prospective participants. However, when the intentions for teaching the class are personal or are not presented in a supportive environment, this can have a negative impact on the participants. This may be the case when an instructor develops the class based on his or her own workout rather than developing a class that is totally focused on success of the participants. Another example would be when the intentions of the instructor are altered in a negative manner due to a nonsupportive environment from management. The theory of planned behavior suggests that instructors need to closely evaluate their intentions for teaching so that the students have a positive perception of the instructor's intentions.

## THEORY OF SELF-EFFICACY

According to research conducted by Bandura (2), self-efficacy is one's belief in one's ability to succeed in a specific situation. Self-efficacy can play a major role in how one approaches challenges, tasks, and goal-setting and is commonly thought to be one of the primary determinants of behaviors related to physical activity. It is also related to motivation and associated with intrinsic (internal) rather than extrinsic (external) motivation. Intrinsic motivation is doing something because you choose to do it (autonomy) rather than for an extrinsic reward. Research (13) has shown that exercise adherence is directly related to exercise self-efficacy, and instructors and their strategies are the key to exercise self-efficacy. Group exercise self-efficacy is defined by Barbara Brehm (3) as people feeling efficacious when they believe they have the knowledge and skills to perform successfully in your class. As we are aware, it takes time to for the positive health benefits of physical activity to occur and many people will drop out because they do not believe that they are capable of completing the work at hand. A person with a high level of self-efficacy believes that he or she can accomplish the work and will be more willing to adhere to the program in order to gain the benefits. It also stems to reason that an instructor with a high level of self-efficacy in his or her ability to teach will inspire participants.

## MOTIVATIONAL READINESS TO CHANGE

One role of the group exercise instructor is to appropriately motivate class participants. Motivation is linked to behavior change and explained in the model, known as the "Motivational Readiness to Change," developed by Prochaska and DiClemente in 1983 (11). The premise of the model was to define five specific stages that individuals progress through as they adopt and maintain a new habit or behavior. Researchers have since adapted the original model to apply specifically to physical activity (5,12). The modified stages with descriptions are provided in Table 4.5.

Group exercise instructors may have any number of class participants at each stage. It is the role of instructors to aid *all* participants toward the maintenance stage. Research indicates that self-efficacy for physical activity increases as people progress through the stages of change. Marcus et al. (12) have proposed numerous behavioral and cognitive strategies that instructors can apply in the course of helping participants increase their overall physical activity levels and maintain physical activity throughout their lifespan. Cognitive strategies

| Table 4.5 | STAGES OF CHANGE |
| --- | --- |
| Precontemplation: inactive and not thinking about becoming active | |
| Contemplation: inactive but thinking about becoming active | |
| Preparation: physically active but not at the recommended levels (30 min or more of moderate-intensity physical activity on most, preferably all days of the week) | |
| Action: physically active at the recommended levels and have been active for <6 mo | |
| Maintenance: physically active at the recommended levels and have been for 6 or more months | |

involve increasing awareness, influencing attitudes, and assisting an individual as he or she thinks through situations, while the behavioral strategies involve changing the actions of the person. Table 4.6 provides examples of both cognitive and behavioral strategies.

The strategies outlined in Table 4.6 can be applied to your group classes with little advanced planning. Cognitive strategies are most useful in the precontemplation, contemplation, and preparation stage (see Table 4.6), whereas the behavioral strategies peak at the action stage. There is also a process known as "decisional balance" that can be helpful as individuals progress through all the stages. This process encourages participants to weigh the "pros" and "cons" for engaging in physical activity. This is an effective method of assisting with positive behavior change in your class.

## FACTORS INFLUENCING ADHERENCE

One common goal for all group exercise instructors, regardless of their specialty, is to increase the likelihood that their participants will become more physically active on a regular basis. According to research published in the Journal of Teaching Physical Education, instructors have the responsibility of teaching not only skills associated with their specialties but also self-management skills such as self-assessment, self-monitoring, planning, goal setting, and how to overcome barriers (12). Brehm has recommended the following behavioral strategies (3) for application in a group setting.

### Problem Solving

Use the time during cool-down to discuss common pros and cons to being active. Have the participants identify their common barriers and then, as a class, discuss possible solutions.

### Self-Monitoring

Encourage students to start an exercise diary to track workouts, including class participation. Discuss specific goals that participants can strive toward and encourage them to participate. Share information in class during warm-up/cool-down or before or after class.

| Table 4.6 | THE PROCESS OF CHANGE — APPLICATION OF STRATEGIES | |
|---|---|---|
| **COGNITIVE STRATEGIES** | | **BEHAVORIAL STRATEGIES** |
| *Increasing Knowledge (example):*<br>· Have articles available describing the specific health benefits for your exercise class topic. | | *Substituting Alternatives (example):*<br>· Participants miss class because they didn't have time to go home to change for class — instructor suggests they place clothes in car the night before so they don't forget in the morning. |
| *Being Aware of Risks (example):*<br>· Have information on the risks of being inactive and relate it to your exercise topic. | | *Enlisting Social Support (example):*<br>· Invite participants to bring family member or friend to class. |
| *Caring About Consequences to Others (example):*<br>· Provide information on how inactivity relates to disease and how it might affect family, friends, and coworkers.<br>· Ask participants what would happen if something happened to their health, making them more dependent on family and friends (valuable tool when working with an older population). | | *Rewarding Yourself (example):*<br>· Discuss positive self-talk that participants can use in class.<br>· Have T-shirts made specifically for class participants (cost involved). |
| *Comprehending Benefit (example):*<br>· Have a participant in class provide a testimonial of benefits in some aspect of his or her life. | | *Committing Yourself (example):*<br>· Encourage participants to make promises, plans, and commitments to be active.<br>· Have poster in class for participants to record their promises, plans, and/or commitments. |
| *Increasing Healthy Opportunities (example):*<br>· Provide suggestions and information on the benefits from other classes or services offered. | | *Reminding Yourself (example):*<br>· Participating in class provides a structure and makes it easier for participants to remember to exercise. |

Source: Marcus & Forsyth (2004). Motivating people to be physically active.

## Managing Stress and Negative Emotions

Discuss the negative physical consequences of stress and incorporate breathing and positive self-talk techniques into your class. Encourage participants to explore various relaxation techniques on their own and provide support information on the benefits.

# UNDERSTANDING THE PROCESS OF LEARNING

Group fitness instructors have a responsibility to "educate" participants on the benefits of pursuing a healthy lifestyle as well as the specific benefits related to the class topic/activity. Education has both a physical and intellectual component. As instructors, we focus on the process of skill development within an exercise class. We often associate skill development with motor skill development or the actual movement. But there are other types of skill development such as cognitive and perceptual/psychological, and a combination of the two that is referred to as psychomotor skill.

A cognitive skill requires a thought process, whereas a perceptual/psychological skill is how the participant interprets the information presented to him or her. Participants will learn those skills at different rates based on their individual motor abilities such as balance, visual acuity, eye hand/foot coordination, agility, response time, and speed of limb movement. Group exercise instructors mostly focus on motor skill development when teaching. (Non-locomotor skills, such as stretching, do not involve movement and are easier to master than locomotor skills, such as walking, biking, and dancing. The most difficult skills to

master are manipulative in nature such as throwing, catching, tracking, or using any type of external implement).

The process of learning involves moving through three stages. Instructors can benefit from understanding the process of learning, as well as the way people prefer to learn (see *Types of Learners* below), in order to apply various teaching styles that will bring success to the participants.

## STAGES OF LEARNING

### Cognitive Stage

Participants will start the learning process in the cognitive stage when learning a new psychomotor skill. They have to first think about how to perform the skill before it becomes automatic. It is critical for them to understand the sequence of movements and gain a mental and visual image of the proper execution of the skill.

### Affective or Associative Stage

One enters this stage once one masters the basic mechanics and fundamentals and can then focus on practice on repetition. The goal of this stage is to refine the performance of the skill. Motivation is also a key component of this stage, and verbal cueing is critical.

### Autonomic Stage

This occurs once the participant can perform the skill without having to think about the physical aspects of performance.

It is important for group exercise instructors to be aware of these learning stages and recognize that each participant may be at different skill levels at any given time. This will influence the amount and type of feedback provided by the instructor. For instance, participants in the cognitive stage need detailed verbal instructions with a physical demonstration. Once they move to the affective/associative stage, the focus should shift to providing adequate time for practice. In this stage, the focus for the instructor is to provide detailed comments on how to refine the skill. A seasoned group exercise instructor will be able to identify which stage each student is in. The instructor can then apply the appropriate teaching strategies to ensure that all participants can progress to the next level.

## TYPES OF LEARNERS

The process of learning is actually a process of self-discovery and therefore will occur differently among participants. Research has shown that individuals possess a preference for how they learn. Rose and Nicholl (15) describe the preferences as three styles of learning: visual, auditory/verbal, and kinesthetic/tactile.

It is noted that individuals may use all three styles to learn, yet there is usually a dominant preferred style for each individual. It is estimated that 60% of American learners are dominant visual, 25% are dominant kinesthetic, and 15% are dominant verbal/auditory (16). Group exercise instructors will benefit from understanding each style in order to ensure that they apply teaching strategies that are the most appropriate for each preference.

### The Visual Learner

The visual learner prefers to learn through sight. This type of learner is often very social and responds favorably to the use of charts, videos, diagrams, articles, etc. They can learn specifics by watching demonstrations and taking notes for review at a later time. Overstimulation from a visual perspective can actually be a deterrent for these individuals. This is something to consider when designing an exercise room. Having too many posters, instructions, and/or pictures can be a distraction for the visual learner.

### The Verbal/Auditory Learner

The verbal/auditory learner prefers to learn through hearing or listening. This type of learner is often analytical and responds to the verbal directions, so the instructor's tone of voice and pace of speech are a major factor to learning. Note taking can also benefit this type of learner. It is critical for the instructor to provide clear and detailed instructions in a logical manner. External noise, such as sound systems, radios, and/or televisions can aid with learning or serve as a distraction if not used as part of a planned routine.

### The Kinesthetic/Tactile Learner

The kinesthetic/tactile learner prefers to learn by doing and practicing the skill introduced. They also benefit from physical assistance from the instructor, so it may be helpful for the instructor to be more "hands on" by actually assisting the participant in order to ensure proper execution of the skill or exercise. It is highly recommended that an instructor always ask the participant for permission prior to providing any physical assistance. This technique is commonly used in order to have the participant palpate various muscle groups while performing exercises.

Research indicates that most individuals don't only use one learning style; they often occur together (15). However, there is always a preferred style for various activities. It is suggested that group exercise instructors apply teaching strategies that address each of the learning styles in order to accommodate class participants' preferences.

It is very common to observe a higher percentage of kinesthetic/tactile learners in athletes. In fact, many instructors find their preferred style to be kinesthetic/tactile. A common mistake many group exercise instructors make is to teach using predominately their personal preferred style. One must remember that the majority of the population prefers visual learning, and instructors should be able to apply various teaching styles to address all learning preferences.

 CLIP 4.3    Figure 4.4 summarizes techniques to address the various learning styles.

## THE PERSONALITY VARIABLE

As a group exercise instructor, it is your responsibility to "lead" the class. One of your main responsibilities is to provide an informative, safe, and supportive environment.

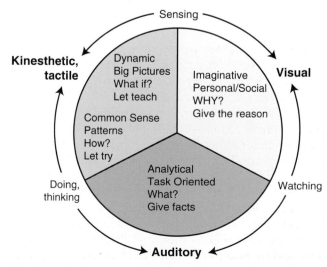

■ **FIGURE 4.4** Techniques to address the various learning styles.

It is important for the instructor to always maintain control within the class. Leadership while teaching group exercise involves being able to influence the behaviors of each individual in the class. Each instructor possesses his or her own style and will have either a positive or negative impact on the participants. But individuals in a group may also have an impact on participants. It is important for instructors to know how to capitalize on the group dynamics to ensure that individual participants do not have a negative impact on the class. One way to maintain control of a class is to provide participants with expectations and class policies. Individuals are less likely to act

out if they clearly know the rules. Participants should know your expectations regarding issues such as talking in class, asking questions, and how to set personal physical limits. A common issue for participants that may result in inappropriate behavior is not being able to hear and/or see the instructor. In order to prevent problems, the instructor should consistently ask if he or she can be seen and heard.

Negative situations can occur even in a safe, supportive, and organized environment. Instructors should be prepared to handle a negative situation in a swift and quick manner in order to prevent the group dynamic to be negatively influenced. The following chart (see Table 4.7) provides a few examples of negative personality traits and suggested strategies for the instructor.

Instructors should have preplanned strategies on how to assist positive behavior change for those who disrupt the class. If strategies do not work, it may be necessary to request that the disruptive participant leave the class (See Chapter 7 for detailed strategies on conflict resolution techniques).

**RECOMMENDED RESOURCES:** Bandura A. *Self-Efficacy: The Exercise of Control.* New York: Freeman and Co.; 1997.

Brehm BA, *Successful Fitness Motivation Strategies.* Champaign, IL: Human Kinetics; 2004.
Fable S. NLP: The "Soft" science of communication. IDEA Fitness J. 2008;5(7). www.ideafit.com
Marcus BH, Rossie JS, Selby VC, et al. The stages and processes of exercise adoption and maintenance in a workplace sample. Health Psychol. 1992;11:386–95.

## Ask the Pro

# What is a quick method of determining the learning styles of class participants?

**AUBREY WOREK, BS, ACSM-HFS, AFAA-GROUP EXERCISE INSTRUCTOR**
*Co-owner*
*Health Solutions at Work, Inc.*
*Pittsburgh, Pennsylvania*

Teach primarily to one learning style, and observe how the class responds. For example, verbally cue an exercise from the back of the room. You will likely notice the auditory learners will understand and perform the exercise without the use of a visual example and the visual learners will be looking for you. You can train your class to adapt to various learning styles by consciously using one style and coaching them through the process. This is especially useful when you need to leave the front of the room to make a correction or adjust the music volume or room temperature.

| Table 4.7 | PARTICIPANT PERSONALITY TRAITS AND THE IMPACT ON THE INSTRUCTOR | |
|---|---|---|
| **PERSONALITY TRAIT** | **CHARACTERISTICS** | **INSTRUCTOR STRATEGY** |
| *The Expressive Participant:* "The Talker" | · Can be distracting<br>· Participant who frequently speaks out regarding his or her individual needs<br>· Has conversations with other participants | · Reinforce the class policies that are either displayed in the class or provided in a handout.<br>· Address situation personally with participant after class. |
| *The Assistant* | · Assists instructor by frequently correcting other participants<br>· Monopolizes instructor's attention | · If they are performing skills correctly, use them as demonstrators where you are in control of what they do.<br>· Position them in class where they cannot see all other participants (class without mirrors). |
| *The Challenger* | · Participant expresses (verbally and nonverbally) disinterest or appears that he or she is not being challenged physically. | · Provide appropriate modifications to accommodate their individual skill level.<br>· Talk with the participant personally at conclusion of class.<br>· Encourage goal setting. |
| *The Emotional Participant* | · Participant seeks constant positive reinforcement.<br>· Participant finds challenges and barriers performing skills or being active. | · Apply "decisional balance" (pros/cons) to the situation and have an empathetic ear.<br>· Encourage goal setting. |

## SUMMARY

*Teaching group exercise is both an "art" and a "science." The research (3) is clear on the numerous benefits, both psychological and physiological, of regular exercise. In addition, there are proven strategies (9) for instruction of all forms of exercise (9). However, success for participants of group exercise is individualized and highly influenced by the environment set by the instructor. Providing a positive exercise environment requires the application of many different skills and strategies by the instructor.*

*Learning the various skills and strategies is a "science;" knowing how and when to apply those skills and strategies is an "art." As an instructor, you need to look for moments when participants are open to your advice — and it begins with your ability to connect with the participants. How will you share your expertise? Will your delivery be the same for each person? What strategies will you apply to ensure individual success for participants? These are just some of the questions you should be able to answer after reading this chapter.*

## References

1. Annes JJ. Effects of minimal group promotion on cohesion and exercise adherence. *Small Group Res.* 1999;30:542–57.
2. Bandura A. *Self-Efficacy: The exercise of control.* New York: Freeman and Co.; 1997:66.
3. Brehm BA. *Successful Fitness Motivation Strategies.* Champaign, IL: Human Kinetics; 2004.
4. Brown S, Vaughn C. *Play: How It Shapes The Brain Opens the Imagination, and Invigorates the Soul.* New York, NY Penguin Group; 2009.
5. Dunn AL, Marcus BH, Kampert JB, et al. Reduction in cardiovascular risk factors: six month results from Project Active. *Prev Med.* 1997;26:883–92.
6. Dunn AL, Marcus BH, Kampert JB, et al. Project active: a 24-month trial to compare lifestyle and structured physical activity interventions. *J Am Med Assoc.* 1999;281:327–34.
7. Hunter M. *Mastery Teaching: Increasing Instructional Effectiveness in Elementary and Secondary Schools, Colleges, and Universities.* Thousand Oaks, CA: Corwin Press; 1982.
8. IHRSA. *The International Health and Racquet Sports Association (IHRSA) Heatlh Club Consumer Report.* 2009;9:14.
9. Kennedy CA, Yoke MM. *Methods of Group Exercise Instruction.* 2nd ed. Champaign, IL: Human Kinetics; 2009.
10. Marcus BH, Bock SC, Pinto BM, et al. Efficacy of an individualized motivationally tailored physical activity intervention. *Ann Behav Med.* 1998;20:174–80.
11. Marcus BH, Lewis BA. Physical activity and the stages of motivational readiness for change model. *President's Council of Physical Fitness and Sports Research Digest.* 2003;4:3–11.
12. Marcus BH, Rossi JS, Selby, et al. The stages and processes of exercise adoption and maintenance in a worksite sample. *Health Psychol.* 1992;11:386–95.
13. Mcauley E, Talbot HM, Martinez S. Manipulating self-efficacy in the exercise environment in women: influences on affective responses. *Health Psychol.* 1999;18(3):56–8.
14. Mehrabian A. *Silent Messages.* 1st ed. Belmont, CA: Wadsworth; 1971.
15. Rose C, Nicholl M. *Accelerated Learning for the 21st Century.* New York: Dell; 1997.
16. Thompson WR. *Amercian College of Sports Medicine, ACSM's Resources for the Personal Trainer.* 2nd ed. Philadelphia, PA Lippincott Williams & Wilkins; 2007.

# 5 Choreography, Music, and Cueing in Class Design and Delivery

KEN ALAN • SHANNON FABLE

## objectives

**At the end of this chapter you will be able to:**
- Describe class formats for cardiovascular and strength workouts
- Identify choreographic options for various class formats
- Analyze effective cueing methods for group exercise classes
- Discuss techniques for synchronizing exercise to music
- Apply elements of change for creative movement drills and patterns
- Describe equipment-based class design and exercise options
- Instruct a variety of movements, exercises, and drills to improve cardiovascular and muscular fitness

Designing and delivering a fitness class was relatively simple in the past. An instructor easily managed the demands because classes were homogenous and participants were a similar demographic: 18- to 34-year-old women. Today, with the diverse amount of program formats and equipment available, creating a class that meets the needs of a much wider and diverse demographic is challenging. To be a successful group fitness instructor, you must first determine which formats you are best suited to lead. Learn all you can about the format and the people who frequent these types of classes. Make sure it blends with your own personal style, as you have to deliver it with a keen eye on movement mechanics, safety, and effectiveness, all conveyed through your personality, framed in your stage presence, inspired by your passion, and fueled by your motivation. It is a tall order, but someone has to make it happen!

In the earlier days of "aerobics" before our profession was known as group fitness, you were primarily skilled in teaching exercise routines. You learned a little about the body and learned a lot about music, choreography, and movement breakdown. Class design simply required you to fit these skills into a high-impact, low-impact, or muscle conditioning class. Classes were "leveled," and your design and delivery matched your current level of instruction and (hopefully) the needs of the participants who came to each particular class. Although your repertoire grew varied over time, the exercises, choreography, music, and class design were predictable, and participants knew what they were getting when they walked in the door making the outcome much easier to control.

Fast forward to today. Although becoming competent in teaching one kind of class is an accomplishment, becoming adept in leading a variety of classes is in high demand (2). A program director might expect you to teach five different formats on the schedule, all with unique end users, expectations, goals, and skill levels. Your ability to get this "right" is much more challenging. You must come armed with a general outline or lesson plan, have a clear-cut method for delivering your plan, and be able to progress or regress the plan so that everyone has the opportunity to feel successful. The work you put into developing your classes prior to teaching is as important, if not more so, as the work you put in during your class.

This chapter reviews cardio and strength classes that populate group fitness schedules. Each of these formats will be broken down by choreographic or class design methods, including suggested movements to consider, creating combinations or drills suitable for a wide audience, and suggestions for effective delivery of your class content. We discuss appropriate music, how best to use your music to support the class goals, and appropriate music tempo for specific formats. We also talk about how your workout environment and equipment availability affect class design.

## CLASS FORMAT OVERVIEW AND ELEMENTS

Schroeder and Dolan report that almost 80% of health clubs and fitness facilities in the United States offer group exercise classes (18). Group exercise has expanded over the years to include a diverse list of class titles, descriptions, and objectives. A majority of classes fall into four broad areas, each with a specific fitness focus:

- Cardio: Choreographed
- Cardio: Nonchoreographed
- Strength
- Cardio/strength combination

## Ask the Pro

# What is a key element to be a successful group exercise instructor?

**CAROL MURPHY**
*Owner*
*Fitlife*
*Rochester, New York 2010 IDEA Instructor of the Year*

Your success as a teacher lies first, in your ability to make that special connection with your class

participants and second, to teach so they succeed. Be well rehearsed; 30% of your time should be spent on what you will teach and 70% on how you will teach it (teaching methods, cueing, variations, modifications).

---

Within these categories, you find

- Self-designed classes in which the instructor is responsible for developing the content of the class within a broad framework
- Prechoreographed classes or branded programs in which fitness companies such as Les Mills, Zumba®, Jazzercise®, and Body Training Systems develop and release new choreography and training routines on a regular schedule. Instructors learn the predetermined class content and teach it as is from start to finish.
- Classes delineated by skill or fitness level, or sport-specific orientation, like an advanced cardio kickboxing class or a ski conditioning class
- Classes targeting specific populations such as kids, teenagers, men, seniors, athletes, or prenatal
- Equipment-based classes that further distinguish one class from another

Let's take a closer look at what types of classes fall under the four broad categories.

## CARDIO CHOREOGRAPHED AND NONCHOREOGRAPHED

Whether choreographed or nonchoreographed, a cardio class is any workout that has a primary goal of performing large muscle, repetitive movement patterns to place an appropriate stress on the heart and lungs (20). Classes range from 30 to 90 minutes, with 60 and 45 minutes being the most popular lengths (18). Classes have become shorter in the past decade to accommodate busier consumers wanting more time-efficient workouts (22). The length of the class may influence the type and intensity of cardiorespiratory exercise (interval training or steady-state endurance training). A variety of cardio class lengths and types can help address participant preferences. There is more information about this as we further discuss class formatting options.

If equipment is used, it could include but is not limited to step platforms, balance trainers, rebounders, gliding discs, jump ropes, slides, rowers, treadmills, and indoor cycling bikes (18). If no equipment is available, your creativity is key to providing variety for participants, no matter what type of class you teach.

Music choices vary greatly depending on equipment used and type of cardio class. For example, a step class might use continuously mixed, moderate speed music with a strong dance beat, while an indoor cycling class might favor unmixed tracks with varying music styles and speeds.

Choreographed classes are music-driven workouts that build exercise sequences around specific songs. Participants learn predetermined movement routines that may or may not link together from start to finish. An element of coordination and musicality is necessary to be successful, and beginners often find these classes challenging until they have learned the movement patterns. In the past, we have had the luxury of "leveling" classes allowing participants an entry into choreographed classes. However, today, schedules may be jam-packed with class variety. It is hard to find enough schedule space to be able to level your choreographed cardio offerings. Offering a weekly, monthly, or quarterly sampler or introduction class provides a nonintimidating and welcoming way for members to learn vocabulary and movements to ensure a more positive workout experience and successful outcome when joining an ongoing class. You can also arrive early and stay after class to help newcomers. If you know the class will be highly choreographed or intense in nature, it is always best to mark it so.

### Examples of Choreographed Cardio Classes

*Zumba®, Jazzercise®, Cardio Dance*

Nonchoreographed cardio options allow participants to elevate their heart rate without necessarily linking movements together or learning combinations. Although low on mental complexity, nonchoreographed classes may still require coordination. Athletes, nondancers, and those lacking rhythm greatly appreciate these options on the group fitness schedule. The music may be used in the background versus coordinating movements to the music beat. Nonchoreographed classes allow people to more easily meet their specific needs as movements are generally easier to modify than those in a choreographed format. There is not as much need to "level" a nonchoreographed class for skill, though the intensity level may need to be specified.

### Examples of Nonchoreographed Cardio Classes

Indoor cycling, rowing, sports conditioning, treadmill (walk/run), boot camp, freestyle cardio, and most circuit classes.

## STRENGTH

Strength formats can be defined as any workout that has a primary goal of increasing either muscular strength or endurance through progressive resistance exercise (20). Strength training formats are typically structured and preplanned, but not necessarily choreographed to specific music (except for prechoreographed programs such as BodyPump and Group Power programs). The length of a full-body strength training class might range from 40 to 60 minutes. A focused core-training class is commonly 15–30 minutes. Resistance exercises can be linked together resulting in a cardio challenge, or there may be rest periods after each exercise. Your movement selection can be functional, static, dynamic, or anything in between. We discuss these options further in the chapter.

A variety of equipment is available for use in traditional or untraditional strength training formats including, but not limited to, hand weights, barbells, weighted bars (i.e., Versa Bars or BodyBars), suspension trainers, resistance tubing (covered or uncovered), gliding discs, soft weighted fitness balls, medicine balls, balance trainers, ballast balls, stability balls, and step platforms. When no equipment is available, bodyweight and/or partner exercises form the basis of a strength training class. Music can help you pace the speed of an exercise for safety and effectiveness. It can help you keep count of repetitions and/or help you be aware of the amount of time a muscle group is under tension, as discussed shortly in the music section. Alternatively, music may be in the background only to help energize your class.

### Class Design Options

- Rotating circuit (performing specific exercises at consecutively arranged stations around the room)
- Unison circuit (one station throughout class with equipment specific to the participant)
- Partner training (teamed up for anchoring solutions or sharing of equipment).
- Focus/emphasis can include the following:
  - One or several specific muscle groups
  - Opposing muscle groups
  - A selected region of the body (upper or lower body strengthening)
  - Functional movements
  - A balance challenge

## COMBINATION CARDIO AND STRENGTH

Since more participants understand the benefits of resistance exercise, cardio and strength combination classes continue to grow in popularity (18). The goal of a cardio and strength combination class is to elevate the heart rate and increase muscular strength or endurance. You can incorporate the same equipment described above in a class that is 30–90 minutes in length. Numerous possibilities exist for combining strength and cardio using a circuit format. For example, a circuit with a 3:1 ratio has 3 minutes of cardio followed by 1 minute of strength to complete one cycle. Repeating the cycle ten times allows ten strength exercises interspersed between cardio segments for an efficient 40-minute cardio/strength workout segment. Using a 2:2 ratio will equally split the time spent on cardio and strength exercises. In these examples, you will want to avoid long or complex combinations for cardio training due to time considerations. Another example is a 20/20 format, with 20 minutes of cardio followed by 20 minutes of strength. With this type of format, the cardio segment can be choreographed to music or you can keep movements straightforward, similar to a nonchoreographed format.

When a class does not seem to fall into one of the four broad categories, it is usually referred to as a "specialty" class perhaps focusing on flexibility, mind-body, or sports skill development. Being able to categorize each of your classes in this manner encourages participants to cross train and helps them make smart choices for their fitness needs. It also helps you to make smart choices about the moves that you choose, the equipment that you use, the cues you deliver, and the motivational environment you create. Each choice made, whether in planning or delivery, must relate back to the overarching class theme or objective to provide safe, effective, and predictable experiences for each person.

Before we break down each category and discuss how classes are designed and delivered, we review universal class design concepts including music, environmental considerations, equipment, ideas for sourcing new moves, and general cueing techniques to help instruct and build your group fitness classes.

# ELEMENTS OF UNIVERSAL CLASS DESIGN AND DELIVERY

## MUSIC MATTERS

Music is a major component of many group fitness classes. Different classes utilize different kinds of music (4). Latin and hip-hop are common in dance-oriented fitness classes. Pilates and yoga favor new age, smooth jazz, chill, and trance. Cardio classes gravitate toward club and top 40 music with strong rhythms. You will find a mixture of music styles for cycling and water fitness programs. No matter what class you teach, if you are not excited about your music, it is hard to get others excited about it. It is important to use music that you enjoy, yet it is more important that participants enjoy the music. Appreciating a wide range of music styles is beneficial as an instructor. The more variety in your music, the more people you attract to your classes. Additionally, when you have a substantial library of songs to begin with, you are less likely to become burned-out on your music. Experiencing other classes is one way to start expanding your musical horizons. Being open to music suggestions from class members is another possibility. Solicit participants for recommendations. Periodically, someone brings in a song that instantly becomes a new class favorite.

Though different classes will incorporate diverse musical styles, there are two distinctly different ways music is actually utilized for exercise. In one approach, music takes on a minor, secondary role in class, contrary to another approach in which music functions in a primary role.

### Music and Exercise: Incidental Role

Music can function in an incidental role as a background audio soundtrack for exercise. When utilized in this manner, it does not mean you can play any type of music you like in class. Even when utilized just in the background, music needs to supply an appropriate energy to support your participant's efforts. Never allow music to be an afterthought. Music should be well planned and carefully chosen to complement the workout and facilitate class objectives. Exercises are not necessarily performed to the music beat; rather, music creates a desired ambiance that allows participants to exercise at a self-selected pace and level. Therefore, it is not critical if the music has a consistent rhythm and evenly phrased counts. You also may find group cohesion is less evident as your class is not always moving in unison. Pilates, yoga, stretch, boot camps, circuit training, sports conditioning, water exercise, indoor cycling, and other machine-based and equipment-based classes frequently use music in this manner.

### Music and Exercise: Prominent Role

The second approach in which music can function is markedly different. Music comes out of the background and moves into the foreground. No longer secondary, it is a primary ingredient of class design. It is prominent. It influences your selection of exercises. It shapes your style of movement. It is beat driven. The rhythm sets the movement cadence or speed. The class moves in unison to the music cadence. Music now has a substantial role in class content and for motivating participants. For many participants, music will make or break their workout. Nowhere is this most apparent than in the cardiovascular section of a class.

There are three methods to maximize music's potential for a class. These methods are also referred to as choreographic styles or choreographic techniques. All three methods share a common characteristic — physical movements are coordinated to match musical cadence — the music speed dictates the movement speed. The other characteristics that define how music is integrated into a class are based upon the attributes of either song structure or rhythm structure.

### Song Structure

In addition to exercise matching the music beat, changes in exercises or movements are coordinated to changes in song structure (verse, chorus, break, etc.). This is known as choreographed exercise. Movements are choreographed or dependent upon the overall structure of each song. With choreographed exercise, music selection always comes first. Once you have chosen your music, you create and build exercise sequences that are specific for each song. This method capitalizes on the popularity of music, based upon the cultural phenomenon that many people find exercise to be more enjoyable when performed to popular songs that are familiar to them.

### 8-Count Rhythm Structure

In addition to performing movements at the same speed of the music, movements or exercises are designed and performed in sets of 8 counts or 8 repetitions, or in a multiple of 8 counts (2, 4, 16, or 32). This choreographic method, known as freestyle, evolved because most popular dance-oriented music is produced or structured in groups of eight music beats or counts throughout the song (more on this in the "Music Count Organization" section). With this method, exercise selection becomes equal to music selection in terms of priority — you can select your music first and create cardio sequences, or you can create cardio movements first and simply choose music with 8-count phrasing to fit the movements.

### 32-Count Rhythm Structure

In addition to exercise and music cadence corresponding, four 8-count movement patterns are combined to form a longer 32-count combination. The combination is generally repeated several times either continuously or in conjunction with other combinations throughout the workout. This is referred to as the 32-count combination or 32-count choreography method. With this method, the cardio combinations come first. You create your combinations, and then you select music to your liking that is phrased evenly in 32 counts to fit your choreography. (Each of these methods is explored further in the chapter.)

What is notable is the outcome you receive from incorporating music in any of these three methods. A dynamic synergy results when exercises synchronize with both music tempo and rhythm structure (8-count or 32-count) or song structure. If there is an art to teaching group fitness classes, this is certainly part of it — the fusion of music and movement. It is a little bit of magic and a whole lot of joy. It is a key feature that distinguishes the group fitness experience from solo exercise. It is what makes group fitness classes unique, energizing, motivating, and fun for millions of people.

Whether used in a secondary or primary capacity, music should work harmoniously with the selected exercise tasks. Effective music choices will help promote the proper movement quality and elicit appropriate energy from participants. Developing a good ear for music is essential for developing your potential as a group fitness instructor.

### Music Research Implications

There is a growing body of research that demonstrates various elements of music such as tempo, type, and loudness do have physiological effects on perceived exertion, heart rate, endurance time, and other measures (10,21). Most studies have looked at music's effects while exercising on cardiovascular equipment (5,9,10,21). Although the findings could be extrapolated to group exercise, we do not know if music's effects in group fitness classes are similar to equipment-based workouts. On cardiovascular equipment, you can control for the biomechanical stimuli (walk on treadmill, pedal on bike, etc.). The locomotor movement does not change. Group fitness uses numerous locomotor movements, making it quite complex to design a study on music's effect on exercise in a group setting.

One element that influences music selection is content. Some tracks may be controversial due to the subject matter or explicit lyrics. Be aware of the content or messages in your music choices. Determine if anything is derogatory or would be disturbing to an individual or group. Visual images associated with music are also a consideration, since new song releases have a corresponding video clip. Avoid music that would offend or alienate participants by screening your selections before using them in class. You want music to create a positive environment, not a disconcerting one. Music that induces positive affect and promotes enjoyment is likely to increase exercise adherence levels (21).

Karageorghis proposes four factors contribute to the motivational qualities of music for sport and exercise (10):

1. Rhythm (music tempo or speed)
2. Musicality (melody, orchestration, lyrics, song structure)
3. Cultural influences (pervasiveness of the music in your region, socioeconomic background)
4. Association (emotional response a piece of music may evoke)

Music tempo seems to be a significant determinant of musical response on cardiovascular equipment like treadmills or indoor bikes (5). Fast tempo and strong rhythms may be linked to physiological arousal. As intensity increases, there will be stronger preferences for fast tempo music (9). This preference is logical, since there are some established relationships between speed and intensity (i.e., as running speed increases, intensity increases). Although some studies extol the virtues of fast music tempo during repetitive exercise, it is currently not known whether continual exposure to such music results in negative affective responses, such as boredom and irritation. Hence, to maximize affective responses to music, variation in music tempo can be an option in cardio formats. This may be novel to some instructors as most premade music downloads and CDs for cardio classes are produced with minimal tempo variation.

Women exhibit a stronger preference than men for the rhythmical qualities of music. Because of greater exposure to dance and movement-to-music, women may show a preference for music with a tempo linked to their exercise intensity (9). This preference may be reinforced just by attending exercise-to-music classes where cardiovascular intensity and music tempo are commonly associated with each other. However, not all fitness classes show this association. Hip-hop classes as an example, frequently use down-tempo music, yet with anecdotal reports of perceived exertion ratings comparable to up-tempo cardio classes. Movement selection observably, is as much a factor influencing cardiovascular intensity as music tempo.

It is important to consider music with reference to participants' preferences and sociocultural background (10). It appears that music popular during one's formative years is likely to be a favored music style throughout the life span. If you grew up in the 1930s and 1940s, Benny Goodman's big band sound and Duke Ellington's swing styles and bluesy ballads are likely still a favorite listening. If your teenage years were in the 1950s and 1960s, the rock 'n roll of Elvis Presley or the soul of Aretha Franklin may continue to rock your world. "Saturday Night Fever" became the biggest selling album ever in the mid-1970s, and disco fever is still here today but under names like techno, rap, house, and Euro. Older adults of today gravitate toward the softer and more melodic jazz and pop music from the era when they were young adults (15).

If the past is any indication of the future, hold onto your hip-hop, rap, and mash-up downloads, playlists, and CDs. It will be your senior music 40 years from now.

### Tempo: Counting Counts

Hearing the rhythm and identifying the count is fundamental in order to coordinate physical movement to music. If this does not come naturally to you, it can be learned, but it will require a diligent effort to acquire this skill. The regular accent or pulse you hear in a rhythmic song is a music beat. Just like counting a pulse for 1 minute to determine heart rate, counting music beats for 1 minute determines music rate, or tempo. Tempo is expressed as beats per minute or bpm, rather than terms like "slow" or "fast" which are subject to individual interpretation. For example, music that is 120 bpm is both slow and fast dependent on its use relative to physical movement. It is very slow for high-impact cardio moves, yet 120 bpm may be too fast for some strength exercises. General music tempo guidelines for various class formats are shown in Table 5.1.

### Music Count Organization

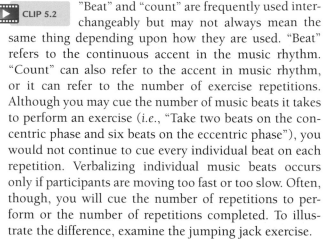 Every 4 music beats or counts is called a measure. Two measures (8 counts) are known as a bar of music. Four bars (8 measures) comprise a 32-count phrase or block of music (see Table 5.2). The term 32-count phrasing identifies a consistent, even number of beats or counts in a piece of music. Music with 32-count phrasing has a steady and predictable rhythm without any extra beats, measures, or bars. Most (though not all) dance-oriented music heard on radio, in clubs, or through the Internet is produced in this configuration.

As you listen closely to music, you will notice that in most songs, every other music beat has a stronger feel or accent to it. This is identified as the downbeat, and downbeats occur on the odd-numbered music beats [1, 3, 5, etc.]. Even-numbered beats [2, 4, 6, 8] usually have a lighter accent and are called upbeats. An exercise or movement should start on the first downbeat (count "one") of a bar or phrase of music. You locate this starting point

by the distinctly stronger emphasis on the first downbeat of a musical bar or phrase. This is a critical first step to matching physical movements to music.

### Differentiating the Beat and the Count

CLIP 5.2    "Beat" and "count" are frequently used interchangeably but may not always mean the same thing depending upon how they are used. "Beat" refers to the continuous accent in the music rhythm. "Count" can also refer to the accent in music rhythm, or it can refer to the number of exercise repetitions. Although you may cue the number of music beats it takes to perform an exercise (*i.e.*, "Take two beats on the concentric phase and six beats on the eccentric phase"), you would not continue to cue every individual beat on each repetition. Verbalizing individual music beats occurs only if participants are moving too fast or too slow. Often, though, you will cue the number of repetitions to perform or the number of repetitions completed. To illustrate the difference, examine the jumping jack exercise.

A jumping jack requires two music beats to perform — jump out on the first beat and jump in on the second beat. You cue the completed jack as count "one" (not "count one, two"). The next completed jumping jack is cued as "two" (not "three, four"). In other words, the counts occur on every other musical beat, not on every beat. If you perform eight jumping jacks, it takes 16 music beats to complete the task, as each jack uses 2 beats of music. If you cued every "beat" as a "count," you would do only four jumping jacks (jump out 1, jump in 2, jump out 3, jump in 4, etc.) (Box 5.1).

### 32-Count Structure

Most pop songs have a similar music structure. There is an opening (usually instrumental), a central part (often vocal), and an ending. The 32-count structure neatly fits into the formation of a musical track. A song might use a 32-count phrase as the opening, have two 32-count blocks for the verse, a 32-count phrase for the chorus, and so on. "Jingle Bells" (see Box 5.2) is an example of a song with a 32-count structure. Note that every other

| Table 5.1 | MUSIC TEMPO GUIDELINES |
| --- | --- |
| **EXERCISE CLASS** | **BPM** |
| Indoor cycling | 60–110 |
| High-impact | 135–155 |
| Low-impact | 120–140 |
| Step training | 118–128 |
| Kickboxing | 126–136 |
| Yoga/Pilates | <110–120 |
| Hip-hop | 90–120 |
| Latin | 110–140 |

| Table 5.2 | MUSIC COUNT ORGANIZATION | | |
| --- | --- | --- | --- |
| 4 counts/1st measure | 1st bar | |
| 4 counts/2nd measure | | |
| 4 counts/3rd measure | 2nd bar | 32-count phrase or 32-count block |
| 4 counts/4th measure | | |
| 4 counts/5th measure | 3rd bar | |
| 4 counts/6th measure | | |
| 4 counts/7th measure | 4th bar | |
| 4 counts/8th measure | | |

**BOX 5.1** Counting Counts or Beats?

When you instruct your class to do 8 counts of squats, does it mean to squat for 8 music beats or to do 8 repetitions of squats? If 8 counts refers to music beats, you have to decide the exercise execution speed to know how many repetitions to perform. For example, you can squat down in 1 beat, come up in 1 beat stopping after you hit the 8th beat, resulting in 4 repetitions. Alternatively, taking 2 beats to squat down and 2 beats to come up would result in 2 repetitions. On the other hand, use 4 beats down and 4 beats to come up for 1 completed repetition.

If 8 counts refers to 8 repetitions, you use 16 music beats when you perform the exercise at a pace of 1 beat down and 1 beat up. If your pace is 2 beats down and 2 beats up, it takes 32 music beats. If the pace is 4 beats down and 4 beats up, it takes 64 music beats to complete the task.

Every count is always a music beat, but every music beat is not always a count. To avoid confusion whenever you give a numerical cue, clearly communicate if you are cueing music beats, music counts (may or may not be the same as beats), or repetitions.

beat is [labeled] a count. Although there are 32 "counts" in the chorus of "Jingle Bells," the number of "beats" is 64, an example illustrating the distinction between beats and counts.

### Using 32-Count Music

Evenly phrased music can help you balance movements and exercises to incorporate both sides of the body symmetrically. It can help track the number of repetitions you do, allowing you to better observe and teach the class members. For example, you decide an exercise will use 8 music beats per repetition with a goal of performing 12 repetitions. Rather than count repetitions, you can count music phrases (32-count). With 4 repetitions per 32-count phrase, you complete 12 repetitions at the end of the third phrase. It is easier to keep track of 3 items (music phrases) than 12 items (repetitions).

Step classes benefit with 32-count music because most step patterns are 4 counts or a multiple of 4 counts to execute, making it convenient for synchronizing to 32-count music. High/low cardio classes often rely on 32-count music, building 32-count combinations to fit seamlessly into the music structure. Not all classes or class segments need evenly phrased music — indoor cycling, water exercise, boot camps, circuit training, Pilates, yoga, stretching, and sports conditioning formats usually accommodate music with extra bars, measures, or the odd extra beat that sometimes occurs in a favorite tune. With

**BOX 5.2** "Jingle Bells" 32-Count Rhythm Structure

(1st 8 counts/1st bar/1st and 2nd measures)

1    2    3    4    5    6 7    8

Jingle Bells Jingle Bells Jingle All The Way

(2nd 8 counts/2nd bar/3rd and 4th measures)

1    2    3    4    5    6    7 8

Oh What Fun It Is To Ride In A One Horse Open Sleigh

(3rd 8 counts/3rd bar/5th & 6th measures)

1    2    3    4    5    6 7    8

Jingle Bells Jingle Bells Jingle All The Way

(4th 8 counts/4th bar/7th and 8th measures)

1    2    3    4    5    6    7 8

Oh What Fun It Is To Ride In A One-Horse Open Sleigh

(Total: 32 counts)

these types of workouts, you have a wider range of music possibilities. You want to have 32-count music when your class design incorporates 32-count choreography.

### Working on the Music Phrase

Though evenly phrased music allows you to match blocks of movement easily into the music structure, you must know the music count in order to "time" your exercises to that structure. You could be off the music count without knowing it when teaching a class. Participants sense when exercise does not correspond to the music. The exercise will not feel right because it is a few beats behind or in front of the music count. Participants respond positively when a series of movements start and end when a music phrase starts and ends. How do you find the beginning of a music phrase? It is characterized by one or more of the following clues:

- A stronger or more powerful accent
- A melodic line begins (or ends)
- Change in orchestration (new instrument sound)
- Change or emphasis in music structure (verse, chorus)
- A big cymbal sound or other percussive sound
- A building crescendo that peaks on the first count of the music phrase

Starting a movement sequence at the start of a 32-count phrase synchronizes movement to music. Your class feels a stronger connection to the music, and that helps to connect better to the exercise. Most participants know when you arbitrarily or inadvertently start an exercise irrespective of the music count. For some, it becomes an irritation when movement and music counts do not match, particularly if it continues for an extended period.

### We've Got the Beat

 CLIP 5.3    You can develop the ability to hear the rhythm in a song, locate the phrases, and identify the counts. Start by listening and identifying the 8-count music bars whenever you listen to a song. Next, locate the 32-count phrases. Ask a friend to let you know whether you are on or off the correct count. Once you can identify 8-count bars and 32-count phrases, begin to practice talking over the music without losing the musical count. This may be one of your bigger challenges as an instructor; to simultaneously provide verbal instruction, track the number of repetitions performed, and match your movements to the music count. Your multitasking abilities are put to the test here.

The minimum musicality essentials are

1. With nonchoreographed cardio formats, be competent in identifying 8-count music bars.
2. In choreographed cardio formats, be proficient in recognizing song structure (verse, chorus, breaks, etc.)

to determine appropriate movements and when to transition to another movement.
3. For 32-count choreography cardio formats, be capable of hearing the 32-count phrase in order to match it to 32-count combinations..

It enhances the workout experience and participant's enjoyment when exercises and movements match your music to a "T"!

> **✔ RECOMMENDED RESOURCES:** *Fitness Music Companies*
>
> *The following companies have music CDs formatted for various fitness classes. They also have exercise videos/DVDs and other associated products.*
>     AeroBeat
>     **www.aerobeat.com**
>     *Burntrax*
>     **www.burntrax.com**
>     *Dynamix*
>     **www.dynamixmusic.com**
>     *Muscle Mixes*
>     **www.musclemixes.com**
>     *Power Music*
>     **www.workoutmusic.com**

### Environment

As a professional group exercise instructor, you may find yourself teaching in less than professional settings; a conference room that doubles as a group fitness room, or a racquetball court that never transitioned into a state-of-the-art studio. Environmental consideration is a two-step process.

1. Assess the exercise area for obstacles, constraints, limitations, sight lines, acoustics, ventilation, and flooring.
2. Adapt your class for safety and effectiveness within the parameters of the environment.

Attention to the following elements help ensure the comfort and safety of participants, no matter where your class is located.

*Floor.* If flooring is a nonresilient surface (*i.e.*, linoleum or carpet on top of concrete), it is a good idea to avoid high-impact activity. Without any "give" in the floor, you subject participants to unnecessarily high impact forces on joints. Almost all high-impact movements have a low-impact alternative. Mode is sometimes mistaken for intensity where some participants think high impact is high intensity and low impact is low intensity. Impact refers to exercise mode, not exercise intensity. You can have a high-intensity, low-impact workout. A low-impact workout is always the best choice without optimal flooring.

*Carpeting.* Use discretion with lateral movements when teaching on a carpeted surface. Shoes can get caught on carpeting while moving laterally. For example, modify grapevines or lateral shuffle steps by turning sideways and walking toward the side of the room. Most turns are difficult to execute on carpet, including pivot turns. Instead of pivoting as some kickboxing movements require, pick up the foot and place it down to help protect the knee.

*Obstacles.* Are there pillars, columns, or other physical obstructions in the room? Prepare for this by positioning individuals where it will least interfere with their workout. Determine if any of your planned movements cannot be executed safely. Modify any exercise or choreography where someone could risk running or bumping into an obstacle.

*Room.* Is class crowded? A buffer zone may form around you, creating distance between you and participants. Yet, there is valuable workout room to utilize. Encourage participants to fill in the empty spaces to give everyone a bit more room for comfort and safety. When the class is small, encourage people to come closer to you, making the class more intimate and personal. There is no reason to have to vocalize as if the room was at capacity when there are a handful of participants. Make it comfortable for everyone, including yourself.

*Movement Selection.* When your room is filled to capacity, you may not be able to do any traveling patterns due to lack of space. In this case, you have an "on-the-spot" cardio class. What you can do for variety is change orientations by regularly facing different walls. Interestingly, when the same movements are performed facing another direction, some participants perceive the change as new exercises. Just a change in orientation can make an exercise feel quite different. For intensity options, incorporate frequent changes in the center of gravity.

*Acoustics.* It is a big room filled with people, no microphone, and poor acoustics. In these circumstances, you have to keep music volume low. It is more important for people to hear you, not the music. You can turn the music volume up for a few moments when repeating movement patterns already learned. To be better heard and understood, face your class. Remember to "mirror" your class anytime you are facing them. Periodically move yourself to each wall, making each wall the front of the room. This gives everyone the opportunity to hear you and see you with greater ease for part of the class time. Another technique is to split the room into two halves — one group facing the other group; you stand near front and center. Have the groups mirror each other for cardio movements. For prone and supine position exercises, position yourself in the center of the room. In supine or prone positions, more people can see and hear you when you are in the center compared to when you are at the front of the room.

## Equipment

Product manufacturers along with fitness professionals create a wide variety of equipment to enhance the exercise experience and broaden class options. Equipment can be a minor or a major component within your class. For example, you might use stability balls for a specific class segment like core training. On another day, you might utilize stability balls for the entire class time, from warm-up through cool-down. Choosing equipment is based upon your inventory, your participant's abilities and preferences, and the versatility of the product. Equipment commonly outfitting group fitness studios includes the following:

*Step Platforms* (Fig. 5.1). Step platforms are the most popular product in the group fitness market. They are versatile and can be used for cardio and strength classes. For cardiovascular training, the platforms are used for stepping up and down in varying patterns and/or at varying heights. Sports conditioning and athletic-based classes use the platforms for cardiovascular, strength, plyometric, and agility training. In strength classes, the step is used as a bench, much as you would use in a weight room for both upper and lower body conditioning. Nearly every class you teach has the potential to make use of this group fitness staple.

*Balance Trainers* (Fig. 5.2). Like the step platform, balance trainers are extremely versatile and used for advancing cardiovascular and strength exercises as they incorporate the element of balance. These are effective tools for core conditioning and balance training. Mind/body classes can incorporate the balance trainers as well. You must thoughtfully introduce this style of training in your classes. Without proper instruction and safety cues, the potential for injury escalates due to the unstable nature of these products.

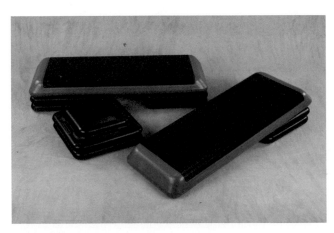

■ **FIGURE 5.1** Step platforms.

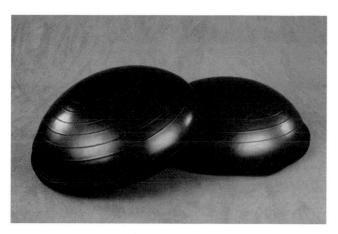

■ **FIGURE 5.2** Balance trainers.

Most participants successfully use the product when you provide thorough directions and select appropriate exercises for your participant's skill level.

*Gliding Discs* (Fig. 5.3). Gliding discs bring a dynamic element to many exercises, providing variety and a greater challenge as a participant's fitness level increases. The discs are placed under the hands and/or feet to increase muscle recruitment by creating a stability challenge. They allow you to create unique exercise sequences and movement patterns. Some common uses for the discs include performing squats, lunges and pushups to add intensity by recruiting many stabilizer muscles. The discs are also used for core work (crunches, planks) and flexibility exercises.

*Weighted Bars* (Fig. 5.4). Weighted bars, such as the BodyBar or VersaBar, are tools for strength training classes. The distribution of weight evenly across the bar allows instructors to create new conditioning exercises involving rotation, twisting, and bending, while classic barbell exercises are readily available (biceps curls, chest press, etc.). The bar is used for bilateral exercises (two arms) or unilateral exercises (single arm). An additional benefit — use the product on end as a balance aid (*i.e.*, holding the bar while practicing a lunge).

*Dumbbells* (Fig. 5.5). Dumbbells are a staple for strength training exercises. Familiarity with the product allows clients to feel successful immediately. Dumbbells are perfect for traditional strength training exercises and can be used in conjunction with steps, balance trainers, stability balls, and ballast balls. A weight range of 1–15 lb allows members the ability to progress. In the group exercise setting, heavier weights may not be feasible or available en masse, which might present a problem when trying to overload larger muscles like the legs, back, and chest. Creative exercise sequencing helps to address this issue.

*Elastic Bands and Tubing* (Fig. 5.6). Elastic bands and tubing have been around nearly as long as dumbbells and are extremely versatile for strength training. One advantage is the ability to quickly increase or decrease the intensity of an exercise without needing to change equipment or look different from anyone else in the classroom. Strength exercises performed with elastic bands or tubing allow you to focus on the eccentric phase of an exercise. Bands and tubing allows you to target the posterior torso area in an upright rather than prone position, a real plus for individuals who have orthopedic/medical issues that make prone-positioned exercises difficult to perform.

*Barbells* (Fig 5.7). A weight room staple, barbells started showing up in workout studios when exercisers

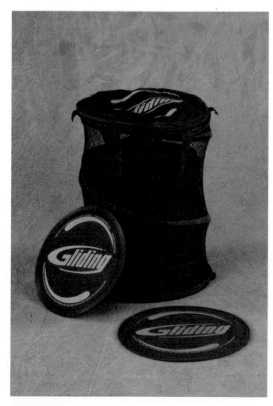

■ **FIGURE 5.3** Gliding discs.

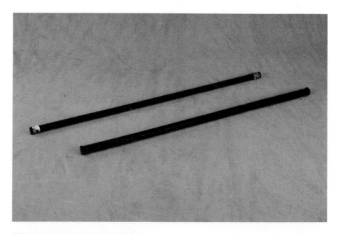

■ **FIGURE 5.4** Weighted bars.

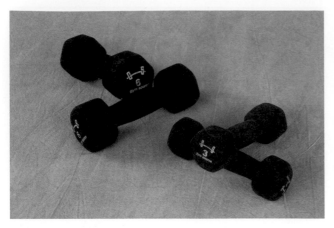

■ **FIGURE 5.5** Dumbbells.

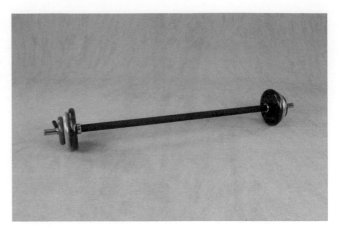

■ **FIGURE 5.7** Barbells.

discovered the motivation inherent in performing resistance training in a group with music. The advantage of a barbell is the ease with which you can adjust the load for a given exercise. With one bar per student, and multiple weights for each bar, the space and time constraints presented by other fitness equipment is minimized. The limited number of exercises, due to the restriction of performing only bilateral exercises, is a drawback.

*Stability Ball* (Fig. 5.8). The stability ball is a popular and effective tool from the physical therapy field that benefits a wide range of populations, from athletes to seniors (14). Available in a variety of sizes to accommodate people of different heights, the ball acts as a bench for strength exercises or as an apparatus for core training by enhancing abdominal and low back exercises. The unstable nature of the ball makes it valuable for balance and spinal stability training (6). The ball offers a number of new stretching exercises, and creative instructors will incorporate the ball into their cardio segments (16).

*Medicine Ball* (Fig. 5.9). Previously utilized in personal and small group training, the medicine ball has made

its way into the group fitness studio. Medicine balls are about the size of a basketball, but weigh much more than basketballs making them a great accessory in strength and core conditioning classes. Storage for stability and medicine balls and choosing appropriate sizes is a consideration, but providing just a few for circuit classes is a great idea.

*Suspension Trainers.* The suspension trainer introduced a new way of thinking about vertical core training alongside bodyweight leverage training. While still primarily used in personal training and small group settings, more facilities are investing in the hardware to outfit a studio with suspension trainers to enhance group fitness programming. Like tubing, the advantage of body weight leverage training is the ease and quickness in changing intensity by small changes in body positioning. Additionally, changing exercises is simple. Stability, balance, and core are challenged on almost every exercise, which makes for an efficient workout.

*Kettlebells* (Fig. 5.10). Another personal training piece crossing over to group exercise is the kettlebell. It is produced in various sizes accommodating the diverse

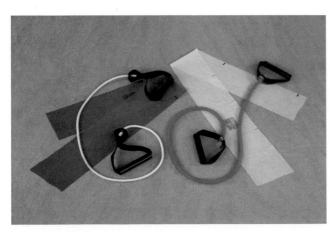

■ **FIGURE 5.6** Elastic bands and tubing.

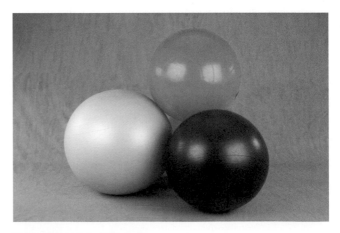

■ **FIGURE 5.8** Stability balls.

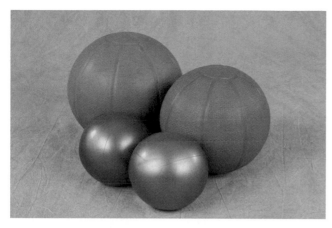

■ **FIGURE 5.9** Medicine balls.

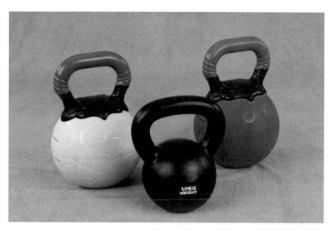

■ **FIGURE 5.10** Kettlebells.

participants in a group exercise setting. The kettlebell can mimic strength exercises that you do with weighted bars and dumbbells, or you can experiment with more traditional kettlebell moves including the swing, clean and press, and windmill. Kettlebells make an ideal addition to a circuit training or small group training environment.

Group Fitness equipment can be purchased through the same channels as personal training equipment. Resources for group fitness equipment are listed in the Recommended Resources box, below.

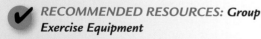

> ✔ **RECOMMENDED RESOURCES: Group Exercise Equipment**
>
> *Perform Better*
> *www.performbetter.com*
> *Power Systems*
> *www.power-systems.com*
> *Spri Products, Inc.*
> *www.spri.com*

## Movement Choices

Each type of class will have its own movements to help you achieve the overall goal of the workout. The list below is not an all-inclusive list but merely a jumpstart to building your choreographic library.

Additional movement ideas come from the numerous commercial exercise DVDs led by reputable instructors. Check your local library for recent additions to their collection. Cable television may have a fitness channel or exercise programming that you can watch on demand. Although a lack of screening protocol means quality can range from the mundane to the profoundly creative, youtube.com (and similar networks) is a resource that instructors draw on to share ideas. When possible, observe other classes in your area and when you travel. Give some brief feedback to the instructor, sharing a few things you liked about the class. Invite him/her to do the same for you. You build a creative network by sharing ideas with other fitness professionals. Lastly, step out of your box and try new activities to jostle your creativity.

- *Dance*: ballet, modern, jazz, tap, folk, social, ballroom, line dancing, street/hip-hop
- *Mind-Body*: yoga, martial arts, bodywork methods like Feldenkrais or Alexander techniques
- *Sports*: observe basketball, soccer, and football drills; track and field warm-ups; tennis drills
- *School*: physical education classes, kids' games, theatrical games, cheerleading drills

Dance training allows you to experience different ways the body can move and travel through space. Jazz dance helps develop movement style; steps and routines learned will help you create cardio combinations. Salsa and Latin dance deliver new moves to segue into dance-flavored cardio segments. Ballet improves posture, alignment, and positioning, enhancing body awareness and how you carry yourself. Line dancing and folk dancing have movement patterns readily adaptable for cardio training.

Turn to sports, especially athletic training drills, for movement and exercise concepts to incorporate into nonchoreographed cardio classes. Even children's interactive games (Gymboree and other programs) have been streamlined into adult classes. Stepping out of your comfort zone and experiencing new physical activities is one of the best ways to get your creative juices flowing. It is enlightening to discover a ballet pas de bourrée, a hip-hop break step, and a ballroom waltz step are essentially the same step. The style simply differs.

## Cueing

In most cardio classes, it is important to get everyone moving in the same direction at the same time to keep the workout safe and motivating. Regardless of the class format, you make this happen with universal cueing strategies. The ability to cue effectively is essential for a successful exercise experience for participants. There are three general cueing categories: movement, safety/technique, and motivation.

### Movement Cues

Have you ever driven along on a road and had to suddenly hit the brakes because another car cut in front of you? There was no warning, no signal, and the driver did not even check to see if it was safe to change lanes. Similar experiences can occur in group fitness classes, and it is just as annoying and dangerous in a class as it is on a road. In a class setting, you are the driver (instructor), hopefully with better driving skills (movement cues) than the person who cut you off on the road! Just like driving, participants need clear, concise movement cues (signals) to be able to follow your directions (road map) and arrive safely (smooth transitions) at your destination (the next exercise).

Movement cues are instructions on what to do and when to do it. You describe the task to perform and give signals, or cues, to indicate when the task will start, stop, or change (2). Explain the action, body parts involved, and direction of movement. You convey this information so participants can prepare for what is going to happen next.

*"Get ready to change the stationary squat."* (cueing which body part will be changing)

*"We will change to a lateral squat."* (cueing what action the body part will be doing)

*"You will be moving side to side, starting right."* (cueing what direction you move)

As you become more adept at cueing, the three pieces above become one succinct cue. For example:

*"Get ready to change to a lateral squat moving side to side; let's go right."*

Cueing helps participants follow you with greater ease and more confidence and facilitates both the learning and performing of exercises (21). The driver who cut in front of you almost caused an accident because there was no signal when changing lanes. When there is an inadequate signal to change exercises, participants experience a similar knee-jerk reaction. Movement cues come before a change happens, not during the change. Cueing 4 to 8 counts prior to the next movement generally allows adequate time to process the information. Properly timed cues remove the "speed bumps" when changing from one movement to the next, facilitating a smooth transition from exercise to exercise. Participants feel lost and frustrated when movement cues are insufficient, poorly timed, or lacking altogether.

Along with verbal movement cues, visual cues and visual previews are part of the signaling system.

### Visual Cue

 CLIP 5.4    Visual cues are hand signals used to enhance communication to your class (Fig. 5.11). For

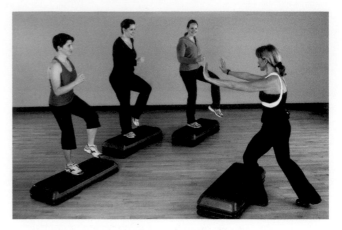

■ **FIGURE 5.11** Hand signal used as a visual cue.

example, pointing right will help your class see which way to move. Holding your hand up can signal to hold or stop. Your fingers can designate the number of repetitions left to perform. Circling your arm above means walk around the room. A small chopping motion with hands in front of you delineates to march or jog in place. The palm of your hand on top of your head means to start again or repeat from the beginning ("take it from the top").

CLIP 5.5    A visual preview is a demonstration of the next movement or exercise. Have your class continue doing the current exercise and explain, "Stay with this exercise, and please watch what you are going to do next." You would then demonstrate the next movement. Visual previews are advantageous when introducing an exercise for the first time and for teaching more complex movements. Emphasize to observe you (not join you), when giving a visual preview. After one or two demonstrations, cue to start the next exercise upon finishing the current one. You increase participant success when the participants can see what they are going to do before doing it. Visual previews ensure better understanding of the next task and should be used as often as needed.

### Safety and Technique Cues

You promote safe and effective exercise by providing safety and technique cues. These cues, both verbal and visual, focus on body awareness by addressing alignment, positioning, breathing, and appropriate technique while performing an exercise. As an example, the movement cue for a squat is to bend at the hips, knees, and ankles. A technique cue might be, "Keep the chest up during the squat." Alternatively, you can give the same cue visually by demonstrating the squat and exaggerating the chest lifted while tapping on your chest.

It is best to show and explain what you want to happen versus what you don't want to happen. To appreciate the rationale, try this experiment: tell someone at home, "Don't look in the refrigerator." What do they want to do? With a cue such as, "Don't drop the chest during the squat," participants have to process "drop the chest" and then put an "X" through it in their mind. This can take several seconds longer and might actually cause the reverse to occur due to the power of suggestion (8). You create a truly positive, motivating class by eliminating the word "don't" from any safety or technique cue. In its place, simply ask for what you do want, such as, "I want you to keep your chest lifted," or, "Be aware of your torso position as you squat."

You should be genuinely interested in helping your participants. When delivering safety and technique cues, you provide feedback to your participants. There are five methods to deliver feedback in a group setting:

1. *General Feedback.* Providing general feedback addresses the entire group with a blanket statement. This is the first level of feedback because it allows those making mistakes to remain anonymous and can potentially correct the problem without drawing attention to an individual. For example, you could say, "I'd like you to keep the weight in your heels on these next few squats."
2. *Indirect Feedback.* Adding body language to feedback allows you to be a bit more specific with the subject of your feedback without verbally identifying or physically walking over to the participant. Through eye contact and your body placement, try to gain the individual's attention and then give the general feedback statement. Using the example from above, you could turn to face the person who is allowing the weight to shift into the front of the foot, lock eyes with him/her, point to your heels, and restate the same cue.
3. *Direct Feedback.* When you address a person by name or point or walk over to a participant, you are using direct feedback. While sometimes the easiest of the five methods (to get a response or correct a mistake), it is used as a last resort if you are concerned for someone's safety at that moment. However, you do not want to unknowingly intimidate a person by correcting him/her when the individual is already concerned that his/her noble attempts will be met with criticism from the teacher in front of his/her peers. When appropriate, gentle humor can lighten the moment when using general, indirect, or direct feedback. Be sure your participants do not misinterpret your humor for laughing at them (18).
4. *Tactile Feedback* (Fig. 5.12). This method is most practical to do in smaller classes although it can be done in any class. It is commonly used in yoga, Pilates, and other mind-body programs. Using a hands-on approach, you passively place a student's limb in a precise position, move a joint through a desired range of motion (ROM), or guide a body part through a specific pattern of movement. You could lightly touch the area of focus to clearly identify the muscle groups to engage or relax. Concurrently, explain where to feel it, how to feel it, and what to

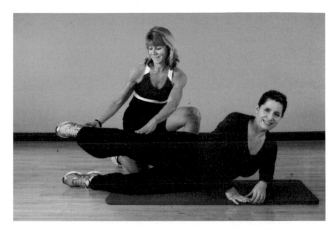

■ **FIGURE 5.12** Tactile feedback.

do if they cannot feel it. A caveat — use discretion with tactile instruction. Although some people learn best with kinesthetic approaches, it is not appropriate all the time or for all participants. Once you know class members individually, you can determine the best feedback technique to use. Always respect your participants' personal space, and never assume you have the right to touch any person. You do not want a participant to respond negatively and pull back from you. Avoid this by asking permission before doing any hands-on assistance, even if you have done so previously with an individual.
5. *Deferred Feedback.* At an opportune time, inform the individual who needs correction that you would like to see him/her after class for a few moments. Once the class is over, you can discuss the exercise, offer more detailed instruction, and provide assistance if needed. Without other people around, you can avoid risking embarrassment to the individual (21).

If a participant is at risk of an acute injury, you need to give feedback promptly. No single feedback method is best to use. Choose the most appropriate method for the participant and circumstances. At times, it may be best to use a combination of feedback methods. Conversely, if there is a way to provide a correction without singling someone out, go there first. No matter which method you select, balance your feedback by following up with a compliment, positive reinforcement, or similar acknowledgement.

## Motivation Cues

Motivation cues are action words that add appropriate energy to classes and provide guidance, encouragement, and reinforcement to participants at selected intervals throughout the class. Cues such as "make it happen, go for it, do it, focus, move it, power-up, push yourself, dare, concentrate, work it, energy, meet the challenge, you've got it" can inspire people when the going gets tough.

Motivational cues not only help your class to work out harder, but also to work out smarter. Cues such as "slow, control it, hold, lighten, easy, listen to your body, calm, still, soften, relax, bring it down, quiet, ease, reduce, it's your workout, notice, diminish, this is for you, gentle" are as essential as the high-energy cues.

Over time, it is beneficial to listen to yourself to be aware of your specific motivational cues (2). Words used too frequently eventually lose their effectiveness. Some cues may simply be misplaced and sound ambiguous, or they lose their authenticity. While being energetic and upbeat is an expectation in a group class, it is not necessary to fill every moment with a "good job," "way to go," "you can do it," or "that's it!" More detailed cues such as, "this is it, come on, only two more," "give it all you got this last time through," or "we're halfway there, give yourself a pat on the back" can register well in class. Choose your words carefully. Remember, people can detect artificial enthusiasm and overhyped comments. Be sensitive, sincere, and genuine as to when your class could most benefit from your words of inspiration.

Now that we have the basics down for universal concerns regarding music, environment, equipment, movements, and cueing, let's move on to specific types of classes including choreographed cardio, nonchoreographed cardio, and strength.

## CARDIO CLASSES: CHOREOGRAPHED

A choreographed workout refers to formally arranged and repeated exercise sequences or movement patterns that are performed in a predetermined order. You select specific songs for specific class segments, and choose specific movements for various parts of each song. You change exercises or movement patterns when there is a change in the structure of the song. For example, during a verse, you do one movement pattern. When the chorus starts, you change to a different movement pattern. During the next verse, you repeat the movement pattern done on the first verse. When the chorus repeats, you revert to the same movements previously performed on the first chorus. Movement patterns or choreography is designed carefully around song structure. The patterns stay consistent from class to class, though you can make minor changes over time as you continue to utilize a song. Generally, though, you stay with the same movements each time you use the song in class.

"Choreography" is a term that can be frightening if you have not had dance experience. This term is associated with programs like Zumba and Jazzercise, as these programs are designed and choreographed around song structure. They also happen to evolve from Latin dance and jazz dance, respectively. Body Pump and Group Strength are also choreographed programs, yet they do not look or feel like dance at all. You do not need a dance background to teach a choreographed cardio class, and a choreographed cardio class does not have to include fancy footwork or clever combinations. As an example, for a selected song you might jog in place during the musical verse, do jumping jacks during the chorus, and perform squats during the introduction and instrumental break. This example of a choreographed cardio routine is composed of athletic movements, not dance moves. A choreographed class does not mean it will be like dancing. You decide if the movement and exercise style is athletic or dance. "Choreographed" only means you change moves or exercises when the structure of the song changes.

A key benefit of choreographed workouts is familiarity. Since the song structure provides the cues to change movements, participants are able to anticipate a transition as they hear the change coming up in the music. Once your class learns the "choreography," it reduces the amount of movement cues needed. Many people like knowing what to do from class to class with each song. Participants can commit to the movement more fully instead of holding back wondering what move you might decide to do next. Typically, there are two, three, or four movements/exercises per song in a choreographed cardio class. Group exercise classes in the 1960s started as choreographed workouts in the United States. Today, when you use music from the 1960s or any music that is not the most current music, it might be considered a theme class (*i.e.*, "oldies-but-goodies" class).

Choreographed cardio classes require considerable preparation before teaching, as you must plan and memorize the entire class, or at least the cardio section, in advance. Here is the process for designing a choreographed cardio class.

1. First, determine your audience. Who is in the class or who do you want to attract to class?
2. Select your music based upon the appeal it has for your audience.
3. Decide the music order — warm-up song, first cardio song, second cardio song, etc.
4. For each song, identify the number of major parts in song structure: introduction, verse, chorus, etc.
5. Design/select movements or exercises to fit the various parts of the song.
6. Develop modifications or alternative movements for different fitness and skill levels.
7. Practice your cardio class, assessing how the music and movements feel and fit together.
8. Replace any movement that does not smoothly transition into or out of another movement.
9. Resequence the song order as needed looking at biomechanical and physiological stresses.
10. Record your class design and choreography to reuse ideas in the future (videotaping is an option).

## CARDIO CLASSES: NONCHOREOGRAPHED

Group exercise classes have evolved to include formats for a wider variety of participants. Previously, people gravitating toward classes were dancers — those with rhythm and coordination. While extremely fun for those individuals, the choreographed format had little appeal to people who were not musically inclined or coordinated but equally interested in participating in a group setting to get cardiovascular exercise. So evolved cardio classes with less emphasis on linking movements together and building complex combinations. This has opened the door for not only new participants but also new instructors with different backgrounds and expertise.

Today, there are many options for cardio classes that are less choreographed than the original "aerobic" format. You may find elements of nonchoreographed cardio included in classes such as sports conditioning, boot camp, or circuit. Often it is easier to find a class that combines nonchoreographed cardio with strength and/or core training, but you may have the opportunity to teach an entire class dedicated to this format. Let's take a look at how these classes can be constructed and delivered to offer the best results for your participants.

### Class Design Methods

There are two primary methods to design nonchoreographed cardio classes.

1. *Circuit.* A circuit class usually has participants performing different cardio drills at designated stations for a specific time. The instructor determines how many stations he/she will use, sets up the stations in the room with enough equipment for anticipated number of participants, and chooses how long participants will spend at each station as well as how many times the circuit repeats. Participants move from station to station around the room during the workout. This is a rotating circuit format. Here is an overview of class design for a circuit class.
2. *Warm Up.* Like any fitness class, a circuit class should begin with a warm-up. As choreography is not a main objective of the class, the warm-up should also be nonchoreographed and less rhythmic. You may choose to warm up within or outside of the circuit. Within the circuit, warm-ups could have participants moving through each station to practice the cardio drill at a slower tempo and smaller ROM. This is an effective way to warm up and introduce the stations. It may be a bit challenging to facilitate, however, as participants are all doing something different right from the start.

More common is to create a warm-up outside of the circuit in a circle formation (around the outside edge of the circuit), line format (traveling down the room in lines), or traditional class format with you at front/center and

participants at their own, individual station (like in a step training class). This is a unison circuit format. The warm-up should last between 7 and 10 minutes.

*Cardio Stations.* Circuits are set up with any number of stations. Typically, 4–10 stations would be both manageable for you and doable for your participants. First, consider space constraints, and then the amount of equipment to determine the number of stations for the class. The fewer stations you have, the more cycles you will be able to have around the circuit. You can do the same exercises or change the exercises each time around the circuit. Also experiment with having cardio activities in the center of the circuit at regular intervals (*i.e.*, perform all stations in the circuit and then have everyone come to the center of the room for 3 minutes of cardio drills).

*Cool-Down and Stretch.* After completing your last station, it is important to take 3–5 minutes to systematically bring the heart rate down toward preexercise levels. You might repeat your warm-up at a lower intensity, or take a few laps around the room to decrease the heart rate. Keep in mind, if nonchoreographed cardio is the nature of your class, the cooldown should follow suit. Finish up with a full-body stretch highlighting the muscles that were used during the cardio stations.

Circuit classes help time pass quickly because each station will not last too long (usually from 30 to 90 seconds). The constant changing of stations and exercises keeps participants distracted and interested, yet provides enough time to learn the drill, perform the drill, and improve the drill. Circuits allow participants to explore higher intensities for short periods. Circuit class structure naturally lends itself to being an interval format with periods of work (the stations) and periods of active rest (moving to and setting up the next station). Built-in recovery time allows participants to push harder to increase cardiorespiratory benefits. With multiple stations, participants can experiment with a wide variety of equipment without having to be perfectly proficient. Circuits are also an efficient way to use equipment of limited quantity and for introducing new equipment into the mix.

*Traditional.* A traditional nonchoreographed cardio class would resemble a kickboxing class, step class, high/low impact class, or dance-based class with you positioned at the front and center of the room and each participant facing you. It is possible to construct the class much like you would a circuit, except participants would stay in their place and move from exercise to exercise without traveling around the room (unison circuit format.)

A traditional nonchoreographed cardio class is usually time driven and linear. In other words, you choose an exercise or drill and determine how long the participants will continue performing it before moving on to another drill. You may repeat the movements, but they would never be linked together in combinations or be repeated from the top as add-on choreography.

Here is an overview for a traditional class. We discuss exercises and delivery method details further in this section.

*Warm-Up.* As with the circuit format, the warm-up should last between 7 and 10 minutes and have a primary focus of elevating the heart rate and gently increasing intensity over time. Straightforward calisthenics or athletic moves combined with dynamic flexibility exercises should make up the warm-up to prepare for the drills you will be performing for cardio training. If any equipment is used during the workout, acclimation to the types of skill needed to safely and effectively utilize the equipment should be included.

*Cardio Drills.* You can choose to create a long list of drills to compose the cardio training or choose a limited number of drills that you repeat throughout the class. Keep in mind, providing an opportunity to repeat drills is always a good idea for nonchoreographed classes. The amount of time you stay with a skill or drill will typically be the same length as a station in a circuit (30–90 seconds). If you are musically inclined, it may be possible to use the music phrasing to determine how long you stay with a drill versus having to watch the clock. Keep equipment to a minimum. Two different pieces combined with the floor is appropriate for one class. Limiting equipment ensures you have enough space to move in a safe and effective manner. ROM is a factor influencing intensity in nonchoreographed cardio classes.

*Cool-down and Stretch.* After your last set of drills, take 3–5 minutes to decrease the heart rate back down toward preexercise levels. You could repeat your warm-up at a lower intensity or walk around the room a few times to decrease the heart rate. If nonchoreographed is the nature of your class, the cool-down should follow suit. Conclude with a full-body stretch targeting muscles used during the cardio section.

Classes like rowing, treadmill, or indoor cycling can be slated into the traditional, nonchoreographed category but exist in separate rooms than your circuit and traditional nonchoreographed cardio formats. Programs such as these do not require coordination, rhythm, dance ability, or memorization, helping to open group fitness to new audiences. Concurrently, if the brain is free to focus on intensity, participants can break through plateaus in cardiorespiratory fitness. Additional training is needed to adequately create and deliver safe and effective rowing, treadmill, or indoor cycling workouts.

## Exercise and Equipment Choices

### Equipment

More equipment than ever is suitable to include in nonchoreographed cardio formats. Below is a list of the most common equipment you may have access to in your studios.

- Steps
- Balance trainers
- Cones
- Agility ladders
- Hurdles
- Kettlebells
- Gliding discs
- Minitrampolines
- Indoor rowers
- Indoor cycling bikes

This is not meant to be an all-inclusive list of the possible equipment. It is always an option to provide exercises and nonchoreographed cardio classes that use no equipment. Removing equipment from nonchoreographed cardio classes can decrease the possible intimidation factor for new participants, increase the number of options you have for traveling movement patterns, and offer a wider range of intensity options for a larger number of participants.

The movements you might choose to include in a nonchoreographed cardio class are limitless. Movements may be shared between choreographed and nonchoreographed cardio formats, but the look and feel of the movements certainly changes. Whether minimizing or maximizing equipment, a nonchoreographed class should be more drill-like than dance-like. Only your imagination and the equipment you plan to use (or not use) limit movement selection.

## Exercises

### Step

Almost any movement you would use in a choreographed cardio class utilizing a step platform are appropriate in a nonchoreographed format that utilizes step platforms. The original moves created for step training form the basis of a nonchoreographed workout. It is perfectly acceptable to perform any (alternating) step pattern repeatedly rather than just once or twice before changing to another pattern. This is appealing to many individuals in whom repetition breeds confidence, not boredom. There are two kinds of step patterns:

- Single lead: The same leg (either right or left) always starts the step pattern
- Alternating lead: The opposite leg automatically starts the step pattern after completing 1 repetition

When performing single-lead step patterns, the starting leg will eventually fatigue as it is carrying your body weight up onto the platform. You should limit a single-lead pattern to about 1 minute and then switch lead legs to prevent overfatigue.

Instead of thinking "choreography," think "drills" without weaving step patterns into complex combinations or adding multiple hops and continuous turns. Those who are experienced and well skilled in step classes can perform complex combinations. Nonchoreographed step training is for those who prefer athletic-oriented workouts. It actually helps new participants find their footing in group fitness classes and serves as a venue to acquire the skills needed to progress to more advanced choreographed step classes. There are six approaches in which you can begin a stepping pattern:

1. From the back. Standing behind the platform, facing front.
2. From the side. Standing sideways behind the platform.
3. From the end. Standing at the end of the platform, facing the platform.
4. From the corner (diagonal). Standing at the back corner of the platform, facing diagonally center.
5. From the top. Standing on top of the platform.
6. From astride. Standing sideways with one foot in front of the platform and one foot behind the platform.

Table 5.3 illustrates common patterns used for step training classes. You can expand these exercise choices and vary intensity by exploring the following options:

*Platform Height.* The beauty of step training is simple: increase or decrease the intensity of your workout by adjusting the platform height. Without changing any movement pattern, stepping at a different height, whether it is lower or higher, will cause a corresponding decrease or increase in intensity (17).

*Amplitude.* Creating distance between your feet and the ground (or your feet and the step) can automatically increase the intensity and impact of a movement. Sometimes known as "power" or "propulsion" moves, you add selected jumps, leaps, hops, or runs into your step patterns. It is a good idea to add these moves only when participants are experienced in step training, exhibit good form, and are ready for an additional challenge. Perform all power moves when moving up to the top of the platform, not coming down to the floor.

*Range of Motion.* Adding arm patterns, extending the levers (arms, legs) in movements, or covering more ground (much like we mentioned in direction), will change the intensity of the exercise. Since arm patterns can be confusing for some participants, it is best to make them optional as performing the correct step pattern is the priority.

Since stepping is an acquired skill, here are two tips for mainstreaming novice participants into a step class or any cardio class.

## Orchestrate the Room

A group exercise class tends to have horizontal divisions in it, with advanced students in the front few rows, intermediate-level participants behind them, and beginners or less skilled individuals in the back rows. Ironically, the people who most need to see you and that you need to monitor are positioned where they are least able to see you! Instead, organize your class by fitness/skill level into three vertical sections with intermediate level in the center, advanced level on one side, and newer exercisers on the other side of the room. A vertical layout makes it easier to address varied fitness levels in the same class. You are more effective providing a modification for novices when they are positioned together on one side of the room rather than scattered all across the back of the room. Additionally, when grouped together, they are less apt to feel pressure from surrounding students to perform more complex or intense exercises. People feed off the physical energy of others, so this actually works well for all participants. Advanced participants like to be next to other advanced participants, and beginners prefer to be next to other novice exercisers (1).

### Be Specific

▶ CLIP 5.6  Incorporate or introduce step patterns as part of the active warm-up. You perform the step patterns utilizing the platform, while participants perform them on the floor as low-impact. For example, transform a grapevine into step-together-step-tap. As the class continues the pattern on the floor, demonstrate it as over-the-top and across-the-top. Another example: with marching in place, add a tap on the 4th count, resulting in march, two, three, tap which you demonstrate as a tap down step and a turn step. A step-specific warm-up lets a novice hear the name and experience the rhythm of a step pattern. He or she gets to see what the step pattern looks like before performing it. This preview creates a better opportunity for success when performing the pattern in the cardio section.

### Balance Trainer

The BOSU Balance Trainer is like a fusion of a stability ball and wobble board. It is a great tool for nonchoreographed cardio workouts and provides unique benefits to classes. Intensity is increased due to balance required in the unstable nature of the product and, like step training, the height of the dome. The surface is pliable, making propulsive movements inviting to explore. The circular design of the product begs you to move in many different directions. Present movements in a "drill" rather than "choreography" format as the neurological system is already challenged with the balancing task. Drills allow participants a better chance to feel successful and get the most out of the workout. Consider incorporating the following movement drills that are unique to the BOSU:

Mountain Climbers — Dome side down, assume plank position with hands braced around the edge;

| Table 5.3 | BASIC STEP PATTERNS AND MOVEMENTS |  |
|---|---|---|

| PATTERN NAME | MOVEMENTS<br>(all patterns start from the back approach unless otherwise noted)<br>(R= right foot, L = left foot) | COUNTS |
|---|---|---|
| Basic Step | R up, L up, R down, L down. | 4 |
| Alternating Tap-Down | R up, L up, R down, L tap down.<br>If performing only 1 repetition of a Basic Step, you tap your foot on the last count rather than step on it. This frees up the (opposite) foot to start the pattern, now called an Alternating Tap-Down step. | 4 |
| Turn Step | Facing sideways at R end of platform.<br>R up, L up wide turning to face opposite end, R down, L down tap facing the opposite direction from which you started. If you gradually begin to face the side walls while performing the Alternating Tap-Down step, it transforms into a Turn Step. | 4 |
| V-Step | R up wide, L up wide, R down narrow, L down narrow | 4 |
| U-Turn | A tight, very small turn step that stays on same end of the platform. | 4 |
| Over-the-Top (Up-and-Over) | From the side.<br>R up, L up, R down on front side of platform, L tap down. | 4 |
| Across-the-Top | End approach (L), facing front.<br>R wide up, L up, R wide down off opposite end, L tap down. | 4 |
| Diagonal (Corner to Corner) | Face (L) sideway at back right corner of platform.<br>R up toward center of platform, L up moving forward at a diagonally to the other end, R down in front of platform, L down or tap. | 4 |
| Rock Step | R up (without stepping all the way up), L down. | 2 |
| A-Step | Start at L side of platform.<br>R up to center of step, L up, R down towards R side of platform, L tap down. | 4 |
| Tap-Up/Tap-Down | R up, L tap up, L down, R tap down. Used mostly in a side approach or end approach. | 4 |
| Lift Steps | Weight is never loaded on count #2 as the leg performs a lifting variation. |  |
| Knee Up | R up, L knee lift, L down, R down. | 4 |
| Front Kick | R up, L kick, L down, R down. | 4 |
| Hamstring Curl | R up, L curl, L down, R down. | 4 |
| Rear Lift | R up, L extend, L down, R down. | 4 |
| Side Leg Lift | R up, L abduct, L down, R down. | 4 |
| **Hop Turns** |  |  |
| Half hop turn | R up, R hop with ½ turn, L down on front side of platform, R down. A half turn to the other side of platform. | 4 |
| Quarter hop turn | R up, R hop with ¼ turn, L down off end of platform, R down. A quarter turn around the platform. | 4 |
| **Repeaters** |  |  |
| 3 –Count Repeater | R up, L knee lift, L tap down, L knee lift, L tap down, L knee lift, L down, R down (knee lift repeats 3 times). Use any lever or combination of levers, such as knee lift, front kick, side leg lift, hip extension, or hamstring curl. | 8 |
| 5-Count Repeater | R up, L knee lift, L tap down, L knee lift, L tap down, L knee lift, L tap down, L knee lift, L tap down, L knee lift, L down, R down (knee lift repeats 5 times). Use any lever or combination of levers, such as knee lift, front kick, side leg lift, hip extension, hamstring curl. Add any 4-count pattern at end to complete a 16-count phrase. | 12 |
| 2-Count Repeater | R up, L knee lift, L tap down, L knee lift, L down, R down, march L & R. | 8 |
| 4-Count Repeater | R up, L knee lift, L tap down, L knee lift, L tap down, L knee lift, L tap down, L knee lift, L down, R down + 6 counts (i.e., rock step, basic step) to create 16-count pattern. | 16 |
| L-Step | Standing toward left end of platform.<br>R up, L knee lift, L down off the L end, R tap, R up from the end, L knee lift, L down behind platform, R down behind platform. Can vary lever on lifts. Forms an "L" shape. | 8 |
| Rear Lunges | Top approach, facing front.<br>R lunge back to floor, R up, L lunge back, L up.<br>Lunge on downbeat to the back tapping the sole of the foot on the floor behind you (the full foot should not make contact with the floor). | 4<br>(2 per leg) |

| Table 5.3 | BASIC STEP PATTERNS AND MOVEMENTS *(CONTINUED)* | |
|---|---|---|
| **PATTERN NAME** | **MOVEMENTS**<br>(all patterns start from the back approach unless otherwise noted)<br>(R= right foot, L = left foot) | **COUNTS** |
| Diagonal Lunges | Top approach, face sideway.<br>R lunge to floor on one side of platform, R up, L lunge to floor on opposite side of platform back, L up. Tap the sole of the foot on the floor (the full foot should not make contact with the floor). | 4<br>(2 per leg) |
| Centered Side Touch | Top approach. Feet together.<br>R touch side, R touch in, R touch back to floor, R up.<br>Alternate touching a toe out to the side and to the floor, then switch to the other foot without any weight going onto the foot on the floor; perform this widthwise or lengthwise. | 4 |
| **Straddles** | | |
| Straddle-down | Top approach, facing sideway.<br>R straddle down, L straddle down, R straddle up, L straddle up. | 4 |
| Straddle-up | Astride approach.<br>R straddle up, L straddle up, R straddle down, L straddle down. | 4 |
| Alternating Lift Straddles | Use any variation to create an alternating straddle step: tap, knee lift, side leg lift, front kick, hamstring curl, and hip extension. The lift variation is inserted on count #2 of straddle-up, or on count #4 of straddle down. | 8 |
| **Pattern Variations** | **Using parts of different patterns to create a new step pattern.** | |
| L-Step | Standing toward left end of platform.<br>R up, L knee lift, L down off the L end, R tap, R up from the end, L knee lift, L down behind platform, R down behind platform. Can vary lever on lifts. Forms an "L" shape. | 8 |
| Z-Step | R up, L tap up, L step wide, R tap, R down, L tap down, L step wide, R tap. Forms a "Z" shape. | 8 |
| T-Step | From the end approach, facing platform.<br>R up, L up, R straddle down, L straddle down, R straddle up, L straddle up, R down off the end, L down off the end. Forms a "T" shape. | 8 |
| Y-Step | R up wide, L up wide, jump in jump out (on top), R walk in (on top), L walk in, R down, L down. | 8 |
| I-Step | R up, L up, one jumping jack on top, R down, L down, one jumping jack on the floor. Forms an "I" shape. | 8 |
| X-Step | R up wide, L up wide, R down, L down. R up wide, L up wide, R down, L down with ½ turn R. Repeat same pattern on the floor facing the back of the room. Forms an "X" shape. (V-step twice on platform and V-step twice on the floor facing back.) | 16 |
| Indecision | R up, L up, R straddle down, L straddle down, R straddle up, L straddle up, R down on front side of platform, L tap down on front side of platform. | 8 |
| Rocking Horse | Same pattern as a 3-count repeater, lever changes to a knee and a curl to create the "rocking" motion. | 8 |
| Horseshoe | From the side approach.<br>R up, L up wide into turn step, R straddle down, L straddle, R straddle up on front side of platform, L up wide turn on top of platform, R down in front of platform, L tap down in front of platform. Forms a "horseshoe" shape. | 8 |
| Split Lunge | R up, L up, R lunge, R up, L lunge, L up, R down, L down. | 8 |
| Weave or Crossback | From the side approach.<br>R up, R hop while L leg swings in back over the platform, L down on front side of platform, R down on front side of platform. This takes the "tap" out of over-the-tops — the trailing leg lands first. Similar to a hop turn in that you need to unload with a hop, but you do not turn; direction will remain the same as an over-the-top with a tap. | 4 |

*Modified with permission from Mary D. Griffin, Gin Miller Productions, LLC.*

begin alternating the knees in towards the dome while you hold the platform still. Vary the tempo from slow to quick.

Burpees — Either with dome side up or down, jump into a squat position, legs jump out behind you into a plank position, jump the feet back in, and stand up. This is modified by walking the legs into these positions instead of jumping. When performing with the dome side up, you can start on top of the dome or with feet behind the dome.

The movement choices highlighted in the step section may also be performed on the BOSU Balance Trainer. Using the same elements we discussed in the step section will increase or decrease the cardio challenge. Another element unique to the balance trainer is the direction from which you approach the apparatus. For example, from the back means you start behind the dome and move forward. A diagonal approach, side approach, or anywhere around the rest of perimeter is game. The top approach means you start or stay on the dome.

### Agility Ladder/Cones

Sports performance equipment is sneaking into non-choreographed cardio classes in clubs around the world. Typically, such products are utilized in a circuit-type format, as the possibility of having a 1:1 ratio of product to participant is highly unlikely. When working with these products, it is important to keep the drills simple and provide plenty of time for the participant to rehearse the drill prior to executing for speed, power, and intensity.

Approach agility ladders (Fig. 5.13) facing forward starting at one end of the ladder and progressing to the other end (front), or facing side on one end of the ladder and progressing to the other end (side). Options include the following:

- Walking down the ladder with two feet in each square (front or side approach)
- Walking down the ladder with one foot in each square (front or side approach)
- Two-footed hops in each square (front or side approach)
- Skips (front approach)
- Up and back like a basic step moving down the ladder (side approach)
- Jump in/jump out, where two feet jump into a square and out of the square, move to next square (side approach)
- Icky-shuffle: you start on side of ladder and pass through to the other side with a 1–2–3 rhythm (front approach)

Cones are small, portable, and affordable. Position the cones in different arrangements to create nonchoreographed cardio patterns that work on speed, agility, and power. Experiment with long lines of cones (spaced appropriately for the drill you are performing) and walk, run, hop, zigzag, or shuffle through them. Use cones as minihurdles (hopping over the cones).

### Kettlebells

Traditionally thought of as a strength product than cardio product, yet, when sequenced appropriately, the cast iron bell provides a two-for-one cardio and strength challenge. Once properly trained on the technique involved, adding swings (double-handed, single-handed) will move right into your inventory of cardio drills. Walking lunges with circles around the lower leg or figure 8s through the legs can cause a cardio push. Kettlebells are likely less accessible in a 1:1 ratio for a group setting, but in a circuit class with adequate prior instruction and experience, they could add variety to your nonchoreographed cardio classes.

### Gliding Discs

Gliding discs are another product commonly thought of as a core or strength product. With the discs under the feet, you can add these movements for cardio exercise:

*Reverse Lunges.* When the ROM is smaller and you pick up the pace a bit on a traditional reverse leg lunge, a strong cardio effect is felt. Think of this like a Nordic skier motion, quickly alternating the feet forward and back, rather than performed as a static strength lunge.
*Side Lunges.* The side lunge used with the disc is much like the centered side touch discussed in the step section, quickly moving from the right leg pushing out laterally to the left leg, then repeating the same movement.
*Lateral Squats.* A traditional squat adding a side lateral movement. Start with feet under hips, toes face forward. As you squat down, slide right leg to the right keeping weight equal over both feet. On the up phase, slide left leg towards right to starting position. Reverse to the other side.
*Jump Squats.* A squat that slides both feet out simultaneously and back in the same manner.
*Lateral Shuffles.* Linking slides left and right, quickly.
*Mountain Climbers.* From plank position, alternating sliding knees in towards the chest.
*Burpees.* Squat down to place hands on the floor, slide both feet back, slide both feet back in and stand up.

### Minitrampolines

Additional training will teach you appropriate movements when utilizing a minitrampoline. Movements are dependent on the type of minitrampoline and the type of mat surface on it. The "basic bounce" forms the foundation of cardiovascular moves on minitrampolines and begins with the feet wide, knees slightly bent, and a slight hinge at the hips. The movement involves pushing down

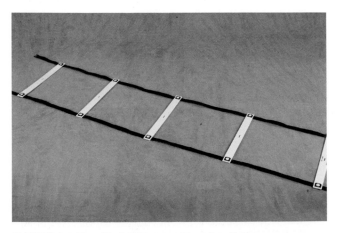

■ **FIGURE 5.13** Agility ladder.

into the mat, rather than jumping far off the mat. From the basic bounce, the feet can move in various directions (wide, narrow, in/out, front/back, diagonal). You can add knee lifts, hamstring curls, or a variety of leg shapes to the basic bounce. Jogging and sprinting are good movement choices. The soft, pliable surface reduces impact on the joints, which can allow exercisers to go longer and harder. The pliability makes the surface unstable, requiring attention to where you land and how you land to keep this a safe, injury-free class. Some trampoline models include attached handrails providing a measure of security for participants.

### Indoor Rowers

Rowing has been around a long time though it has never achieved the popularity as other cardiovascular equipment like treadmills or elliptical trainers. Rowing offers some superb benefits — it is truly a full-body workout, it is non-impact, and there is simplicity. Like cycling, you can do one movement only; in this case — row! Specialty training helps you to design and implement classes for rowing machines. Rowing combines three movements most everyone needs to combat the effects of gravity and daily life biomechanics — shoulder girdle retraction, shoulder joint extension, and spinal extension while simultaneously providing active stretch to the anterior shoulder and chest area. The learning curve is quick and there is a wide range of intensity levels.

### Indoor Cycling

Indoor cycling (Fig. 5.14), like rowing, is a long-time staple for cardiovascular training. Even if you are an avid bicyclist, additional training is required prior to teaching indoor cycling classes. Indoor cycling is another great, nonchoreographed cardio format due to the simple execution and easy-to-master movement. You are seated, standing, or doing a combination of both positions during a cycling class. The intensity is determined when speed and resistance are combined (not simply one in exchange

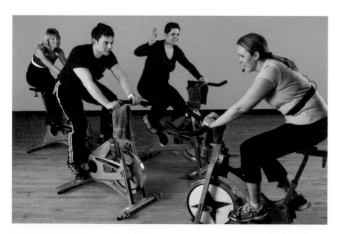

■ **FIGURE 5.14** Indoor cycling.

for the other). Indoor cycling has the best opportunity to attract not only new audiences but also new exercisers. It has a quick learning curve and is the least intimidating activity for a novice exerciser. Intensity level is invisible. In a step class, you can see the height of the platform. You can see how high someone kicks in kickboxing. No one can see how much tension there is on your wheel in a cycling class, eliminating the "sticking out like a sore thumb" feeling that can occur when a novice enters a group exercise class. With minimal skill and coordination required, indoor cycling is the most accommodating and welcoming exercise class for people new to exercise.

### No Equipment

Any movement that we explored for use in nonchoreographed classes using a step platform or the BOSU Balance Trainer can be performed without the product on the floor. The same elements of change are used to progress, regress, or change the movements. Teaching non–equipment-based cardio classes is sometimes called "floor-based cardio." If you have not had the experience of utilizing just the floor space without equipment, this approach may seem a little scary at first. However, no equipment is the way to take away a bit of intimidation that equipment can bring. Now you explore ROM of movements and the creative use of space. It can help grow classes that might be encumbered by equipment taking up too much space or lack of equipment for the desired number of participants. Here are some ideas for manipulating movements previously discussed for a floor-based cardio class:

*Basic Step.* The up-up-down-down pattern that you do on a step platform can be transferred to the floor; use the same foot pattern focusing on the forward and back of the movement to increase intensity. You can also choose to focus on the speed or changing the center of gravity elevating up to the toes on the forward step and flexing the knees and lowering on the backward step.
*V-Step.* The foot pattern stays the same as in step training, but you would shift focus to how far forward and back you can go, how wide you can go, how low you can go, or the speed.
*Step Touch.* Stepping right and left on the floor is transitioned into several exercises on the floor when you use the elements of change, such as focusing on the ROM (how far you can step side to side) is a great option to increase the intensity of the exercise. At times, this might lead to slight hopping from side to side (often referred to as 'skaters' or 'speed skaters'). You can also link two or more step touches together moving to the side and change the tempo to transition it into a shuffle or a 1–2–3 rhythm shuffle.
*Alternating Taps.* Without the need to step up and down, more directions and bigger ROM are quickly available.

*Repeater Taps.* As with Alternating Taps, explore different directions and bigger ROM for a cardio challenge.

*Squats.* Whether single squats, in place and traveling, or multiple squats that move, the squat can quickly elevate the heart rate while increasing lower body strength.

*Lunges.* Lunges without equipment can move around the room and in multiple directions. Walking lunges are effective in building lower body endurance and strength, as well as challenge the cardiorespiratory system.

*Centered Side Touch.* Without using a step platform, coordination demands are reduced for the centered side touch. ROM options are greater though, for increased cardiovascular challenge.

*Carioca.* Moving laterally across the floor, the trail leg alternates between crossing in front of the lead leg and crossing behind the lead leg.

*Mountain Climbers/Burpees.* Mountain climbers and burpees become more challenging from a core conditioning perspective because of the body position relative to gravity.

*Marching.* As simple as it is, marching is one of the most versatile and useful exercises on the floor. Using elements of change, marching can become jogging, high knees, or 'butt' kickers (all three can be done stationary in place or moving around the room). You can also transform marching by moving forward into a "hustle" (walk 3 counts forward and then tap on the 4th count; walk 3 counts backward and tap on the 4th count). You can experiment with the foot pattern of a march and take the feet out wide and then back in close together. Play with speed and turn the move into a double-time "fast feet" drill. Marching forms the foundation of cardio class choreography, and may be the epicenter of creative movement. Almost all cardio moves are a derivation of a march. Let's explore this concept more to identify the elements involved developing cardio steps, combinations, routines, sequences, and drills. It is the architecture of creating a floor-based cardio class.

## Locomotor Movements and Elements of Change

The steps and patterns used in floor-based cardio classes evolve from basic locomotor movements. How you manipulate the rhythm, intensity, and movement dynamics together determines the type of class you create. The following five locomotor movements form the basis of choreographed and nonchoreographed cardio classes:

1. Walk or march: continuous low-impact transfer of body weight from one leg to the other
2. Run or jog: continuous high-impact transfer of body weight from one leg to the other
3. Leap: same as a run, except a pause after each transfer of weight
4. Hop: continuous jumping on one leg
5. Jump: propelling upward with both feet off the ground simultaneously and landing on both feet

For example:

*Locomotor move: Jog.*
*Movement cue: Jog in place for 5 minutes.*
*Results: No change in movement makes it easy to follow, but it becomes boring for some individuals. Rather than a long, extended segment of one locomotor movement, consider doing a series of locomotor movements. Perform sufficient repetitions of each movement to allow everyone to be successful in performing the move. Here is an example of a cardio sequence:*

> *March in place 30×*
> *March with wide stance 30×*
> *Jog in place 30×*
> *Leap side to side 20×*
> *March in place 30×*
> *Left leg hop 10×*
> *Right leg hop 10×*
> *Alternating front kick 20×*
> *Alternating side kick 20×*
> *Alternating side heel dig 20×*
> *Alternating front heel dig 20×*
> *Alternating front double heel dig 10×*
> *Alternating side double heel dig 10×*

The sequence is for a nonchoreographed cardio class (i.e, boot camp or sports conditioning) where music is used in the background, or there is no music at all. Depending on the speed, repeating the sequence two or three times would take ~5 minutes. Compared to jogging in place for 5 minutes, this sequence provides a lot of variety with an adequate amount of repetitions for learning and performing each movement.

Here is the same sequence for a nonchoreographed cardio class that uses the music count:

> *March in place 32×*
> *March with wide stance 32×*
> *Jog in place 32×*
> *Leap side to side 16×*
> *March in place 32×*
> *Left leg hop 8×*
> *Right leg hop 8×*
> *Alternating front kick 16×*
> *Alternating side kick 16×*
> *Alternating side heel dig 16×*
> *Alternating front heel dig 16×*
> *Alternating front double heel dig 8×*
> *Alternating side double heel dig 8×*

Instead of performing 10, 20, or 30 repetitions, you perform 8, 16, or 32 repetitions. This allows you to unite movement counts to music counts. Each move transitions easily and smoothly into the next move. Planning a minimum of 8 repetitions per move the first time through (or 16 or 32 repetitions) provides a sufficient learning curve before changing to another movement. You retain the simplicity inherent with jogging in place for 5 minutes, but without the redundancy of performing only one locomotor movement. You may repeat a movement you already performed whenever you like. The examples above are known as a linear progression, and it is the essence of a freestyle cardio class.

Freestyle choreography is a series of cardiovascular movements that change at no specific time interval. Movements are generally performed in sets of 8 counts or a multiple of 8 counts (4, 16, 32 counts) and coordinate to the 8-count phrase of your music. Freestyle choreography is not dependent upon song structure to designate a movement change or to start or end an exercise. Instead, you spontaneously select your moves and sequence them as you go along. The movements may vary from class to class rather than adhering to the same pattern in each workout. Freestyle cardio classes do not require the amount of preparation needed for teaching choreographed classes. However, you do need a sufficient library of cardio moves to draw from in order to have a continuous cardio section without having to stop and think of what move to do next. Freestyle is the simplest choreographic technique used in cardio classes and accommodates groups with the following characteristics:

- New to exercise-to-music
- Low coordination ability
- Don't want to think too much
- Prefer simple moves/drills
- Prefer cardio without dance steps or routines to remember

## Combinations

Two (or more) movements put together sequentially that repeat are a combination. Combinations take the locomotor moves and start to add structure to the cardio section. Without combinations, you have a long, unbroken sequence of locomotor movements. Here is an example of a combination:

*Locomotor movements: Jog, alternating front kick.*
*Combination:*
*Jog 16×*
*Alternating front kick 8×*

*Repeat.*

*Results: By taking two movements and assigning a number of repetitions to perform of each, you introduce an element of change called cardio combinations rather than performing each locomotor move separately.*

The above combination is simple, and it is an example of 32-count choreography. This choreographic method is an extension and progression of freestyle choreography. Freestyle choreography encompasses 8-count blocks of movement that correspond to most dance-oriented music. Four sets of 8-count movement blocks create a 32-count

block of movements that also corresponds to the structure of most dance-oriented music. If the same 32-count block of movements is repeated within the workout, it is now a 32-count combination. Cardio movement sequenced in blocks of 32 counts is one of the most popular choreographic formats for cardio classes. You may perform a combination a few times, then "delete" it (not perform it anymore in that class) and begin to teach another combination. This cycle can be repeated for the entire cardio section. Another option is to build a second combination and then perform both combinations one right after the other. You can repeat this cycle for the entire cardio section, developing a growing list of combinations that repeat after learning each new combination. This is known as an add-on progression. The following are some examples for building and sequencing very simple cardio combinations (all combinations begin with right leg).

### Building Cardio Combinations (R = Right, L = Left)

#### Combination A
*16 cts. Jog 16×*
*16 cts. Alternating front kick 8×*

*Repeat.*

*To build: 32 cts. Jog 32×*
*32 cts. Alternating front kick 16×*
*Then cut each movement by ½ to create final combination.*

#### Combination B
*16 cts. Grapevine R&L 4×*
*16 cts. Alternating hamstring curl 8×*

*Repeat.*

*To build: 32 cts. Grapevine R&L 8×*
*32 cts. Alternating hamstring curl 16×*
*Then cut each movement by ½ to create final combination.*

#### Combination C
*16 cts. Alternating double hamstring curl 4×*
*8 cts. Single ham curl R, single ham curl L, double ham curl R*
*8 cts. Single ham curl L, single ham curl R, double ham curl L*

*Repeat.*

*To build: 32 cts. Alternating double hamstring curl 8×*
*8 cts. Single ham curl R, single ham curl L, double ham curl R*
*8 cts. Single ham curl L, single ham curl R, double ham curl L*
*8 cts. Single ham curl R, single ham curl L, double ham curl R*
*8 cts. Single ham curl L, single ham curl R, double ham curl L*

*Then cut the two patterns by ½ to create final combination.*

### Combination D
*8 cts. Hop R 8×*
*8 cts. Hop L 8×*
*4 cts. Hop R 4×*
*4 cts. Hop L 4×*
*2 cts. Hop R 2×*
*2 cts. Hop L 2×*
*2 cts. Hop R 2×*
*2 cts. Hop L 2×*
*Repeat.*
*To build: This combination can be taught in its final form.*

### Sequencing Cardio Combinations

*Linear sequence example:*
*Build and teach combination A.*
*Repeat combination A two times.*
*Build and teach combination B.*
*Repeat combination B two times.*
*Build and teach combination C.*
*Repeat combination C two times.*
*Build and teach combination D.*
*Repeat combination D two times.*

*Add-on sequence example:*
*Build and teach combination A. Repeat the combination one time.*
*Build and teach combination B. Repeat the combination one time.*
*Perform combination A followed by B one time.*
*Build and teach combination C. Repeat the combination one time.*
*Perform combination A, B & C one time.*
*Build and teach combination D. Repeat the combination one time.*
*Perform combinations A, B, C, & D one time.*

The first option for sequencing combinations is a linear format; teaching a combination, performing it a few times, then teaching a new combination. You may or may not repeat a combination after you have performed it a few times. The second option for sequencing combinations is an add-on format, continuing to add on to the combinations already taught. Add-on sequencing is more advanced as participants need to recall the previously learned combinations. Whether you choose the linear or the add-on approach, upon completing the 4th combination (combination D), you would be able to begin combination A again if you choose. Alternatively, you can create a new combination and perform it in either a linear or add-on sequence.

Song structure (verse, chorus, bridges, break) is not involved in developing 32-count combinations. Evenly phrased music rhythm is important though, and you want to use music that stays consistently phrased in 32-count blocks. The beginning of a combination should always coincide with the beginning of a 32-count music phrase in order to optimally merge movements to your music.

## Traveling

Traveling involves movement that dissects space, and it is very useful in the choreographic mix. Cardio classes in a previous era used to be taught mostly in place, with marches, hamstring curls, knee lifts, etc. Yet, you can move with those movements rather than stay in one spot. Travel as much as possible in various directions and patterns.

- Forward/backward
- Left/right lateral
- Diagonal front/back
- Geometric designs: circles/squares/rectangles/triangles/diamonds/figure 8/free-form snake

Adding travel into the mix:

*Locomotor Moves: Jog, jumping jack.*
*Combination: Jog 8×, jumping jack 4×.*
*Traveling: Jog forward 8×, jumping jack moving back 4×.*
*Results: Traveling results in a shift of musculoskeletal stress compared to staying on the spot, and you avoid boredom associated with stationary positions. You need adequate space to be able to do travel patterns in your class.*

## Directional Orientation

Which way the participants face determines the directional orientation.

- Participants face forward toward the front of the room
- Participants form half-circle facing instructor
- Participants turn at 90 degrees from instructor
- Participants turn 45 degrees at a diagonal
- Participants form a circle facing in

Split the room, with the left and right halves of the room turning to face each other. For example:

*Locomotor movements: Front kick, march.*
*Combination: Alternating front kick 4×, march in place 8×; repeat.*
*Traveling: Alternating front kick moving forward 4×, march moving backward 8×, repeat.*
*Directional orientation: Kick to the right corner 4×, march traveling back 8×; Kick traveling forward 4×, march moving back 8×; Kick to the left corner 4×, march moving back 8×.*
*Results: Directional changes combined with traveling, begins to form patterns. Patterns are an efficient way to keep cardio segments fresh by changing the orientation (or which way your participants are*

facing). This element of change allows movements to be repeatable without feeling repetitious to participants. Adding another element of change begins to add complexity to the cardio segment.

## Geographic Options

Geographic options refer to the participant's position relative to the room. For a moment, visualize cookies on a square plate. Think of the plate as your room, the cookies are participants. Consider the different ways to arrange the cookies:

- Horizontal lines
- Vertical lines
- A big circle or several smaller circles, either around each other or separated
- Lining the perimeter of the plate
- Groups of cookies in each corner
- Lined up in alphabetical patterns: x-formation, u-formation, t-formation

Positioning participants in various geographical locations is an effective technique to add freshness to movement. Some individuals will feel you have new choreography when the reality is you have only changed their orientation by varying spatial positioning. You gain a lot of mileage from locomotor movements by incorporating geographical design concepts. It is also the essence of another type of choreography known as organized-action.

Organized action is similar to freestyle choreography, but it utilizes geographical options for variety rather than many different locomotor movements. You only need four to six moves for an entire cardio section. There are no combinations combining two or more moves together. The objective is to keep it simple, and it is quite effective for boot camp and sports conditioning classes. There is an athletic orientation and feel to it. Music is used sometimes only in the background to energize the class, and at other times it is used to set the exercise cadence. Here is a closer look at developing an organized-action class:

*Establish the Movements.* Select four cardio movements. Introduce them one at a time. Label each move with a number. For example:
- March in place ("move #1")
- Step touch ("move #2")
- Knee lift ("move #3")
- Hamstring curl ("move #4")

*Embed the Number to the Move.* Once you introduce your moves, cue the move by number rather than by its name. For instance, you say, "Number 1," then march in place for 16 counts. "Number 2," then step touch for 16 counts, and so on. Once everyone understands what move goes with what number, switch the order randomly for a few sets to truly embed the number to the move. These are the only cardio moves you do for the cardio section, and it fits the bill for anyone who does not care for the complexity found in other types of cardio classes. Work your way down to performing 8 counts of each move, then 4 counts of each move. This is called numerical reduction, a choreographic technique to enhance the learning curve when introducing physical movements. Start with a high number of repetitions to give participants the opportunity see a move, practice it, and master it. Progressively reduce the number of repetitions performed when the class demonstrates proficiency.

*Introduce the Walls.* You likely have four walls in your room — front, side, back, and side. Assign each wall a number, such as the front wall is "#1." The right wall is "#2." The back wall is "#3," and the left wall is "#4."

*Match Moves to Walls.* When you cue, "Number one," participants march in place (move #1) and face the front wall (wall #1). When you cue, "Number two," they turn to face the right wall (wall #2) and perform step touch (move #2). "Number three" means to turn and face the back wall (wall #3) and change to knee lifts (move #3). Upon cueing, "Number four," turn to face the left wall (wall #4) and perform hamstring curls (move #4). They not only change movements as you cue numbers one through four but also change orientations to face the corresponding wall (see photos 6.13–6.16). Use numerical reduction starting with 16 repetitions and then reduce to 8 repetitions. If you get down to 4 repetitions, it will be fun! After performing this in numerical order, switch it up by randomly calling out numbers one through four. You find out who is paying attention in class with this variation!

*One Movement, add Travel.* Bring everyone back to move "Number one," marching in place and facing front. Add travel to the march by walking forward 4 counts and walking back 4 counts. Repeat a few times. Have participants march in place again.

*Split the Room.* Divide your class in half. Instruct the left half of the room to continue marching in place. Instruct the right half of the room to get ready to walk front and back on 4 counts each direction. When ready, cue the right half to begin walking front and back. Instruct the right half to continue walking front and back. This will orient the class to their group and the basic patterns we will expand on using the following patterns:

*Zig-Zag.* Cue the left half of the room to get ready to do the same pattern, a 4-count walk forward and back. Cue the left half to start moving forward but not at the same time the right half is moving forward. As the right half is walking backward, cue the left half to start walking forward. You have created a zigzag effect — as half of the room walks forward, the other half is walking backward. The locomotor movement has not changed, but a very different dynamic is born with splitting the room and staggering the walks. You may be surprised at the enthusiasm generated from this relatively simple geographic option.

*Push-Pull.* As the zigzag walk continues, you are going to change the orientation and have the two groups face each other. Remind your class to continue the forward and backward walk in their group while you give the next instructions. The forward/backward walk never stops, just make it smaller, covering less space. Cue your class to slowly face the opposite group while continuing to move forward and backward. Each group slowly turns 90 degrees toward the center of the room, ending up facing the opposite group. Once everyone catches on, you have a push-pull effect — one group walking toward the second group that is backing up. Then, they switch directions, and the other group is now chasing the opposite group. There may be more vocal reaction from class members because inconspicuously, you formed two teams in the room, and teams always produce a synergy amongst its members.

So far, you have a few minutes of playful variations with one movement: marching. There are more variations, but while the two groups are facing each other, here is another idea.

*Mirror-Mirror.* Cue your class to stop walking forward and backward, but to continue to march in place still facing the opposite group. Cue everyone to perform "move #3" (knee lift). Next, cue to perform "move #4" (hamstring curl). Repeat as needed to ensure that everyone recalls these two moves. Instruct the right half to continue performing "move #4." Instruct the left half that when you give the cue, they are to change to move "#3." At the appropriate time, give that cue to the left group. Half of the room is performing knee lifts and the other half is performing hamstring curls (photo 6.17). Instruct your class that when you cue to change, they switch movements. Direct your class to look across the room. The movement the other group is performing is the next move they will start doing. They look at the opposite group, not you, for a visual cue of the upcoming move. Use numerical reduction starting with 32 counts and then 16, 8, and 4 counts. Next, bring everyone back to "move #1" and face front for the next geographic option.

*Split-the-Room.*

*Squad Lines.* Form four squad lines vertical to the front of the room. One line should be close to the side wall, another line close to the other side wall, and the two other lines equal distance from each other in between. Use nonintimidating methods to form the lines, such as, "What is your favorite snack — apples, bananas, cantaloupe, or donuts? Apples form "line 1" close to the side wall; bananas form another line in towards the center of the room for "line 2." Cantaloupes form another line next over from the second line for "line 3," and donuts over by the other side wall to form "line 4." Once everyone has selected a line, perform "move #1" (march). Instruct line #1 to keep performing move #1.

Ask line #2 to start performing move #2. Line #3 performs move #3. Line #4 is instructed to perform move #4. Four lines; a different movement for each line.

*Stationary Line Circuits.* Instruct participants when you cue to change, they are to look to the line to their right and change to that movement. Line #1 changes from marching in place to step-touch. Line #2 changes from step-touch to the knee lift. Line #3 changes from the knee lift to a hamstring curl. It is best to position yourself by the fourth line so they can follow your cue to change from hamstring curl to marching in place (Line #1's move). Each time you are about to cue to change, remind the class to look to the right to get their next movement instead of looking at you (you cannot do all four movements at once)! This is an example of a nonrotating (stationary) line circuit. Start with a high number of repetitions, and use numerical reduction to lower the amount of repetitions on each cycle (*i.e.*, 32, 16, 8).

*Rotating Line Circuits.* After a few rounds of nonrotating line circuits, you are ready to introduce a rotating line circuit. It is the same setup as stationary line circuits, except when you cue to change, not only do they look to the right to see the next move, they shift to the right and move over into the next line to perform the next move. Line #1 moves over to line #2 and then performs move #2. Line #2 moves over to line #3 and performs move #3. Line #3 shifts over to line #4 and performs move #4. Line #4 does an about-face, runs to the back of the room behind the other lines and to the opposite side of the room where line #1 was standing and begins move #1 (marching). The person who was standing at the end of that line will now be standing at the front of the line. It is a rotating line circuit where you change moves and change line positions. After a few rounds of this, bring everyone back to move #1. Again, use numerical reduction to ensure everyone understands the concept.

*Perimeter Wall Stations.* Remember wall #1, #2, #3, and #4? Ask line #1 to move to wall #1, line #2 to move to wall #2, and so on. Have participants face the center of the room as they are lined up along the perimeter walls. Instruct your class to perform their corresponding moves. Perimeter wall circuits work the same as line circuits. When you cue to change, they look to the right and whatever move the group on the right is doing, they switch to that move. Although the tendency is to look at you when you cue to change movements, participants must look to the next wall to receive their visual cue of the upcoming move. Use numerical reduction beginning with 16 counts, then 8 counts, perhaps try 4 counts if they are up for a challenge. This is known as a nonrotating (perimeter) wall circuit.

*+Rotating Wall Stations.* Same as above, except when you cue to change, not only do they look to the right

to get the next move, they rotate positions and move to the right going to the next wall and perform the move associated with that wall. Because of the additional travel involved with rotating line and rotating wall circuits, you will need to stay at the station for a longer period than when conducting a nonrotating circuit. (Performing just 4 repetitions of a movement before rotating is too short a period to be at the station.)

*Traveling Wall Circuits.* Bring everyone back to his or her original starting wall. Cue everyone to perform move #1 (marching) facing the center of the room while lining up around the room perimeter. This circuit involves moving one line at a time. Instruct lines #2, #3, and #4 to continue to march in place as you cue line #1 to walk to the opposite side. When they reach the opposite side, they do an about-face and walk back to their original wall. As soon as line #1 finishes, instruct lines #1, #2, and #4 to continue to march in place as you cue line #3 to walk to the opposite wall, turn around, and walk back to their original wall. Continue this traveling pattern with the two remaining lines (#2 and #4). Repeat the sequence if you like.

*Square Dance Circuit.* This circuit moves two lines simultaneously. Participants continue to perform move #1 (marching) as you instruct lines #2 and #4 to stay in place. Cue lines #1 and #3 to walk to the center of the room simultaneously. When they meet in the center, turn around, and return to their original wall. Repeat one time. Next, have the two other lines do the same thing while lines #1 and #3 march in place.

*Opposites Attract.* Participants continue move #1 (marching) as you instruct lines #2 and #4 to stay in place. Cue lines #1 and #3 to simultaneously walk to the center of the room and continue walking past the other line as they walk to the opposite side of the room. They switch sides. Repeat with lines #2 and #4. Repeat this a few more rounds. Participants usually get fired up from this one!

*It's Only the Beginning.* When everyone is back at their original wall, change to move #2 (step-touch). Here is where you begin to receive a big increase in mileage from your moves. Insert move #2 into geographical options #11 to #15 above. For instance, line #1 performs step-touch traveling to the opposite side of the room, followed by line #3 doing the same thing, and so on. After completing steps 11–15 above with move #2, insert move # 3 and then move #4 if you have time — your cardio training segment may be over before then!

Organizing movements into various geographic formations increases the mileage you get out of every cardio move. There are no combinations whatsoever, fulfilling the mandate of nonchoreographed cardio class formats. Teaching an organized-action class requires you to be a "coaching" instructor rather than a "follow-the-leader" instructor. Although movements are simple, it does require preplanning (see Table 5.4). You do not want to have your class divided into groups or teams, and then forget what to do with them. A simple march can take you to quite a few places through organized-action.

### Modifications

Up to this point, choreographic concepts present the body as one entity, creating form by moving through space. Divide the body transversely and you have two

| Table 5.4 | COMPARING CHOREOGRAPHIC STYLES | | |
|---|---|---|---|
| **FREESTYLE** | **CHOREOGRAPHED** | **32-CT. COMBINATIONS** | **ORGANIZED-ACTION** |
| Calisthenics/sports/athletic-oriented movements | Possibly more dance-oriented steps or style | Can be dance, calisthenics, or athletic-oriented moves | Simple locomotor moves, no dance style or cardio combinations |
| Easy to follow and perform, simple combinations | More musicality, maybe more complex | Can be mentally challenging and complex | Requires good coaching and verbal directions |
| Good for "unmusical" individuals | Attracts those who like music and dance | Requires well-developed movement-to-music skills | Good for sports/athletic-oriented workouts |
| Exercises can change spontaneously | Music structure dictates movement changes | Combinations build progressively and are usually repeated | Simple movements, variety achieved through use of geographic positioning |
| Coordination demands are low | Moderate coordination skill necessary | High coordination skill needed | Minimal coordination required |
| Requires the least amount of preplanning | Initially, substantial preparation is required | Requires planning, or extensive teaching experience | Requires preplanning |
| Relies on music tempo, energy, and 8-count phrasing | Relies on song structure and music energy | Relies on 32-count music phrasing and music energy | Music used as background energy or to match with movement tempo |

## Ask the Pro

# How do you extend the life of your choreography?

**JUNE KAHN**
*BeamFit Director of Education*
*Broomfield, Colorado*

Avoid the temptation to give all the magic at once.
You receive a lot of mileage from your moves by

utilizing various elements of change such as rhythm,
directional, intensity, levers, and geographic
changes. The magic is to milk the moves.

separate entities, the upper and lower body, for creating movement options. Example:

1. Locomotor movement (step-touch)
2. Add travel (move forward 4×, move back 4×)
3. Stay stationary; add upper body movement (alternating uppercut)
4. Stay stationary; add upper body movement (alternating uppercut)
5. Travel again, with arm movement (move forward 4×, move back 4×)
6. Stay stationary; change lower body movement (low kick), no upper body movement
7. Add travel (move forward 4×, move back 4×)
8. Stay stationary; add upper body move (alternating front jab)
9. Travel again, with upper body movement (move forward 4×, move back 4×)

**CLIP 5.7**    There are numerous possibilities. The upper body movement stays the same while you change the lower body movement. The lower body movement stays the same while you change the upper body movement. Arm patterns can confuse some participants. Encourage people to do only the lower body movements if upper body movements are too complex to perform concurrently. It is a good idea to change only one element at a time, such as traveling, direction, locomotor move, or lever variation. Not everyone can handle two or more changes simultaneously. Providing manageable challenges leads to the concept of intensity modification. Theoretically, it is ideal if every class is attended by people of the same skill and fitness level. The reality is, this rarely occurs. Even if a class is targeted and designed for beginners, everyone starts at a different level of fitness and acquires physical skills at varying rates. Participants receive permission to "work at their own level" and "listen to their body" when you grant them the license to modify: "There are 22 people in class today. It is perfectly fine to see 22 different variations of this movement." Your goal is to create — in all classes, for every person — a

feeling of success by including moves that everyone can perform safely (3). Modifications are best provided without judgment or inference that a person is unskilled, uncoordinated, or unfit. Instead of labeling an exercise beginner or advanced, use terms like option A, option B, option C, or level 1, level 2, level 3. Participants can then choose the level or option that is best for them.

There are both psychological and physical modifications. Psychologically easy movements allow participants of all fitness levels but low skill levels to feel successful in the cardio section of class. In general, athletic or sports-oriented individuals, older adults, and a majority of men prefer mentally easy movements. Freestyle and organized-action classes accommodate this preference. You increase the psychological challenge by increasing the frequency of applying an element of change (*i.e.*, locomotor move, rhythm, etc.). A change in movement style can also create a mental challenge. The interplay in combining upper and lower body movements also affects complexity.

Physical modifications are variations in movement intensity that increase or decrease the cardiovascular demand or muscular load. Physically easy movements involve exercises that require low muscular or cardiorespiratory effort. Sedentary individuals should begin activity with low-demanding movements to avoid excessive muscular soreness, a major deterrent to adherence for the novice exerciser. Physically challenging movements are appropriate for experienced exercisers with no apparent orthopedic limitations or medical considerations.

It is important to understand the difference between physical and psychological intensity to apply the right kind of manageable challenges in class. When you receive feedback such as, "That was a hard workout," find out what that means — was it hard because it was complex or because it was physically intense? Participating in group exercise helps people develop better kinesthetic awareness as they become accustomed to moving to music. This improves coordination and the ability to handle more complex movement demands (or greater psychological challenge) over time. To continue to enhance coordination and movement skills, gradually increase psychological complexity in class design. Challenging the brain creates new neural pathways, makes the brain more versatile, and improves the brain's multitasking ability (11). You will maintain not only physical fitness but also mental fitness.

### Instructional Tips

- Teach one movement at a time, if many movements are involved.
- Teach one combination at a time, if multiple combinations are involved.
- Break down each combination or routine into individual parts.
- Determine the elements of change to use to build into the finished product.
- Change or add one element at a time.
- Take time to build combinations piece by piece. Repeating it is essential. You build confidence and ease of movement, and it is much more fun for the group.
- Create names for your combinations. Choose a name that relates to the combination. Names should provide clues to help participants remember the movement sequence. For example, if your third combination has a number of shuffle steps, you might call it the Shuffler. If there are rhythm changes in the fifth combination, you can name it Rhythm. Compare the following cues: "Get ready for combination #3 followed by #5," and, "Get ready for the Shuffler followed by Rhythm." The former offers no help in remembering what to do, while the latter triggers memory recall.
- If a cardio movement or pattern involves upper and lower body, teach the lower body movement first.
- Except for a natural arm swing, adding arm movements in cardio training often results in missteps for some individuals. Deemphasize arm movements before it becomes frustrating for a participant.
- People like to participate in activities that they can do successfully. Build opportunities for success into your choreography and movement drills. Anything requiring high skill, coordination, or style should be mixed with "no-brainer" moves that are easy to learn and feel playful or fun to do.
- Manageable complexity and intensity challenges in cardio training is valuable, yet just as vital is the chance to experience flow, a state of being when participants are swept away in the music, movement, and motivation as they temporarily leave their world and lose themselves in the workout and in the moment.
- If participants converse during cardio exercise, it usually means they want to socialize with each other. Turn a potential disturbance into a happy occurrence by giving opportunity for interaction. Try a cardio mixer using two moves, *e.g.*, hamstring curl and low kick. While performing hamstring curl 16×, find a partner. Next, perform low kick 16× facing your partner. On the next set of hamstring curls, find a new partner; repeat low kick 16× with your new partner. The two cardio movements are simple, and the number of repetitions stays constant. Now they have a chance to talk to other participants during cardio training. Interactive line dances like the "Cotton-Eye Joe" or the "Bar Dance" also provide a chance to socialize.
- Be able to teach freestyle cardio choreography. Choose some music and practice freestyle where one movement leads into another movement continuously in a linear manner.
- Be able to teach a choreographed cardio segment. Choose a popular song. Create specific moves to specific parts of the song. People usually like to do a learned routine to a favorite song — they find it is fun.
- Select music tracks with even 32-count phrasing and design 32-count combinations to match the music phrasing. When you are able to teach all three choreographic methods, you can provide participants with a vast library of choreographic variations over time.
- Be your own team teacher. Show various intensity levels and options for cardio movements.
- Then stay at the level appropriate for the less-fit individuals. The fit people know how to work out intensely. The less-fit participants need to see you as a role model.
- When facing your class, you have to mirror your class, which means to move and cue directions from their perspective, not yours. If you cue to "walk right 8 counts," you walk to your left in order to move in the same direction as your class.
- Observation is how you assess your movement cues. If participants did not change movements when you wanted them to change, you need to tweak your cueing.
- Think consistency with cues. Use the same words and terminology as other instructors use.
- When doing a pattern that travels, everyone should move to the right, left, or other direction together to prevent people from bumping into each other. When standing in place, it may not be critical that everyone be on the same limb together.
- A workout is for the participants, not for you. It is beneficial to remind your class it is their workout so they eventually take ownership for their effort.
- A possible resource for movements is your participants. Solicit them for ideas. You may discover some very creative and usable ideas have been in hiding all of this time.
- Cardio choreography is a dynamic process of change and evolution. You do not necessarily need new moves or combinations frequently. Class members often interpret the slightest element of change as new

choreography. How often should you change your choreography? There is no correct answer. Ask your participants — they will let you know.

- Good choreography is choreography your class members can do and, most of all, enjoy doing. Great choreography is the same, except they tell you how much they enjoy doing it.

**RECOMMENDED RESOURCES:**
*Web-based Choreography Resources*

*www.ballroomdancers.com — Video clips, terminology, choreography notes, and breakdown of popular social dances like the rumba, samba, salsa, cha-cha, mambo, tango, lindy, jive, and more.*

*www.ideafit.com — Articles, publications, sample classes, downloadable videos, exercise clips, fitness DVDs, and more from respected fitness educators to help you with your classes.*

*www.jumpybumpy.com — Downloadable fee-based subscriptions and free choreography resource with clips from renown presenters across the globe.*

*www.turnstep.com — An instructor-populated choreography exchange; instructors around the world post their favorite tunes, exercises, combinations, and choreography for different class formats.*

### Sequencing and Transitions

Sequencing and transitioning in nonchoreographed cardio formats is easy. Exercises should be considered drills versus choreography. Oftentimes, the drills that make up your classes will exist independently. For example, if you were using step platforms as your equipment, you may choose to provide the basic step (up-up-down-down) as Drill A and execute for a pre-determined time period (as determined by the number of drills you will introduce and the goals of the class). Next, you would discontinue the basic step and move on to alternating knee lift as Drill B. Choosing how to sequence drills could depend on the equipment, space constraints, or directional approach to the equipment (such as back, side, or top).

To decide how many drills to include in class, first determine how long the warm-up and cool-down will be. Then, divide the remaining time by how long you would like to perform each drill. The number you find is how many opportunities you have to introduce a drill. Keep in mind, allowing participants to repeat the drills is always an effective way to increase success for your participants. Additionally, build in downtime between drills for possible setup, changing equipment, moving stations, and rehydrating.

Sequencing should take into consideration the equipment you are using, how often you change equipment, and the types of drills (or focus) you are planning (i.e., plane of motion, direction, speed, power, or agility). Easier than linking together movements to create 32-count combinations, you simply need to have a plan that efficiently, effectively, and safely moves people toward the overall goal of increasing their heart rate and challenging their abilities. A few points of consideration are as follows:

*Mix and Match Speed, Power, and Agility.* Not everyone is adept at all of these abilities. Allowing everyone to have an opportunity to shine is a great strategy in challenging classes. When you alternate blocks of drills (i.e., choose three drills that focus on speed, repeat once, and then shift the focus to power), there is a better chance of allowing each participant to excel and be less judgmental on himself/herself during challenging drills.

*Avoid Frequent Changes of Equipment.* Design the class so you perform 3–5 drills on one piece before transitioning to another (i.e., perform 5 drills (which will take about 10 minutes) on the BOSU Balance Trainer, then transition to the floor for 5 more drills). Limiting the number of pieces of equipment will free up more floor space for moving around with floor drills and minimize downtime during the workout.

*Consider Direction and Plane of Movement to Ensure a Multidirectional, Multiplanar Workout.* By encouraging participants to break out of their everyday routine, you help bring balance to muscle activity. Most daily movement leads forward in the sagittal plane.

| BOX 5.3 | Sample Circuit Class Time Outline | |
|---|---|---|
| **Total Class Time:** | 60 minutes | |
| **Warm-up Time:** | (−) 10 minutes | |
| **Cool-down Time:** | (−) 10 minutes | |
| **Drill Time Allotted:** | 40 minutes/1.5–2 minutes (length of time for each drill) | |
| **Number of Drills:** | 20–25 (If you choose to do each drill more than once, you will only need 10–12 drills) | |

Changing the orientation of drills to move sideways, diagonal, and backwards will both challenge participants and improve their performance in everyday life. *Alternate Between Single Movement Drills and Multiple Movement Drills.* Nonchoreographed cardio classes should already be limited in complexity. However, in order to challenge coordination, it may be appropriate to sequence two exercises or movements together at times. For example, performing a basic step (on a step platform) directly followed by a knee lift will cause a different physiological and psychological response without being considered overly complicated or complex. However, doing an entire class of combination drills might not be the best idea as it would elevate the mental complexity for some individuals to the detriment of the cardiovascular challenge.

*Transitioning in a Nonchoreographed Cardio Class is Simply How You Choose to Change to the Next Drill.* You may choose to link drills together if you are providing a steady-state cardio experience (*e.g.*, in a cycling class, you would not stop in between each drill) or you might create downtime between the drills if you are providing an interval, or mixed-intensity, cardiovascular workout.

When downtime is included between drills, it may be different for each type of class you teach and last from a few seconds to a few minutes depending on the cardiovascular demands of the previous drill and the overall class goal. During downtime, plan active recovery to minimize standing still. This could be introducing the next drill at half tempo or with less ROM. Here are two scenarios:

1. *Intervals:* If you are teaching an interval class (regardless of the equipment), present Drill A by introducing the drill and rehearsing it for 10–30 seconds. Then, begin showing options to increase the intensity of the drill. This may include using the elements of change to introduce what you will do for the last 15–30 seconds of the drill to increase the intensity. Cue the last push for Drill A and move on to Drill B using the same protocol. After completing the first drill, you can take a few seconds to march in place, preview the upcoming drill, rehydrate, but keep participants moving if you can. The timing will be dependent on how many intervals you plan to perform in your allotted time frame, as well as the cardiovascular response you are looking to produce. Furthermore, timing and drills should reflect the ability level of your participants.

2. *Steady State:* When you want to keep the intensity levels relatively steady throughout the class, plan your transitions with more structure to avoid downtime between the drills. Movements such as marching in place, step-touch side to side, or similar will assist you in keeping participants in a challenged, but comfortable state. Unlike choreographed class, there is no need to emphasize which leg starts. It is unnecessary

to insert clever transitions to get you to the other leg. In nonchoreographed formats, remember to keep the choreography out of the workout! Keep it simple when planning your drill sequences.

## Instructional Tips and Delivery

The secret to a successful nonchoreographed cardio class lies in the delivery, in other words, how you explain and cue the workout. The ingredients of a well-run nonchoreographed cardio class are as follows.

### Broadcast the Big Picture

First, explain the overall goal of the class concerning cardiovascular conditioning. This will require a bit of education about the heart as a muscle and how it needs to be subjected to a wide variety of stimuli, just like skeletal muscle to acquire optimal benefits. Factors include aerobic and anaerobic bouts, steady-state and mixed-intensity segments, and a varying degree of duration. Explain the nature of the class in regard to these factors. Participants are more willing and inspired to do different types of exercise when they understand the reasons behind it.

### Highlight the Hard Parts

In any class, participants want to mentally prepare for the upcoming energy demands. How much effort will they have to exert? Where will the hard parts be? How many are there? Will there be recovery breaks during the workout and if so, how long and how often? This information is significant for class members. It provides them a blueprint to psychologically preplan for the physical requirements. Giving an overview of the planned intensity profile helps participants to know how to ration their energy. Announce how many sections, stations, or drills are planned and how long they will last. Describe what will happen in the cardiorespiratory system. For example: "We have five cardio sections today; there will be three drills in each section that will last 2 minutes each. All of the drills start easy, progress to moderate, build to intense, and push to breathless. You will never have to be breathless for longer than about 15 seconds, and you will always get at least 30 seconds of recovery before starting again."

### Break Down the Big Picture

For each individual drill, break down the exercise and expectations. Use the first part of the drill to acclimate participants to technique and proper execution. With drills being uncomplicated, it is easy to preview the drill. Do it and then cue it. In other words, announce a change is coming, start to show the movement, have the class start the movement, and then provide relevant safety or technique cues. Begin to introduce progressions and regressions to challenge each individual. Along the way, it is imperative to break down the expectations for intensity and the amount of time in each progression. Continually reinforce what intensity level they should be experiencing by describing what they should be feeling. Example: "As you get started, I want to make sure you are at an intensity where you can talk to me in sentences. Now, for the next 30 seconds increase your ROM to move into a level where you can only say a few words. Okay, here you go — for the last 30 seconds, increase the ROM enough to go breathless."

Like organized-action classes, drill-based classes provide an opportunity for substantial interaction with your group as your teaching style is more characteristic of an athletic/sports coach versus a follow-the-leader type instructor. The drills should be easy enough to understand that you do not need to be a physical representation for 100% of your teaching time and you certainly do not need to work to the intensity levels that your participants are experiencing in order to still coach, motivate, and remember what is going to happen next. You should be able to face your class for a majority of the time and walk around to help when needed. Just as the best coaches in the world do not physically perform the training regimen they give their athletes, the best group exercise instructors do not physically perform the entire class they give to their participants. A coach's job is to bring out the best in his or her athletes; your job is to bring out the best in the people in your class.

## Music

Music for nonchoreographed cardio classes can range from 124 (when performing drills on a BOSU Balance Trainer) to 136 bpm and above (floor-based drills that are not using the beat for direction). Music between 126 and 130 bpm provides a midrange tempo to follow when needed. Music can also be used as background energy without regard for tempo or phrasing in some nonchoreographed cardio classes.

## STRENGTH-BASED CLASSES

The evolution of strength training in group fitness is a varied one. In the 1940s and 1950s, exercise advocates Jack LaLanne and Bonnie Prudden practiced high-repetition calisthenics to "tone" and "firm" the body. Dr. Kenneth Cooper's research in the 1960s along with his new term aerobics propelled a running boom and the birth of aerobic dancing to get everyone "in shape." In the next decade, physique muscled its way back in when Arnold Schwarzenegger brought bodybuilding into the cultural vernacular to "develop" the body. High-repetition calisthenics returned in the 1980s as Jane Fonda and others popularized dance-based exercises to "sculpt" and "define" the body. "Muscle conditioning" and "body sculpting" began to appear at the end of all-inclusive aerobic classes. Ten to fifteen minutes of no-frills floor work and abdominal exercises rounded out each class. Fifteen minutes was not enough time for strength work, and full-hour classes were soon on the schedules. No equipment was used, and muscular conditioning was, more often than not, muscular endurance training. A myriad of resistance equipment is currently available, and our knowledge of exercise has caught up with our enthusiasm. We can now provide effective, efficient, evidence-based strength training in group exercise classes.

Today, review any group exercise schedule, and you find hundreds of descriptions for strength-focused formats that promise various results to various participants who frequent classes. Many of these classes were born from the "sculpting" concept, a marketing term that caters to people interested in toning and shaping versus building and bulking (primarily women). High repetitions, low resistance, and targeted toning exercises were (and continue to be) the basis of many strength classes. Classes have now evolved to include different strength classes to suit the needs of more people, including those in need of increased functionality.

## Ask the Pro

# What is a primary role of an instructor?

**LYNNE BRICK**
*Owner*
*Lynne Brick's Women's Health and Fitness*
*Cockeysville, Maryland*

A main role of a professional fitness instructor is to create awesome, world-class fitness experiences in every class. This is accomplished with high energy, professional knowledge, a seamless flow of movement, and coaching participants in such a way that each person feels as if they are the only person in the studio.

Regardless of age, gender, or ability level, everyone can improve his or her strength. Your leadership along with the group dynamics, camaraderie, and social support afforded by group exercise provide many people the inspiration to strength train that they otherwise do not get on their own. In addition to the physical improvements a participant will experience, the psychological shift is also compelling. A subtle change of emphasis in your instruction from highlighting cosmetic changes (*i.e.*, "This will make your arms look great in your tank top") to a focus on the intrinsic value and/or functional benefit (*i.e.*, "This will make you feel much stronger," or "Glad to hear you can hold your baby in your arms for a longer time now") helps participants understand and appreciate the significant benefits besides improved appearance.

There are both men and women who question if a strength training class is an appropriate addition to their workout program. Some women might be concerned about bulking up or may be only interested in working on their "trouble spots." Men may think group exercise does not have sufficient weights for what they need, or they have a preconceived belief that only certain body parts are important to work on, usually in a methodical never-changing manner they have always done in the past. Marketing terminology such as "tone," "firm," "tight," "chisel," "define," "sculpt," "lean," or "shape" is used to appeal to those who, for one reason or another, are not drawn in by the word "strength," which, admittedly, sounds unexciting compared to the emotional pull of the Madison Avenue terminology. Understand if participating in your class is going to result in toned legs, firm rears, defined arms, sculpted backs, chiseled abs, and lean, tight body, it is the same thing — a strong body. Our job as educators is tested in strength training formats to dispel myths and misconceptions, and design safe and effective workouts that maximize the equipment we have while meeting the needs of a diverse clientele. To help participants develop a strong body, help them develop a strong body of knowledge about what strength training is all about. Let's take a look at how we can make this a reality.

## Class Design Methods

There are three broad categories of strength training.

1. Endurance — characterized by higher repetitions, lower resistance, and frequently zone-specific targeting; sometimes referred to as sculpting or toning classes
2. Strength — characterized by lower repetitions and higher resistance; uses straightforward exercises to increase muscular strength and endurance
3. Functional — characterized by moderate resistance and moderate repetitions; multijoint, multiplanar, multidirectional exercises that work on balance, coordination, and increased strength and endurance

It is possible that a strength class can combine the three categories into one class or cycle through these different goals on different days or weeks. It is valuable if all three are represented on a class schedule to be equally represented in participants' fitness regimes. However, equipment availability often dictates what it is possible to accomplish in a class. We will address equipment challenges in the group exercise setting to be able to provide, on some level, each type of workout.

You can design strength training to be interspersed with cardio training creating circuit/interval-style classes to address both components of fitness in an hour (or less). While combining strength moves with cardio moves is not recommended (*i.e.*, performing a jumping jack while doing an overhead press), alternating cardio bouts with strength bouts is an effective way to challenge participants. Sometimes known as a combination class, you can design specific intervals such as 3 minutes of cardio followed by 3 minutes of strength. A circuit class can alternate between cardio and strength exercises. It can alternate cardio exercises only (for a cardio circuit class) or exclusively strength exercises (for a strength circuit class). Another option is to divide the time into separate blocks (*i.e.*, 20 minutes of cardio, 20 minutes of strength).

Strength classes can either be self-designed (where the instructor is responsible for the content of the class) or prechoreographed (where the instructor is supplied the content of the class). In either situation and regardless of the overall class goal (endurance, strength, or functional), your class will have three main sections.

### Warm-up

Class warm-up should be specific to prepare for the upcoming strength exercises. It should increase core temperature, involve motion of the major joints, promote spinal mobility, and apply core stabilization techniques to use throughout the class. The warm-up can be performed without equipment, or it can involve a prominent piece of equipment used in the main workout, if the resistance is adjustable. ROM generally starts small and increases over the course of the warm-up. No resistance should be used if incorporating equipment. Finally, introduce technique skills and provide appropriate safety guidelines. See Box 5.4 for additional recommendations.

### Strength Exercises

The main section of class consists of strength exercises that can be introduced in several ways based on your overall goal. A class can target all major muscle groups, but the order of the exercises will vary depending on equipment, the type and amount of resistance available, and the goal of the class. In order to make the best use of your time and determine what exercises to include, you need some important information. You have to know

---

**BOX 5.4**  **ACSM Recommendations for Warm-up Exercises**

Perform 12–15 repetitions with no resistance before the workout set, with 30 seconds or more rest before the workout set.

A specific warm-up is more effective for strength training than a general warm-up.

No warm-up set is required for high-repetition exercises which are not as intense and serve as a warm-up in themselves. Example: 20–50 repetitions for abdominal training.

Perform a longer warm-up if the muscles and joints involved may be more susceptible to injury. Example: squats or chest press may require a longer warm-up.

---

what other training and exercise your participants do outside of your class. If, *e.g.*, some individuals strength trained upper body yesterday, that may affect your choice of exercises. If their workout yesterday involved only pulling exercises, you can include pushing exercises in your class. But, if you indiscriminately have everyone do upper body pulling exercises in class, you have not allowed adequate recovery for individuals who trained the same muscle groups yesterday. Knowing what strength training they participate in outside of your class is necessary for you to make appropriate exercise selections and to have alternative exercises planned for the varied responses you are likely to get.

With this information in mind, consider how you can design your strength classes so participants can better fit other training they may partake in around your classes. For example, Monday and Thursday classes could be upper body strength training. Tuesday and Friday classes would be lower body strength training. This type of

design makes it easy for participants to plan their workouts with you and other workouts they may do without risking overtraining and/or insufficient recovery time.

For specific exercises, upcoming is a grid providing numerous exercise and equipment options to consider for this main section of class. Guidelines and recommendations for strength training exercise are listed in Box 5.5.

### Cool-down/Stretch

Once muscles have been sufficiently challenged, a stretching section can bring a calming balance to the intense efforts exerted in the workout. A dedicated cool-down period may not be necessary. Heart rate may have already diminished by the end of the main section. It decreases as exercises shift to smaller muscle groups, common toward the end of most strength workouts. However, do keep the head above the heart when the heart rate is significantly

---

**BOX 5.5**  **ACSM Recommendations for Strength Training Exercise**

Perform a minimum of 8 to 10 exercises that train the major muscle groups.

Workouts should not be too long. Programs over one 1 hour are associated with higher dropout rates.

Perform 1 set of 8–12 repetitions to the point of volitional fatigue.

More sets may elicit slightly greater strength gains, but additional improvement is relatively small.

Perform strength exercises at least 2 days per week.

More frequent training may elicit slightly greater strength gains, but additional improvement is relatively small.

Adhere closely to the specific exercise techniques.

Perform exercises through the full ROM.

Participants, especially elderly, should perform exercises in the maximum ROM that does not elicit pain or discomfort.

Perform exercises in a controlled manner.

Maintain a normal breathing pattern during exercises.

Exercising with a partner can provide feedback, assistance, and motivation (participants can pair up in class).

elevated, and take participants to the floor after the heart rate has decreased.

In general, participants enjoy stretching for the chance to relax as much as to increase flexibility. Stretch the areas that were targeted, maintaining a static stretch for 15–30 seconds to promote a relaxation effect and improve joint flexibility.

## EXERCISE AND EQUIPMENT CHOICES

### Equipment

The equipment choices available for strength-based classes has substantially increased in recent years. Listed are the most popular equipment choices being used in strength classes. Equipment offers various types and amounts of resistance for different exercises and allows you to use a choice of positions to train with more comfort and/or effectiveness. For example, to strengthen the posterior torso with hand-held weights, you need to be in a prone position in order to apply resistance to the back muscles. With elastic tubing, you can target the posterior torso in an upright position as well, a more comfortable position for some participants. TRX equipment allows you to train the posterior torso in semirecumbent to nearly supine positions.

There can be disadvantages to relying on equipment. The amount of equipment may limit class capacity. There is setup and transition time to consider. Additionally, even simple equipment can be intimidating for individuals. Consider using body weight exercise to counter potential disadvantages of utilizing equipment. Manipulating variables such as sequencing, exercise execution speed, and lever length can increase intensity. The angle or position of the body allows body weight and gravity to supply sufficient overload for some exercises.

Equipment is divided into two categories for strength classes: resistance and props. Resistance equipment encompasses all products that create overload on muscles. Props include products that act as an accessory for resistance training. A step platform, *e.g.*, acts as a weight bench to sit, to lie, or to stand on. With many products to choose from, it is easy to want to use as much as is available. Be thoughtful about the number of products used in a class. It will minimize intimidation, allow more room for people to attend, and you can make the most out of your class time. A good rule of thumb is no more than two pieces of resistance equipment and one prop (if necessary) for a class.

A certified exercise instructor is responsible for providing safe and effective exercise. This responsibility includes upkeep, maintenance, and evaluation of equipment used in class. Make sure all equipment is safe to use by inspecting it before your class begins. Remove equipment that is worn, frayed, or exhibits other signs of possible breakage or failure. A safe environment is also your responsibility. Ensure hand-wipes or other disinfectant is available for participants to use before and after handling equipment.

### Exercises

There are numerous exercises you can use in a strength training class. You are limited only by the equipment available, possibly by the abilities of your participants, and maybe by your imagination! When selecting exercises, you want the most effective choice that offers a manageable challenge and participant safety and success. Use the following filter to start the critical thinking process:

- What muscles am I working? When? Why? How?
- Does the movement achieve the stated goal of the exercise?
- Does the exercise train the primary function of the muscle?
- Does the movement compromise the safety of other body parts?
- How can the exercise be modified to meet the needs of all participants?
- Are you performing the exercise at a pace that can be controlled through a full ROM?
- Have I addressed the line of pull (TRX, elastic tubing) and body position relative to gravity (weighted resistance) for appropriate setup?
- Does a risk of injury outweigh the benefit of performing the exercise?

### Sequencing and Transitions

Depending on the overall goal of your class, there are many ways you may choose to sequence your classes. The following steps will help you select the best method.

#### Step 1: What is the goal of your class?

You must begin by determining what the goal of your class will be (if it is not defined by the title of the class). For example, are you interested in strength, endurance, functional or a combination of all three?

❑ Strength
❑ Endurance
❑ Functional
❑ Combination: _____ and _____

Once you determine the overall goal of the class, you will have a better idea of how long each exercise (or combination of exercises) should last. For example, if you are trying to create muscular strength gains, it's important to fatigue the muscle (or muscle group) within the anaerobic energy cycle (less than ~90 seconds). If you were trying to provide a muscular endurance experience, you would want to continue with an exercise for longer than the anaerobic energy cycle (more than ~90 seconds). Functional exercises may be any length of time.

*Step 2: How many exercises do I need?*

Based on how long you need to spend with each exercise, you can start to determine how many exercises you need to plan.

How long is the class? _____ minutes

How long will the warm-up be? _____ minutes

How long will the cool-down be? _____ minutes

How many minutes remain? _____ minutes (subtract warm-up and cool-down time from total class time; this will be how many minutes you have for exercises)

How many minutes to perform each exercise? _____ minutes (based on the goal of the class)

How many exercises can I do? _____ exercises (divide the number of minutes left by number of minutes to perform each exercise)

Once you know how many exercises you can do, you will need to decide if they will all be unique or if you will do sets (or repeat exercises). Consider performing exercises more than once to provide time to learn the movement and then perform the movement.

*Step 3: What muscles will I work?*

Next, determine which muscles you would like to work during your class. There are times when you might choose a specific focus (*i.e.* upper body or lower body), and there may be times where you choose to focus on the entire body. Your choice may be determined by the name of your class or how you organize your weekly workouts. Although it's not necessary to target every muscle in every workout, if you do not have a system to ensure the participants will experience exercises for all muscle groups in a week's time, you will want to provide at least one exercise for all major muscle groups. List the muscles (muscle groups) you would like to work here:

_____

_____

_____

*Step 4: What equipment will I use?*

As mentioned earlier, it is important to limit the amount of equipment you introduce to one class to maximize participation and minimize intimidation. The less equipment you use, the more people you can have in class and the less time you will spend changing equipment and explaining its use. You should be able to plan an effective class with two pieces of equipment for resistance and one prop (if necessary) (Tables 5.5 and 5.6).

Resistance Equipment:
❏ Dumbbells
❏ Weighted Bar
❏ Barbell
❏ Gliding Discs
❏ Tubing
❏ Suspension Trainer (TRX)

Prop:
❏ None
❏ Step
❏ BOSU Balance Trainer
❏ BOSU Ballast Ball
❏ Stability Ball

*Step 5: What Methods Should I Use?*

Depending on the equipment you use and the amount of overload you have, you will need to experiment with different types of sequencing to achieve the goal you desire for the class (*i.e.* strength, endurance, functional, combination).

**STRENGTH**    Strength is the most challenging. Chances are, the amount of weight you have available is not enough to fatigue every muscle within the anaerobic energy cycle (which is necessary). You will need to experiment with the following:

*Prefatigue*: exercising the assistor muscles first, before exercising the primary muscle (*e.g.*, performing triceps push-ups first, then overhead presses, and finally performing chest presses). When the assistor muscles are fatigued first, then the amount of weight necessary to fatigue the bigger muscle can be far less.

*Reverse Ordering*: reverse ordering works in similar fashion to prefatigue. You simply begin with all of the smaller muscle groups first, and then progress to the larger, which should make the amount of weight necessary for the larger muscles far less (*i.e.*, begin with shoulder exercises, then biceps, then triceps, then back and finally chest).

**ENDURANCE**    Endurance classes can generally use any type of sequencing because the time you spend in an exercise (longer than the anaerobic energy cycle) requires you to use less weight for all exercises. It is not necessarily the amount of weight you lift, but the amount of time you can 'endure' the weight you choose. It is a good idea to begin with larger muscle groups and progress to smaller when doing an endurance class to help sustain form as the core begins to fatigue. For endurance, you may experiment with the following:

*Super Setting*: alternating exercises to allow muscles to rest between sets; you may choose to do push/pull sets or upper body/lower body sets (*i.e.*, push-ups and then bent-over rows or overhead presses and then lunges).

*Cluster or Giant Setting*: choosing more than one exercise for a muscle group and performing them one after the other with little to no rest between exercises (*i.e.*, a chest press followed by chest fly and finishing with push-ups).

Or, you can simply choose to focus on one muscle group at a time and then move on to the next. Again, progressing from larger to smaller is the best option for an endurance class to ensure safety and effectiveness.

**FUNCTIONAL**    Functional classes should focus on multi-directional and multiplanar movements that are designed

| Table 5.5 | COMPARING TYPES OF RESISTANCE | |
|---|---|---|
| **RESISTANCE** | **ADVANTAGES** | **DISADVANTAGES** |
| Dumbbells | Offers bilateral and unilateral upper body exercises<br>Small increases in weight are possible<br>Familiar to most participants<br>Unobstructed ROM (can rotate wrists)<br>Core engaged in most exercises to stabilize body | Amount of weight available<br>May need several sets of dumbbells if working the entire body<br>New participants need close monitoring to ensure safety |
| Weighted bars (*i.e.,* BodyBars) | Bilateral and unilateral upper body exercise possible<br>Movement can involve rotation and twisting<br>Use as a balance support for lower body exercises<br>Variable positioning including off-center to produce core challenges<br>Padded for comfort<br>Minibars and flexible bars offer additional exercise options | Available in weight from 3 to 36 lb.<br>3-lb increments up to 18 lb; 6-lb increments up to 36 lb.<br>Heavier bars increase in diameter and could be more challenging to handle |
| Barbells | Wide range of weight available Small, incremental changes in weight possible<br>Small diameter of bar is easy to grasp | Only bilateral movements possible<br>Fixed wrist/hand position (no variation)<br>No padding (towel may be needed to pad the neck)<br>Adjustable barbells require clamps to secure weights to the bar |
| Elastic/rubber tubing (regular, covered, or cushioned) | Wide range of exercises possible<br>Able to focus on concentric and/or eccentric action<br>Unrestricted ROM<br>Subtle to substantial intensity changes are easy and quick to do<br>Partner training exercises possible<br>Tubing available from light to heavy resistance | Longevity of product (watch for wear or purchase covered tubing if possible)<br>Fear of elastic breaking<br>Can be uncomfortable when wrapped against skin<br>Learning curve for optimal use |
| Kettlebells | Unique exercises<br>Functional aspect of controlling<br>Momentum<br>Amount of weight available<br>Can challenge advanced exercisers<br>High metabolic demand | Requires thorough directions and explanation of technique<br>Requires close monitoring of movement execution<br>Adequate space required for safety<br>Weight and storage logistics may limit equipment availability<br>Learning curve for optimal use |
| Medicine balls | Unique exercises including partner training<br>Rotation, twisting, and PNF patterns<br>Easily integrated with lower body movements<br>Valuable for sports/athletic drills | Range of weighted balls required<br>Storage logistics when not in use (during class) |
| Soft weighted fitness balls | Unilateral and bilateral movements possible<br>Easy to grip and release at any time<br>Unrestricted ROM<br>Good for beginners and older adults | Amount of weight limited |
| Suspension Trainers (TRX) | Wide range of exercises possible<br>Unique exercises available<br>Core stability required to execute most movements<br>Positioning easily and quickly changes the intensity of exercise<br>Beneficial for sports and athletic conditioning<br>Exercise progression/regression easy to implement | Set-up requirements including anchoring space logistics<br>Amount of units available for the amount of participants<br>Equipment may not be convenient to utilize (set up in another area)<br>Learning curve required for optimal use<br>Requires thorough instruction and close monitoring for safety and effectiveness |
| Gliding discs | Unique sliding property creates dynamic exercise challenge<br>Wide variety of exercises possible<br>Balance and stability challenges<br>Portable, affordable<br>Beneficial for cardio and strength training | Limited for upper body exercise<br>Learning curve required for optimal use<br>Moderate skill required |
| **Props** | | |
| Stability ball | Acts as a bench (head and shoulder support for chest press, triceps, etc.)<br>Use as a chair (for seated curls, shoulder exercises with resistance)<br>Concurrent balance and stability training while performing other Exercises<br>Beneficial for posture, core strength, and coordination<br>Can also be used for cardio and flexibility exercise<br>Many unique exercises possible | Storage logistics<br>Unstable surface creates risk of losing balance<br>Requires slow, careful progressions<br>Difficult to monitor many people at once<br>Various sizes needed to accommodate all participants |

*(Continued)*

| Table 5.5 | COMPARING TYPES OF RESISTANCE *(CONTINUED)* | |
|---|---|---|
| **RESISTANCE** | **ADVANTAGES** | **DISADVANTAGES** |
| BOSU balance trainer (BT) | Acts as a bench (head and shoulder support for chest press, triceps, etc.)<br>Use dome side up as stability ball without the instability<br>Use dome side down as a balance board<br>Ability to perform a wide range of exercises standing, kneeling, seated, prone, or supine<br>Concurrent balance and stability training while performing other exercises<br>Can be used for cardio, strength, and flexibility exercise<br>Beneficial for sports/athletic conditioning and drills<br>Unique exercises possible | Unstable surface creates risk of losing balance<br>Learning curve required for optimal use<br>Storage logistics<br>Maintenance logistics (prone or supine positions on possible dirty surface after stepping on dome) |
| BOSU ballast ball | Acts as a bench (head and shoulder support for chest press, triceps, etc.)<br>Use as a chair (seated curls, shoulder exercises with resistance)<br>Use as a weighted resistance tool like a medicine ball with dynamic load<br>Simultaneous balance and stability training while performing various exercises on the ball<br>Beneficial for posture, core conditioning, and coordination<br>Unique exercises possible including cardio and flexibility exercise | Unstable surface creates risk of losing balance<br>One size, one weight may not comfortably accommodate some participants<br>Storage logistics |
| Step platforms | Stable surface<br>Use as a bench for strength training exercises<br>Use as a bench for cardio training and drills<br>Can use to elevate a leg during lower body exercises<br>Effective tool that offers low-, moderate-, or high-intensity cardio training in a low-impact mode | Requires proper storage for longevity<br>Learning curve possibly needed for cardio exercise |

ROM, range of motion.

to enhance core control as you move through space. You may choose to add the following:

*Balance:* adding balance movements (*e.g.,* reverse lunge to knee lift) or props that require balance to your exercises (*e.g.,* squatting on a BOSU Balance Trainer)

*Movement:* instead of performing stationary exercises, add movement such as forward lunge instead of stationary lunge

*Spinal Actions:* adding lateral flexion, spinal flexion, rotation, bending and twisting to exercises to challenge the core to control movement in and out of neutral spinal alignment (*i.e.,* adding rotation towards the front leg as you move into a forward lunge)

*Combinations:* linking exercises together increases the intensity and functionality of exercises (*e.g.,* squat to overhead press as you stand up)

*Multijoint Movements:* executing two movements simultaneously requires enhanced core control (*e.g.,* squat with an overhead press as you travel back and down)

Transitioning between movements will be different for each type of class you teach. In endurance and functional focused classes, you will most likely try to eliminate downtime by linking your exercises together (*i.e.,* after performing 16 lunge to knee lifts, you may hold the knee lift up and go into single leg squats with no break) or minimizing the time between exercises by previewing

the next move as you're finishing your current one (*i.e.,* "We are getting ready to move into push-ups after this last lunge; take the bar down and position yourself on your mat"). In strength classes, it is appropriate to take breaks between sets and allow time for the class to grab a drink of water, change weights, or reset for the next exercises if you'd like.

### Instructional Tips and Delivery

There are many cues available to help participants execute exercises with precision. A seven-step instructing process organizes cueing for strength exercise.

Step 1. Directions — The cueing of the movement. Identify the exercise by name. Describe how to execute the exercise. Directions are similar to movement cues discussed previously. You verbally describe the exercise task and/or physically demonstrate it (8).

Step 2. Explanation — Explain the purpose of the exercise. What muscles are involved? What are the joint actions? What should the participant be feeling? Explanations educate your class with a reason for doing the exercise.

Step 3. Body Awareness — Body awareness is everything that happens to support and facilitate execution of the primary action safely and effectively. This includes alignment, positioning or placement,

| Table 5.6 | SELECTING EQUIPMENT TO MATCH CLASS GOALS | | |
|---|---|---|---|
| **EXERCISE** | **AREA OF FOCUS** | **EQUIPMENT** | **NOTES** |
| Squats | Legs | Dumbbells, weighted bars, barbells, soft weighted fitness balls, medicine balls, gliding discs, BOSU, tubing, TRX, bodyweight, step platforms, BOSU ballast ball | Squats can be performed stationary (narrow, wide) or moving laterally. It is a multijoint exercise involving gluteals, quadriceps, hamstrings, gastrocnemius, tibialis anterior, and other muscles as assistant movers and stabilizers. Considered one of the most effective functional exercises for the lower body. Upper body exercises can be added for additional challenge (*i.e.*, squat — overhead press). |
| Lunges | Legs | Dumbbells, weighted bars, barbells, soft weighted fitness balls, medicine balls, gliding discs, BOSU, tubing, TRX, bodyweight, steps, BOSU ballast ball | Lunges can be performed stationary, moving forward, moving back, moving side to side, or traveling. There are endless possibilities for adding lunges to a strength training class. Upper body exercises can easily be added to lunges (*i.e.*, lunge — biceps curl). |
| Deadlift | Legs | Dumbbells, weighted bars, barbells, soft weighted fitness balls, medicine balls, kettlebells, tubing | Deadlifts can be performed with two feet on the ground (narrow or wider), staggered stance, or balancing on one leg. Depending on the equipment used, variations for the balance challenge |
| Plie squat | Legs | Dumbbells, weighted bars, barbells, soft weighted fitness balls, medicine balls, gliding discs, BOSU BT, Tubing, TRX, bodyweight, steps, BOSU ballast ball | Plie squats can be performed with two feet on the ground, moving side to side, or one foot elevated on top of a prop (BOSU balance trainer or step) |
| Bridging | Legs | Gliding discs, step, BOSU BT, BOSU ballast ball, stability ball, tubing, weighted bar, TRX, body weight | Bridging can be performed with feet hip distance apart, together, elevated on a ball, platform, BOSU balance trainer (either side). You can perform with two legs or one leg. |
| Hamstring curl | Legs | Gliding discs, BOSU BT, BOSU ballast ball, stability ball, tubing, weighted bar, TRX | Hamstring curls require the beginning position of a bridge to be elevated or on the gliding discs. You can perform with two legs or one. You can also perform a hamstring curl standing. |
| Knee extension | Legs | Body weight, weighted bar, tubing | Knee extensions can be performed standing on a solid surface or an unstable BOSU balance trainer. |
| Abduction | Legs | Body weight, weighted bar, tubing, BOSU balance trainer, TRX | Abduction can be performed standing or side lying. |
| Adduction | Legs | Body weight, weighted bar, tubing, BOSU balance trainer, TRX | Adduction can be performed standing or side lying. |
| Bent over row | Back | Dumbbells, weighted bars, barbells, tubing | Bent over rows can be performed bilaterally or unilaterally, with feet hip distance, wider or staggered. |
| Lat pull down | Back | Tubing | Lat pull down can be performed standing or kneeling. |
| Scapular depression | Back | Tubing, body weight | Scapular depression can be performed standing or kneeling. |
| Scapular retraction | Back | Tubing, body weight | Scapular retraction can be performed standing or kneeling. |
| Back extension | Back | Body weight, BOSU balance trainer, stability ball, BOSU ballast ball, TRX, gliding discs | Back extension can be performed with a variety of arm positions (the longer the lever, the harder the back extension). |
| Chest press | Chest | Dumbbells, weighted bars, barbell, tubing, TRX, soft weighted fitness balls | Chest press can be performed bilaterally or unilaterally (when using tubing, dumbbells, or soft weighted fitness balls). If using tubing, the chest press can be performed standing or lying. You can use the floor, a step, a ball, or BOSU balance trainer as the surface for the chest press. |
| Chest fly | Chest | Dumbbells, weighted bars, barbell, tubing, TRX, soft weighted fitness balls | Chest fly can be performed bilaterally or unilaterally (when using tubing, dumbbells or soft weighted fitness balls). If using tubing, the chest fly can be performed standing or lying. You can use the floor, a step, a ball or BOSU balance trainer as the surface for the chest press. |
| Push-up | Chest | Body weight, TRX, gliding discs, BOSU balance trainer, BOSU ballast ball, stability ball | Push-ups can be performed with a variety of hand positions (narrow, wide, staggered) and be done stationary or moving side to side. Using a balance trainer or ball increases the balance challenge. |
| Biceps curl | Biceps | Dumbbells, weighted bars, barbell, tubing, TRX, soft weighted fitness balls | Biceps curls can be performed bilaterally or unilaterally (if using tubing, dumbbells, or soft weighted fitness balls). The hand position can be palms up, palms down, or palms in. You may experiment with the angle of the biceps curl, as well (straight front or angled on the diagonal). |

*(Continued)*

| Table 5.6 | SELECTING EQUIPMENT TO MATCH CLASS GOALS *(CONTINUED)* | | |
|---|---|---|---|
| **EXERCISE** | **AREA OF FOCUS** | **EQUIPMENT** | **NOTES** |
| Triceps press | Triceps | Dumbbells, weighted bars, barbell, tubing, soft weighted fitness balls | Triceps press can be performed bilaterally or unilaterally (if using dumbbells, tubing, or soft weighted fitness balls). You can use the floor, a step, a ball, or BOSU balance trainer as the surface for the chest press. |
| Triceps extension | Triceps | Dumbbells, weighted bars, barbell, TRX, soft weighted fitness balls | Triceps extension can be performed bilaterally or unilaterally (if using dumbbells, tubing or soft weighted fitness balls). A triceps extension can be performed lying down, standing or kneeling. You can use the floor, a step, a ball or BOSU balance trainer as the surface for the chest press. |
| Triceps kickback | Triceps | Dumbbells, weighted bars, tubing, TRX, soft weighted fitness balls | Triceps kickback can be performed standing (feet hip distance or staggered stance) or kneeling (on mat or unstable surface). You can perform the exercise bilaterally or unilaterally (if using dumbbells, tubing, or soft weighted fitness balls). |
| Triceps push-up | Triceps | Body weight, TRX, BOSU balance trainer, BOSU ballast ball, stability ball | Triceps push-ups can be performed on a mat or BOSU balance trainer or using a ball as a prop. |
| Overhead press | Shoulders | Dumbbells, weighted bars, barbell, tubing, soft weighted fitness balls | Overhead press can be performed standing or kneeling, unilateral or bilateral (if using dumbbells, tubing, or soft weighted fitness balls). The palms can be facing forward or in or rotate as you press up. |
| Front raise | Shoulders | Dumbbells, weighted bars, barbell, tubing, soft weighted fitness balls | Front raise can be performed standing or kneeling, unilateral or bilateral (if using dumbbells, tubing, or soft weighted fitness balls). The palms can be facing down, in or up. |
| Side raise | Shoulders | Dumbbells, weighted bars, tubing, soft weighted fitness balls | Side raise can be performed standing or kneeling, unilateral or bilateral (if using dumbbells, tubing, or soft weighted fitness balls). The palms can be facing down or straight forward. |
| Reverse fly | Shoulders | Dumbbells, weighted bars, tubing, soft weighted fitness balls | Reverse fly can be performed standing (feet hip distance or staggered) or lying, unilateral or bilateral (if using dumbbells, tubing, or soft weighted fitness balls). The palms can be facing in, back or forward. |
| Upright row | Shoulders | Dumbbells, weighted bars, barbell, tubing, soft weighted fitness balls | Upright row can be performed standing or kneeling, unilateral or bilateral (if using dumbbells, tubing, or soft weighted fitness balls). |
| Shoulder extension | Shoulders | Dumbbells, weighted bars, tubing, soft weighted fitness balls | Shoulder extension can performed standing or kneeling, unilateral or bilateral (if using dumbbells, tubing, or soft weighted fitness balls). |

breathing, technique, and form. You want to consolidate oft-repeated body awareness cues for easier assimilation. For example, *"Bend the knees, brace your core by pulling in and tightening the abdominals, shoulders back and down, weight slightly forward over the toes, hands up in front of you in a light fist,"* can be condensed to, *"Athletic stance, ready!"* (12).

Step 4. Stimulation — Imagery and visualization. When verbal instructions provide a strong visual image that participants can associate with performing an exercise, learning the coordination required by the skill becomes much easier (12). Stimulation includes goal-oriented cues (numerical or timed, *i.e.,* *"I'd like you to go for 12 repetitions"*) and process-oriented goals (internal focus, awareness of sensations, quality of movement, breathing pattern, *e.g.,* *"Feel like you're melting into the ground with every exhale,"* or, *"Notice how your back feels during the exercise. Maintain this awareness as you continue to move."*)

Step 5. Action Words — The motivational words and phrases to promote desired movement quality or to facilitate the appropriate effort from the participants.

This includes numerical countdowns selectively placed to inspire and push through a challenging effort (e.g., *"You have just four more, three more…"*).

Step 6. Evaluation — Observe, assess, correct, assist, and adjust. Every repetition matters. Provide feedback and modifications either individually, to the group as a whole, nonverbally through body language, using hands-on assistance, or helping an individual after the workout finishes. A common misconception is that the more often you give feedback, the more effective it is in helping participants learn a movement. Feedback provided less frequently than every practice attempt is more beneficial than feedback during or after every attempt (12).

Step 7. Acknowledgments — Recognize participant efforts with compliments, encouragement, and positive reinforcement. An acknowledgement is more meaningful when it has a participant's name attached to it (7).

Theoretically, you go through the seven steps for each strength exercise you perform. In reality, this does not, and should not, always happen. It is easy to overcommunicate when teaching strength exercise (19). However, if the participant rarely gets to move, he/she will not have much opportunity to get it right or be able to put your great cues to use (23). The following cueing strategy will prioritize the seven-step teaching process: *preview, do, cue.*

A. Preview — Identify the upcoming exercise, muscle groups targeted, and how to adjust resistance. This means verbalizing what is about to happen in as few words as possible to get them headed in the right direction (23). It is also helpful to provide suggestions for the amount of resistance to use based on your desired outcome and the number of sets and repetitions you have planned. Example, "*Next will be overhead press for the shoulders* (direction). *It requires less weight than what you're using now. You're doing one set, 16 repetitions maximum* (stimulation).

B. Do — Explain the major joint actions with an economy of words (explanation) and demonstrate the movement to help participants understand the exercise (13). It is helpful to demonstrate at half tempo if you can. When you take time to do the movement slowly, participants (whether they know the exercise or not) have a better chance of doing it correctly in the upcoming set (19).

C. Cue — Focus on the most crucial elements to perform the exercise safely and effectively (13). Avoid the temptation to give every possible cue for the exercise you are performing. By highlighting one or two areas of focus, participants will have a better opportunity to get it right and feel successful (19). For example, you may focus on keeping the shoulders down and maintaining core stability (body awareness). Next week, change the emphasis to another element (*i.e.,* breathing or alignment).

Within the *preview, do, cue* strategy, you mix in the last three steps of the seven-step teaching process — appropriate action words, evaluative feedback, and acknowledgement of effort. People find motivational words/ phrases are helpful especially when nearing muscular fatigue. Constantly be scanning your floor for safety and effectiveness. Participants are motivated by genuinely positive feedback for their genuinely dedicated effort.

### When Failure is Success

We have talked about the importance of participants feeling and being successful in an exercise class, both in cardio exercise and strength exercise. For strength exercise, there is a paradox. You should avoid exercises so complex that participants fail to be able to do them. However, you want participants to use sufficient resistance on strength exercises to come close to achieving momentary muscular fatigue or experiencing temporary muscular failure. Muscular fatigue or failure is an indication there was enough overload to stimulate a strength training effect (23).

A goal-oriented cue helps to motivate individuals by defining the amount of work to do to complete a task. Achieving the goal will result in a feeling of success. When you give a goal-oriented cue such as, "*You have one set of eight repetitions,*" you can acknowledge the completion of the task. Some individuals may be unable to complete the stated goal (number of repetitions) because they hit muscular fatigue. They also deserve compliments as you would bestow upon those who complete the task. In this sense, "failure" *is* success, as long as failing is a result of overload in contrast to the inability to do an exercise because it is too difficult or complex to learn. The difference is important. Some participants may perceive an inability to perform all repetitions of a strength exercise as a weakness. Yet, those individuals received more of a strength stimulus from the exercise set than the others in class who were able to complete the set with ease. By educating participants about the objective in strength training, you can foster self-efficacy as they "fail" during specific exercises (23). Be certain everyone receives positive feedback, not just the individuals who are able to achieve a stated amount of repetitions to perform.

## Ask the Pro

# What are some teaching tips for group exercise?

**SHERRI MCMILLAN**
*Director, Northwest Women's Fitness Club,*
*Vancouver, Washington*

Cue regularly and with enough prewarning. Use inspirational cueing whenever you can. Have fun with countdowns by having your class join in — and not timidly either — their vocal intensity can effectively energize the group. Make every class manageable, success-oriented, and option-oriented. The next hour should be the best part of your participants' day — you make the difference.

With this in mind, mix in process-oriented cues intermittently with goal-oriented cues. Process-oriented cues downplay or exclude numerical goals altogether and ask participants to direct their focus inward on the quality of movement and awareness of how the body feels during the exercise. This type of cue works well with different ability levels in the same class because it does not push individuals to work beyond what is safe for them (2). With a process-oriented cue, prepare as you would for any strength exercise except to state how many repetitions to do. Maintain count of the repetitions performed to yourself, knowing that you will stop at a predetermined amount depending on your specific objective (strength, endurance, etc.). Reinforce their goal is to achieve muscular fatigue rather than perform a certain number of repetitions. Once they can no longer perform the exercise with correct form, they should stop (23). You should acknowledge this point with copious amounts of positive feedback (*e.g., You had to stop? Way to go — excellent.*") As you are nearing the end of the set, cue for the last few repetitions so participants can make the most out of those final repetitions (*i.e., "For those who can, you have a few more reps — make each repetition count. If you have to stop, yes, that's great*").

Upon completing an exercise set, inquire about the intensity level your participants selected and give appropriate guidance based upon the responses you receive. For example, when you have finished a shoulder exercise ask, "Who could have done a few more repetitions?" Suggest a small increase in resistance for the next time. Also inquire about who was unable to complete at least a few repetitions, and recommend to lower the resistance in the next attempt. Educate participants about the value of achieving momentary muscular fatigue (within a certain time period and repetition range), and give positive feedback when that occurs. Encourage participants to use sufficient overload so they will succeed in obtaining the multitude of benefits from strength training.

### Music Suggestions

Strength classes typically require slower tempo music than cardio classes. Music from 110 to 128 bpm is used, with 120 to 124 bpm being the most common tempo range heard. This tempo range has been used for strength exercises for many decades, yet there is no research to support or oppose it. It happens to be the most popular tempo range in commercially produced pop and dance music. There is more music in this tempo range than any other speed, giving you more music to choose from for your strength classes. Here is an application example of music tempo for an abdominal curl:

- Beginners: Curl-up for 2 counts, lower down for 6 counts

- Intermediate: Curl-up on 4 counts, lower down on 4 counts
- Advanced: Curl-up on 6 counts, lower down on 2 counts

All levels take 8 counts to complete 1 repetition, with beginners spending more time on the easier eccentric phase, while advanced participants spend more time on the more challenging concentric phase of the exercise.

It is not only the speed of the music that is important, but also the speed at which you decide to execute the exercise. It is a primary variable you control for adjusting exercise intensity. Of course, it may be necessary to allow participants to move off the beat to maintain form. Keep in mind, slower tempos ensure momentum is minimized thus allowing the muscles to do more work.

## SUMMARY

*Class design and delivery is a multifaceted concept. It entails establishing a class goal or objective, assessing participant abilities and preferences, a determination of equipment availability, and how such equipment will be utilized. Cardio training can be presented in a nonchoreographed or choreographed format, including freestyle, 32-count combinations, organized-action, or choreographed methods, all closely linked to how music is utilized in class. Elements of change allow you to develop numerous cardiovascular movements, routines, patterns, and drills for participant variety and motivation. Elements of class delivery including movement, safety, technique, and motivational cues enhance participant success by providing the information needed to perform an exercise safely and effectively.*

*You have a wide variety of exercises available for strength training in group exercise. Determine the muscle groups to target, select the equipment to use, decide on the exercises to do, and incorporate the appropriate training techniques to facilitate your goals. As important as planning and selecting exercises is how you teach them. You have to provide the right amount of instruction to understand what to do without causing information overload for participants.*

*In the end, you are not just teaching exercise. You are teaching people. You teach people how exercise will positively impact their lives. You are not just instructing how to do a lunge. You instruct people on how a lunge is important for activities of daily living. You are not just leading an exercise class. You are leading people on a journey where they reconnect with their bodies and experience how good they can feel with the right kind of physical movement. You are the catalyst that helps them feel better about themselves. That, in turn, makes them feel better about the world around them. You have a lot of power and influence in front of the class. It is extremely rewarding when used wisely.*

# References

1. Alan K. Step by step instruction. *American Fitness*. Sherman Oaks, CA Aerobics and Fitness Association of America, 1994.

2. Alan K, Jones C. Teaching and leadership skills. In: Jones C, Rose D, editors. *Physical Activity Instruction of Older Adults*. Champaign (IL): Human Kinetics; 2005. p. 301–5.

3. Biscontini L. Reaching out to newcomers. *IDEA Fitness Edge*. 2002;3(5):1–4.

4. Brick L. *Fitness Aerobics*. Champaign (IL): Human Kinetics; 1996.

5. Brown P. An enquiry into the origins and nature of tempo behavior: II. Experimental work. *Psychol Music*. 1979;9:32–43.

6. Carter JM. The effects of stability ball training on spinal stability in sedentary individuals. *J Strength Cond Res*. 2006;20(2):429–35.

7. Clark J. Designing and managing group conditioning classes. In: Jones C, Rose D, eds. *Physical Activity Instruction of Older Adults*. Champaign (IL): Human Kinetics; 2005. p. 317–33.

8. Graniel L. The cuing connection. *IDEA Health and Fitness Source*. 2004;4 [Internet] San Diego (CA): IDEA [cited 2011 Jun 21]. Available from: http://www.idrafit.com/files/pdf/fitness-library/cuing-connection.

9. Karageorghis C, Jones L, Low D. Relationship between exercise heart rate and music. *Res Q Exercise Sport*. 2006;77:2:240–50.

10. Karageorghis C, Terry P, Lane A. Development and validation of an instrument to assess the motivational qualities of music in exercise and sport: The Brunel Music Rating Inventory. *J Sport Sci*. 1999;17:713–24.

11. Lee I, Jones J. *In Full Bloom: A Brain Education Guide for Successful Aging*. Sedona (AZ): Best Life Media; 2008.

12. Magill R. Augmented feedback in motor skill acquisition. In: Singer R, Hausenblaus H, Janelle C, editors. *Handbook of Research on Sport Psychology*. New York (NY): Wiley; 2001. p. 86–114.

13. Magill R, Grodesky J. Applying motor learning principles to program design. In: Jones C, Rose D, editors. *Physical Activity Instruction of Older Adults*. Champaign (IL): Human Kinetics; 2005. p. 284–99.

14. Nichols J. *The Effects of Stability Ball Training on Functional Strength and Balance of Older Adults*. Abstract presented at the Southwest ACSM, November 1999.

15. Priest D, Karageorghis C, Sharp N. The characteristics and effects of motivational music in exercise settings: The possible influence of gender, age, frequency of attendance, and time of attendance. *J Sport Med Phys Fit*. 2004;44:77–86.

16. Biscontini, L. Resist-a-ball. Creating Cardio Combos with Resist-a-. Ball. *CanFitPro*. September/October 2010; 42–4.

17. Scharff-Olson M, Henry N. The energy cost associated with selected step training exercise techniques. *Research Quarterly for Exercise and Sport*. American Alliance for Health, Physical Education, Recreation and Dance (AAHPERD). 1996.

18. Schroeder J, Dolan S. 2010 IDEA fitness programs & equipment trends. *IDEA Fit J*. 2010;7:7:22–31.

19. Simmons R. The critical loop in quality instruction. *IDEA Fitness Edge*. 1998;1:5:1–6.

20. Thompson WR, ed. *ACSM's Resources for the Personal Trainer*. 3rd ed. Philadelphia (PA): Lippincott Williams & Wilkins; 2010. p. 124–53.

21. Vlachopoulos S, Karageorghis C. Interaction of external, introjected, and identified regulation with intrinsic motivation in exercise and the relationship with exercise enjoyment. *J Appl Biobehav Res*. 2005;10:113–32.

22. Vogel A. Future deliverables in the fitness industry. *IDEA Fit J*. 2007;4:5:2–7.

23. Williams-Evans K. When teaching 'failure" leads to success. *IDEA Fit J*. 2004;1:5:78–81.

# 6

# Teaching Your Class: A Quick Guide

TERI L. BLADEN • LIZA FORSTER

## Objectives

**At the end of this chapter you will be able to:**

· Apply concepts presented in chapters of this manual to a "day-of" scenario for teaching a group exercise class
· Troubleshoot barriers to effectively teaching a group exercise class
· Take theoretical concepts described in this manual and put them into practice
· Understand and execute use of the "I'm OK" rule

In this chapter, we pull together the concepts used in other chapters to explore the "day of" aspects of teaching an effective and enjoyable group exercise class. Think of this chapter as a summary and guide for your very first class or a guide that you come back to as a refresher. This chapter also features the "I'm OK" rule that is unique to this chapter and this publication.

Chances are you became a group exercise instructor, or aspire to become a group exercise instructor, because you had an incredible experience as a participant. Do you remember what it was about the class(es) that made it a great experience? Was it the instructor? The format? The environment? It was likely all of the above and other intangible elements. A truly great group exercise instructor goes beyond facilitating exercise by creating a great experience for all participants and makes it look effortless. Participants don't generally think about how it happens; they just know they had a great experience. Recall the factors that motivated you to get involved with group exercise and channel that great energy as you head in to teach your class.

## PLAN YOUR WORK AND WORK YOUR PLAN

Have your class plan ready and commit it to memory (see Box 6.1 for a sample class plan). Know:

· The goals and objectives of the class (what do you want participants to perform, know, and feel after the class? What are their desired results?)
· The music you will use (if any)
· Your choreography and sequencing of the choreography (the overall routine)
· How much time you will allot to each section of the class

· What equipment you will use and how to use the equipment properly
· How you can modify the plan based on "last minute changes"

Safety begins with the instructor having a solid knowledge of how the body moves and how it responds to exercise (you'll cover this in Part III of this book), as well as how to put together exercises and choreography that meet the physiological goals of the class format while effectively communicating that information to participants (Chapters 3–5). You should also be familiar with the emergency action plan designed for the facility at which you instruct, as well as your role in that emergency action plan (are you a first responder to an accident in your class or do you recruit the assistance of other facility staff to handle the accident?). As for "day-of" safety, consider the following items.

## CLASS ENVIRONMENT

Ensure you have appropriate space to conduct your class format (a traditional high/low-impact format most likely requires traveling and more space than a step format). A general strategy you can employ is to envision participants standing with both arms out in a "T" formation to allow them (at a minimum) that amount of space. Ensure the floor is clear of debris or objects that can be tripped over. Ensure the floor has adequate traction for movement (not too slippery). A carpeted floor may add too much traction; be prepared to modify pivot turns (Fig. 6.1) and quick lateral moves.

The space should be well lit, unless the format calls for lower lighting (a yoga or Pilates class might use lower lighting than a Zumba® format) The ACSM's Health/Fitness Facility Standards and Guidelines recommend a lighting level of 50 ft candles at eye level for

| BOX 6.1 | *Sample Class Plan* |
|---|---|

**Class Format:** Step

**Class Time:** 60 minutes

**Class Goals:** Cardiovascular endurance, coordination, core endurance, flexibility

## WARM-UP

**Duration:** 7 minutes

**Instructer Interaction:** In front of room, facing participants

**Equipment:** Step platforms and risers

**Music:** Energetic, upbeat; ~125 beats per minute (bpm)

**Notes:** Gradually prepare body for activity using large dynamic movement and dynamic stretches; incorporate rehearsal moves

## CARDIO

**Duration:** 30 minutes

**Instructer Interaction:** Move to side and back of room as determined by choreography; exercise with participants (not facing them) during more complicated moves

**Equipment:** Step platforms and risers

**Music:** Energetic, upbeat; does not exceed 128 bpm

**Notes:** Begin with simpler, lower intensity moves and gradually progress to more complex and/or higher intensity moves; follow a bell curve of intensity and stop the group at the peak for a water break and intensity check; continue at higher intensity encouraging participants to modify as needed; gradual decrease in intensity progressing to cardio cool-down

## CARDIO COOL-DOWN

**Duration:** 6 minutes

**Instructer Interaction:** In front of room, facing participants

**Equipment:** Step platforms and risers

**Music:** Energetic, upbeat; ~125 bpm

**Notes:** A noticeable change in energy, still strong but gradual decrease in intensity and movement moving to smaller ranges of motion and stationary movement; end with brief standing isometric stretches for muscle groups worked most during routine; includes 1-minute transition: drink water, put away steps, get mats

## CORE

**Duration:** 10 minutes

**Instructer Interaction:** Demonstrate moves at front of class, then walk around monitoring form and giving feedback

**Equipment:** Mats

**Music:** Strong beat, ~128 bpm

**Notes:** Begin with exercises that engage multiple muscle groups and wrap up with exercises that isolate a muscle group more specifically, *i.e.*, begin with plank, then do sit-ups and back extensions

**BOX 6.1, cont.**

**FINAL STRETCH**

**Duration:** 7 minutes

**Instructer Interaction:** Face the class as much as possible, mirror stretches for students.

**Equipment:** Mats

**Music:** Relaxing, mindful

**Notes:** Focus on all major muscle groups, especially ones worked during cardio section; lengthen to the point of slight discomfort, not pain

**BOX 6.2  Teaching your Class Checklist**

- Arrive 10–15 minutes before your class starts.
- Check the audio equipment (stereo and microphone) to ensure it is working properly; set up your music, check volume of music and microphone (stay within industry guidelines for sound levels); play inviting music while students are coming in and you are finishing setting up.
- Check facility safety: Walk the exercise space for tripping/slipping hazards, ensure space is adequate for the activity, ensure temperature/humidity is comfortable, lighting appropriate for activity.
- Set up equipment needed for class; check for any damaged or worn equipment.
- Greet participants as they enter the room, let them know what equipment they will need, ask if they need assistance with how to use or set up equipment. Visit with new comers. Use the ACSM Quick Screen described in Chapters 2.
- Check participant attire as they come in; attire and footwear should allow for safe movement appropriate to the activity.
- Begin class on time.
- Welcome the group and thank them for coming, introduce yourself, and give a brief overview of the class.
- Inform participants of classroom safety procedures, point out location of water fountains, intensity monitoring charts, methods etc.
- Ask if anyone is new to this activity, give them permission to modify movement and go at intensity that is challenging yet doable for them; ask if participants have any conditions that may require movement or intensity modifications, and generally share those modifications.
- Ask if there are any questions before getting started.
- Conduct warm-up, stimulus, cool-down, and final stretch: throughout each section of the class, demonstrate proper form and technique, incorporate verbal and nonverbal instructional cues to optimize communication/safety/motivation, monitor participants' performance using observation and participant feedback techniques, offer exercise modifications based on individual and group needs, educate participants on health and fitness-related information to enhance knowledge, enjoyment, and adherence.
- As you end the class, congratulate the group on a good workout and ask them to let you know if they have any questions or feedback.
- Respond to participants' concerns professionally incorporating conflict management and customer service strategies as needed.
- Instruct participants how to properly put away any equipment.
- Be available after the class to answer any questions individuals may have.
- Thank participants for joining you, and let them know you hope to see them again soon.
- Properly put away your own equipment, ensure audio equipment is off and properly stored/secured, secure room as needed following that facility's policy.

## CREATE A SAFE ENVIRONMENT

Safety should be a paramount concern for the group exercise instructor. While a participant may be more concerned about how effective the class is in meeting their fitness goals or how much fun they are having, it is the responsibility of the group exercise instructor to provide a safe experience.

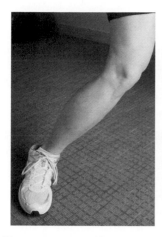 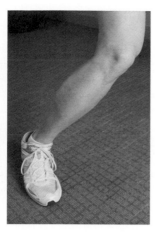

■ **FIGURE 6.1** Avoid pivot turns on carpet. Activities that require pivoting movements — dance-based styles, boxing, and kickboxing are not good choices on carpet; avoid or modify.

most activities (1). Make certain it is not too hot or too cold in your workout space (see environmental concerns, Chapter 3 for details). If you have no control over the temperature, be prepared to modify or even cancel the activity. Any facility or equipment concerns should always be brought to the attention of the facility maintenance or management staff, preferably in the form of a "Facility Maintenance Request Form" for easy tracking. Confirm equipment/facility protocols with your supervisor or the facility's management.

## EXERCISE EQUIPMENT

Make certain the equipment used in the format you are teaching is free from defects. Steps should be checked for tripping hazards and traction, resistance tubing and bands should be checked for tears or fraying, indoor bikes should be checked for pedal/seat/handlebar integrity, dumbbells or weighted bars should be checked for cracks or loose heads, etc. As noted above, report any facility or equipment concerns to facility maintenance or management staff, following established facility protocols.

## AUDIO EQUIPMENT

Ensure your microphone and music are at appropriate auditory levels, as noted in Chapter 3. It is good practice to be prepared with more than one form of music, *e.g.,* an MP3 player and a CD.

## APPROPRIATE ATTIRE

Participants should wear clothing that allows them to move comfortably and safely. Instructors should maintain a professional appearance and avoid provocative or sloppy gear. Keep in mind workout attire that shows a lot of skin (short shorts, sports bras only) can be intimidating to participants who have body image sensitivity and detract your credibility as a leader. Most formats require

an athletic shoe that fully encloses and supports the foot, while other formats (aqua fitness, yoga, and Pilates) may not require shoes at all. More formal dance formats (ballroom, tap, or salsa), may call for footwear specific to that activity rather than a traditional athletic shoe.

## KNOW YOUR PARTICIPANTS

Per Chapter 2, Profile of a Group Exercise Participant: Health Screening Tools, be aware of participants' health issues that may impact their ability to perform the class format, and be prepared to offer exercise modifications. Use appropriate motivational strategies covered in Chapter 4.

## CREATING A WELCOMING ENVIRONMENT

Have you ever approached a receptionist at a business and just stood there waiting for him or her to acknowledge you? It can be an awkward and frustrating experience. Keep this in mind as you prepare the environment for your group exercise classes. In the case of novices who have recently made the commitment to get healthy, joining a group exercise class for the first time can be an overwhelming situation. Do your best to make them feel included and welcome. Consider the strategies discussed in Chapter 4, "Communication Skills: Adherence and Motivation, as you review the "day-of" items listed below.

**Be available before class.** Arrive 10–15 minutes before your class starts in order to set up but also to interact with participants and answer any questions they may have. This is also a good time to apply cognitive and behavioral strategies that enhance motivation and adherence, as addressed in Chapter 4.

**Be prepared.** As mentioned earlier, be very comfortable with your class plan. Practicing your choreography as participants are entering your class is unprofessional and impedes your ability to interact with them.

**Greet participants as they enter your class.** Remember the receptionist example above? Acknowledge participants as soon as they enter your class. You do not need to stop what you are doing as you are setting up your class, just be sure to look up and make eye contact, smile, say "Hi!" and "Thanks for coming in today." This is also a good time to let them know what, if any, equipment is needed for the class.

**Acknowledge the "newbies."** If you notice someone new to your class, spend a little extra time with them. Introduce yourself and ask them their name. Introduce them to other participants in the class. Employ the use of the ACSM Quick Screen. Inquire if they've done this format before, and let them know what to expect. Give them an opportunity to ask questions in this one-on-one setting before the class gets started. This is why it is important to be prepared for your class, so you can take a little time to make new participants feel welcome.

**Introduce yourself and give a class overview.** As you begin to teach your class, introduce yourself and briefly explain the class format. Review and explain the "I'm OK" rule described later in this chapter.

**Face the class where appropriate.** Your participants will feel more connected and engaged if you face them rather than facing the mirror and "performing." Facing the group during the warm-up is a great time to make that connection. You may need to face away from participants during more complicated exercise segments, but try to reconnect with them during the cardio cool-down and final stretch.

**Avoid negative speak and competition.** While some participants thrive on competition and may appreciate a "drill sergeant" approach from the instructor, many participants can be intimidated or "turned off" by those tactics. Keep the atmosphere positive and supportive. Avoid cues such as "Don't do this…" and replace instead with "Try this…" Be encouraging and patient.

**Create group cohesion.** Refer to communication strategies discussed in Chapter 4. Learn your participants' names and call them by name throughout the routine. Within reason, get to know your participants so the group can sing "Happy Birthday" or wish someone happy anniversary on those special days. Create choreography that allows the group to interact (form two lines across from each other, have participants jog toward each other, give a "high five" in the center, and then jog back) or choose partner exercises for muscle conditioning. These activities allow participants to have fun and feel part of the group, which can keep them coming back. This will have a positive impact on their exercise adherence.

**Thank participants for coming to your class.** As you wrap up your class, a little "Thanks for coming to class today" and/or "Hope to see you next week!" shows that you appreciate participants' efforts in getting fit and that you care enough to hope you will see them again. Small, genuine expressions of this kindness can really make a difference in a participant's experience.

**Be available after your class.** Make time for a short while after your class to answer any questions participants may have. This demonstrates that you care about their success in your classes.

**Do your best to make participants feel welcome and a part of the group.**

## SET THE EXPECTATION/GOAL

Another method to ensure participant success in your group exercise classes is to let them know what to expect.

As part of your introduction, give a brief overview of what the class will entail (*e.g.*, a warm-up, the specific class format, a bit of core training, and a final stretch). If the class is focused on cardio, explain how to get the desired cardiovascular response (*e.g.*, "Our goal today is to really get the heart rate up, so be sure to use full range of motion, cover large distance when traveling on the floor"). For a muscle conditioning class, let participants know that muscular fatigue or endurance is the goal and to use resistance accordingly. In an indoor cycling class, give participants an overview of the ride profile; let them know if the focus is on endurance, speed, strength, or a combination of the aforementioned. For aqua fitness classes, let participants know that even though cardiovascular training may be a goal, they can also expect a certain amount of muscular conditioning due to the viscosity of water. In a flexibility class, inform them to strive for length in the muscle fibers and to hold the stretches with patience. You do not have to go into great detail; a simple overview will suffice. Then throughout the workout, be sure to reiterate or revisit the goals you stated in your introduction. If you have newcomers, be sure to remind them to work at their own pace as they develop their level of fitness.

## GIVE PERMISSION

So often the fitness realm is permeated with a "harder, stronger, faster" mentality. Some participants still function under a "no pain, no gain" premise. It is your responsibility as the group exercise instructor to lead participants safely through the exercise class, and this includes giving participants permission to modify movement as needed so that they get the desired physiological response within their individual parameters. If someone is recovering from a cold, give them permission to work out at a lower intensity. Encourage individuality within the group while letting them know that you will coach them to do their best. A responsible group exercise instructor shows high-intensity options, but generally performs at moderate intensity while instructing so participants do not feel obligated to perform at the higher intensity.

## SET THE GROUND RULES

Most often, group exercise classes are a fun and engaging experience. As with any group of people, distractions or disruptions can occur, and it helps to have some basic ground rules to assist with smooth operations. The facility in which the class is held may have specific policies and procedures you need to enforce. If working independently, you may need to develop your own policies and procedures. Be tactful and supportive when reminding participants of the rules, and help them understand why the rule or policy exists. There may also be less formal policies that will assist you in facilitating a smooth class.

You may want to have a "warm-up rule" or a "10-minute rule" whereby if a participant misses the warm-up or first 10 minutes of class, they are not allowed to enter. While this appears contrary to creating a welcoming environment, missing the warm-up can be a safety issue if the person jumps into the activity without properly warming up, and they may have missed important choreography review in the beginning. Tactfully enforce facility policies and protocols, and confirm any less formal yet helpful expectations with your supervisor or the facility's management.

## TEACH YOUR PARTICIPANTS THE "I'M OK" RULE

**CLIP 6.1** During your preclass announcement or during your warm-up, explain to your students that if they leave class for any reason, they need to let the instructor know they are "OK." If a student does not feel well, instruct them to sit down (on their step or on a chair, etc). This is known as the "I'm OK" rule (2) (Figs. 6.2 and 6.3). The purpose of this rule is to share the responsibility of the well-being of the student. The instructor educates students on common responses to exercise so they understand what to expect. This can be done quickly and easily. For example, "If you feel lightheaded or mildly nauseous, sit down." Often, when a participant doesn't feel well, he or she becomes embarrassed and doesn't want his or her classmates to know that he or she isn't "able to keep up." This can become quite serious if the participant leaves the classroom, and the instructor is not alerted to assist the participant in the event of a medical emergency. With the "I'm OK," rule, the instructor is empowered to handle a situation before it gets worse, helping an ill person to the floor to rest and calling help if needed, or feeling confident that the participant simply had to leave early for reasons other than injury or illness.

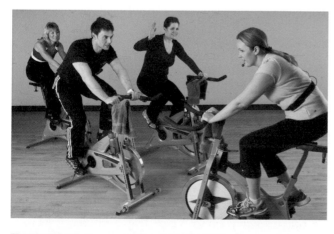

**FIGURE 6.2** Demonstration of the "I'm OK" rule.

# "I'm OK!"

When you are leaving a group fitness class at any time, please let the instructor know you're feeling OK by **raising your hand or making eye contact**. This lets the instructor know you're feeling fine.

If you are not feeling well, **please sit down**. Not only will this alert the instructor that you're not feeling well, it places you in a better position should you become dizzy or faint.

**Please inform your instructor of any changes in your medical condition** including if you become pregnant.

## Taking Care of You Is What We Do!

**+1**
safety first

**FIGURE 6.3** I'm OK marketing sample. (Reprinted with permission DeSimone G. Plus One Health Management Group Fitness Policies and Procedures, 2011.).

## TEACHING STRATEGIES: PROGRESSION/ REGRESSION/MODIFICATIONS

For participant safety and success, plan to incorporate exercise progression (Figs. 6.4–6.6), regression (Fig. 6.7), and modifications (Fig. 6.8) each time you teach a class. Progression can be defined as a gradual change or advancement from one state to another, and as it pertains to your group exercise class, you will want to focus on class structure progression, choreography progression, and exercise intensity progression (Table 6.1).

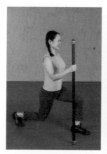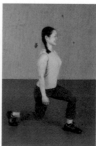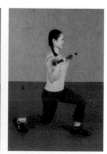

**FIGURE 6.4** Example of progression of a spilt squat (or standing lunges). Exercise moves from supported to unsupported (body weight only) to loaded (with weight).

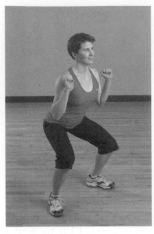
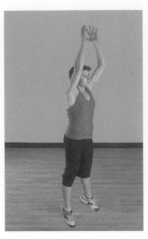

■ **FIGURE 6.5** Progression of a squat using body weight only (dynamic to explosive, *i.e.*, plyometric).

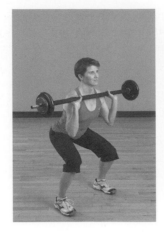
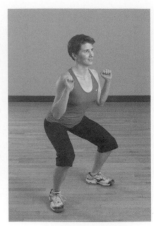

■ **FIGURE 6.7** Regression of a squat from loaded to unloaded.

## CLASS STRUCTURE PROGRESSION

Review "Designing Your Exercise Class" section of Chapter 3 for details, keeping in mind the following progression in your class structure:

- Cardiovascular warm-up specific to the format you are teaching (a muscular conditioning class warm-up will look different from a cardio kickboxing class warm-up)

- Cardiovascular aerobic and/or anaerobic exercise followed by a cardiovascular cool-down (if this is the format you are teaching that day)
- Muscular conditioning (at a minimum, focus on the muscles of the core; if you are teaching a cardio "express" class, you may not have a muscular conditioning component)
- Final stretch with a focus on flexibility gains and relaxation

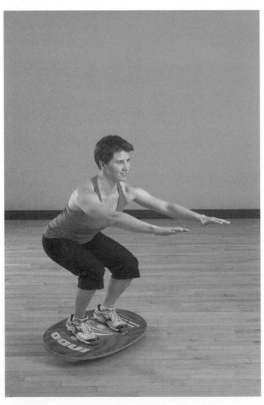

■ **FIGURE 6.6** Progressing a squat using instability (balance board).

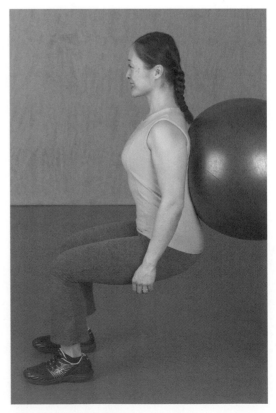

■ **FIGURE 6.8** Modification of a squat.

| Table 6.1 | MOVEMENT PROGRESSION/REGRESSION EXAMPLES | | | | |
|---|---|---|---|---|
| **BASE MOVE** | **CHOREOGRAPHY PROGRESSION** | **CHOREOGRAPHY REGRESSION** | **INTENSITY PROGRESSION** | **INTENSITY REGRESSION** |
| Grapevine (high/low impact format) | Three-step turn | Two side steps | Increase travel distance/cover more ground | Small travel distance/cover less ground |
| Basic step, right lead (step format) | Alternating basic (right, then left lead) | March in place | Leap up, step down | Perform basic at half speed or on floor without step bench |
| Alternating jabs (cardio kickboxing format) | Alternate jab with another punch (jab, hook) | Single jab | Add power and speed to jab without compromising form, more range of motion on pivot into jab | Reduce power and speed, less range of motion on pivot into jab |

## CHOREOGRAPHY PROGRESSION/REGRESSION

**CLIP 6.2** Building choreography and breaking it down is key to the success of your participants. A skilled instructor (seemingly without effort) leads participants through exercise choreography and leaves them feeling accomplished and triumphant, not frustrated. When preparing your choreography, do your best to anticipate where participants may struggle with the moves and plan how you will progress into those moves (see Chapter 5, "Choreography, Music, and Cueing in Class Design and Delivery"). Analyze a move for its most basic components and practice breaking down moves (or regressing them) so that you can seamlessly introduce the moves to your participants. Continue to develop your choreography and cueing skills so that you do not have to rely on a "watch me, then do" approach. See examples in Table 6.1 for progression and regression of popular choreography moves. In our "day-of" scenario, use the following tips:

- Plan to preview more complicated moves during the warm-up section of your class (this strategy is commonly known as providing "rehearsal moves").
- Plan to spend time on the easiest or easier version of an exercise or move and ensure participants accomplish the move before progressing to a more challenging exercise or modification.

### Intensity Progression/Regression

The ultimate goal of exercise classes is for participants to gain health and fitness benefits. For gains to be accomplished, the current condition of an individual needs to be challenged (see the section "Exercise System Adaptations" in Chapter 11). Structure your choreography and exercise selection to follow a bell curve of intensity starting at lower intensities, progressing to a peak, and then regressing intensity as you move to the muscle conditioning or final stretch section of your class. When teaching your class, incorporate the following tips to progress intensity:

- Increase range of motion (*e.g.*, increase from arms moving naturally at sides to larger pumping action).

- Increase lever length (go from a knee lift to a front kick).
- Add traveling moves (go from a stationary march to a march forward).
- Add propulsion or impact (power squat vs. regular squat, high-impact jumping jack vs. low-impact jack).
- Add speed: for a cardio class, use music that gradually increases in tempo, challenging participants to perform movement at a faster pace; remember to stay within industry guidelines for a particular class format, and *never* go at a tempo that compromises the participants' ability to perform movement in a biomechanically sound manner; a solid strategy is to rely more on larger range of motion than faster speed in order to increase intensity.

Incorporate the following tips to regress intensity:

- Decrease speed of movement (as mentioned above, some commercially produced exercise music will gradually slow down beats per minute of the music; however, you can also maintain the same speed of music, yet perform the movement at half time to regress intensity).
- Move from propulsion or high-impact moves to low-impact moves (one foot stays on the floor at all times).
- Decrease movement range of motion.
- Regress from traveling to stationary moves (grapevine to a step touch).

### Movement Modifications and Variations

A challenge with teaching group exercise classes is that participants are at different levels of ability in many aspects (level of fitness, coordination, experience, etc.). When teaching your class, plan to demonstrate easier as well as more challenging options (modifications) in addition to various exercises with similar levels of difficulty (variations) for your exercise moves (review Chapter 5 for more details regarding modifications and variations). Yoke and Kennedy (3) devised a method of categorizing exercises based on a continuum from easiest (1) to hardest (6), a tool that can help you think through

| Table 6.2 | MODIFICATIONS FOR COMMON EXERCISES | |
|---|---|---|
| **BASE MOVE** | **MORE CHALLENGE MODIFICATION** | **LESS CHALLENGE MODIFICATION** |
| Push-up (on knees) | Full-body push-up | Table-top push-up (on knees back parallel to floor) |
| Stationary lunge (single leg, no equipment) | Dynamic lunge, alternating legs | Stationary, single leg lunge using step/bar/wall for balance |
| Squat (lower to 90 degrees at knee, arms out front for balance) | Slide one leg out to side for balance, performing a single leg squat | Perform regular squat, keeping hands on thighs to support the back and staying higher than 90 degrees at knee |

modifications as you create your class plan. Generally speaking, always have an easier option and a more challenging option for your exercise moves, and plan to show movement variations in order to reduce overuse injuries and boredom. Table 6.2 provides examples of modifications for common moves used in group exercise classes.

## BE PREPARED TO ADAPT

You have prepared well for your class, you know the routine and the equipment you are going to use, your music is rockin,' and it is going to be the best class ever. Then you get to the studio and realize you forgot your workout shoes. Or you cannot get your MP3 player to work. Or the participants are not understanding the choreography you worked so hard on. A skilled group exercise instructor plans for glitches that may arise when teaching a class and ultimately recognizes the need to be flexible and adapt to situations as they occur. See Box 6.3 for "What If?" strategies.

## PROVIDING FEEDBACK

A competent group exercise instructor gives participant feedback throughout the workout (see Chapter 4). Feedback on form and safety is imperative, as is feedback on modifying intensity. The key is to provide constructive feedback in a positive, nonthreatening manner. Try these tips:

- Begin your statement with "Please;" a request is less threatening than a demand.
- Avoid singling out an individual, it could embarrass the individual and make him or her not want to return; instead address feedback in general terms: "I see some knees going beyond the toes on that squat, let's keep the knee aligned over the ankle to protect that knee joint."
- Share the rationale behind your feedback; let participants know why the correction will be safer or more efficient for them (as noted in the previous bullet point).
- Demonstrate desired form near an individual who needs adjustments without specifically singling the individual out.
- If you absolutely must physically adjust a participant's form, ask permission before touching the participant.
- Celebrate when participants get it right; if you know it will not embarrass a participant, point out the participant's accomplishments: "Hey, look how Ken keeps his shoulders pulled back on that bent-over row!"

---

| BOX 6.3 | "What If...?" Strategies for Troubleshooting Glitches |
|---|---|

Even the best laid plans can go awry. Know your facility's operational and emergency action plans so you can best respond to the multitude of situations that may occur in the scope of teaching your group exercise class. A few of your own personal contingency plans can also be helpful when the unexpected happens. What if

...*You forgot a piece of your workout gear?*

Be in the habit of keeping backup music and a backup pair of shoes and shirt/shorts in your car (locker or back pack). Rest assured, that is better than canceling a class or borrowing someone else's shoes!

...*You are running late and won't be able to start the class on time?*

Call the facility and let them know you are running behind. See if there is someone who can open the studio, prepare the audio equipment and other equipment, greet the participants, and let them know you will be there shortly; if another qualified instructor is available, they may even be able to start the warm-up for you.

**BOX 6.3, cont.**

*...The audio equipment is not working?*

Check the "on" buttons, function buttons, and cord connections; perhaps someone last used a CD and you might just have to switch to the iPod function. You might call the front desk or send a regular participant to let a manager know about the issue and see if he or she can come and assist. Use a backup "boom box" if it is available. Be willing to teach without the mic as long as it will not compromise the participants being able to hear you.

*...There is a slip or trip hazard on the floor?*

It is imperative you remove the hazard before starting the class. Clear any objects from the area that may impede movement. Many studios have brooms or mops nearby to handle spills or trash.

*...It is too hot/cold in the room, or the lights are not working?*

Contact facilities staff to rectify the situation. You may have to cancel the class if the lights aren't working, or maybe you could take them outside or elsewhere in the facility as long as it is safe to do so and you are not displacing other facility users. If it is warm in the room but safe enough to continue, modify your moves to lower intensity options, and give more water breaks and intensity checks.

*...The equipment you intended to use is broken or otherwise unavailable?*

Plan to have options for the exercises you have chosen. For example if a resistance tube is not available, is there a way to work the same muscle group using body weight or a dumbbell? If a step bench is unavailable, ask if the participant wants to mimic the moves on the floor without the step.

*...No one shows up at the time class is supposed to start?*

Perhaps you have a new format and are trying to build a participation base, or maybe the weather is bad — for whatever reason there may be times when participants are a "no-show." Be familiar with facility protocols for this situation. The expectation may be for you to remain in the studio for a certain amount of time before leaving. It is better if you remain in the room than traveling to the locker room or weight floor; you want to be there if participants show up.

*...Someone comes to class with inappropriate footwear?*

Be tactful and supportive while educating the participant on the necessity for appropriate footwear. Emphasize the importance of their safety and ask if they have other shoes available to change in to. If not, direct them to other cardio options that may be available to them in the facility (perhaps their footwear would be okay on a rower machine or stationary bike). In any case, apologize and empathize, and encourage them to come back.

*...Your planned choreography is complex, and you have a room full of "newbies"?*

Always be prepared to adapt to your group. For each move you put into your routine, have an easier and a more difficult option so you can modify as needed to fit your group. Have a backup combination in case you need to scrap an entire block of choreography.

*...A participant twists an ankle or gets dizzy or actually passes out during your class?*

Group exercise instructors should have nationally recognized safety certifications in the areas of Cardiopulmonary Respiration with Automated External Defibrillator (AED). Make sure you know where your facility's AED machine is and how to use it. Respond to any emergency or injury situation by following established standards of care and facility policies.

*...There is a fire, earthquake, hurricane, or other natural disaster?*

Different parts of the country/world are prone to certain naturally occurring events that are potentially life threatening. Again, be aware of your facility's protocols and procedures so that you can react in a calm, collected manner and keep yourself as well as your participants safe. Participate in safety drills.

## SUMMARY

*This chapter strives to provide insight into a day in the life of a group exercise instructor. A successful instructor thinks quickly on his or her feet, anticipates issues, and is able to teach to and for the participant rather than rigidly adhering to a class plan that may not be suitable. More so than many other professionals in the fitness industry,* *a group fitness instructor has the potential of influencing many participants at one time. Instructors may be asked to teach in all types of conditions, in all types of facilities, or lack of facilities. With proper training, foresight, and attitude, an instructor will always be able to deliver a safe, results-driven, empathic, creative, and scientifically based program.*

## References

1. American College of Sports Medicine. *ACSM's Health/Fitness Facility Standards and Guidelines*. 3rd ed. Baltimore (MD): Lippincott Williams & Williams; 2006.
2. DeSimone G., Group Fitness Policies and Procedures, Plus One Health Management, 2011.
3. Yoke M, Kennedy C. *Functional Exercise Progressions*. Monterey, CA Healthy Learning Publisher; 2004.

# Hospitality and Conflict Resolution for Group Exercise Instructors

## DAVID MILANI • CAROLINE MILANI

7

Objectives

**At the end of this chapter you will be able to:**

- Understand the importance of conflict resolution in the group exercise instruction profession
- Explain how hospitality helps to avoid conflict in the classroom
- Define keys to creating a hospitable environment
- Identify common sources of conflict in the group fitness setting
- Recognize conflict when it happens
- Know the steps to take to resolve conflict (SAFE)
- Know what you need to do to document conflict for liability purposes

To be a successful group exercise instructor, you'll need to develop and apply a unique set of skills that extend beyond your clinical capabilities. The dynamics found in group exercise classes are as unique and variable as the people who take them. It is up to the instructor to manage those dynamics to create an environment that's nourishing and encourages a sense of belonging and shared purpose. While this may sound simple, it's not always easy. Conflicts are certain to arise in any group setting, and group fitness classes are no exception. As an instructor, it is your responsibility to resolve any issues. Not doing so will create barriers to your participants receiving the full benefit of your classes. As such, the goal of this chapter is to prepare you for the challenges you will face in the personal, nonclinical aspects of group fitness instruction, specifically, conflict resolution.

## HOW HOSPITALITY HELPS

The best way to resolve a conflict is to avoid the conflict in the first place. The instructor has a big role in doing that. In addition to being an exercise expert who coaches form and function, the instructor also acts as a host or hostess for the class (and for the club or business as a whole). No single skill set that you master will serve you better than becoming a personable, approachable host who can set his or her class members at ease when they arrive. Setting clear expectations for class participants will prevent misunderstandings down the line. Proactively engaging new participants, explaining what to do and how, sets realistic expectations and sets a tone for a smooth-running class.

## SETTING THE STAGE FOR A CONFLICT-FREE CLASSROOM

Think about the last time you found yourself at odds with someone else. Was the conflict a direct result of a particular argument or situation? Perhaps, but just as likely, your conflict may have arisen out of (or been exacerbated) by a feeling of discomfort or general tension perceived by you, the other individual(s), or both.

An important point to remember is that when people are feeling tense or uncomfortable, they are likely to find conflict. Also, more importantly, the opposite is true: when people are at ease, conflict is far less likely. That's where hospitality comes in.

We all have emotional baggage. Your students will be no different. They will arrive at your classroom door after fixing a flat tire, arguing with their teenagers, paying their bills, or perhaps even more serious issues. For many, especially beginners, the act of walking into the facility and a classroom where everyone else already seems to know one other, the teacher and the class format can be stressful in and of itself.

The solution isn't to solve your students' problems. It's to ease your students' entry into the classroom in a way that helps them shift their focus from any outside stressors so they can actively engage in the class. Doing so will set a tone of respect, teamwork, and shared purpose. It will help your students achieve the best possible results while paying tremendous dividends to you in the form of a harmonious classroom.

Essentially, hospitality is making them feel welcome, setting someone at ease, and anticipating their needs to allow an optimal experience. But, how exactly do you do that?

**BOX 7.1   Seven Keys to Achieving Hospitality in the Classroom**

1. **Arrive Early.** It is difficult to welcome your students if you aren't there. When a student walks into an empty classroom, it's analogous to walking into to a restaurant without a host. *Where do I sit? What's on the menu today?* Arrive for your class a few (~10) minutes early. Be the leader. Your demeanor, positioning, and location during this preclass time are all important. Stand in the front of the room or in a visible place that shows you are the instructor. Be confident and inspiring. Answer questions and give guidance.
   Everyone — you, your students, the club — will benefit from this one simple act. How? It will increase participation and communication levels in your classes.
2. **Welcome *Everyone*.** Say hello to all students entering the room, but pay particular attention to new members or students taking your class for the first time. Introduce yourself, and if possible, introduce them to other students. Chances are that if they are coming to a group class, part of what they are looking for is social interaction with other students. A brief introduction can facilitate this.
3. **Learn Names.** Remember your students' names and use them the next time you see them. Nothing sets someone at more at ease then being greeted by name. One of the basic principles in Dale Carnegie's book, *How to Win Friends and Influence People* is "Remember that a person's name is to that person the sweetest and most important sound in any language" (7).
4. **Be Curious.** Learn the class participants' interests and goals. Then use this information to help determine which students might get along with one another. Stack the deck in your favor by helping establish bonds between people with common interests. Once you do, these members are more likely to work together and form a trusting relationship.
5. **Be Practical.** Use these friendly interactions to help manage your classroom. Guide your members where to set up and, possibly more importantly, where not to. This is your chance to teach members not to set up near the door or in front of the equipment being used for the class. It's also your chance to manage the use of your classroom space by helping members to space themselves in ways that will be most efficient.
6. **Be Available.** Rather than quickly gathering your belongings and leaving right after class, spend a few minutes being available to answer questions, give encouragement, and explain what else you and your club can offer. Many times, a simple "great job today" can make the difference between a one-time student and a regular.
7. **Be Considerate.** Changeover times between classes can be tight, especially during prime-time hours. Designate an open space just outside the classroom or near the front entrance where students can congregate before and after classes. If necessary, encourage your students to clear out of the room to make room for the next class and to reserve socializing to a designated area in the club.

**BOX 7.2   Rules of Hospitality Adapted for Fitness Professionals (1)**

- Speak in public areas. When you are in an area populated with members, guests, or students, speak to them. Look approachable and professional. Wear your smile. Acknowledge everyone including team members and address them whenever appropriate. "Good Morning, Sam!"
- Speak first and last. Start conversations with a greeting and a statement of helpfulness. End conversations with a confirmation that the student, guest, or member's needs have been met and you know what needs to be done for any follow-up to ensure that the person's expectations have been exceeded.
- 10 & 5 Rule. When a student, member, or guest comes within ten feet [10] of a fitness professional(s), the team member(s) should acknowledge the approaching student. (Cease conversations with team members, cease activities, look at member and smile.) At approximately five [5] feet fitness pros should acknowledge the member with a nod, smile and/or greeting, whenever appropriate. "Good Morning!"
- Use the Student's Name. Fitness pros should always try to use the name of the person they are addressing. When we do this, we are recognizing the student as an individual.
- Hospitality Zones. A hospitality zone is any place where a line is likely to form. At these times, students, guests and team members in line should be acknowledged and greeted. Those standing second and third in line should be courteously acknowledged to ease the anxiety of the wait time.

Known for its 5-star hospitality, The Ritz-Carlton organization keeps their approach simple with a three-tenet mantra, as part of their "gold standards," which they call the three steps of service (5):

- A warm and sincere greeting. Use the guest's name.
- Anticipation and fulfillment of each guest's needs.
- Fond farewell. Give a warm good-bye and use the guest's name.

Translating this approach to the world of the group exercise instructor, it is important to note that the goal in delivering these three steps is how students feel throughout their experience in the classroom. A warm and personal greeting helps the class participant to feel welcome and comfortable. Facilitating the participant's access to equipment, providing adequate space, acknowledging any unique needs of the participant, and providing positive feedback throughout the class, among other proactive interactions by the instructor, keep the participant engaged with a feeling of belonging. A fond and personal farewell and simple "thank you" for attending class will help make the participant feel appreciated and accomplished. This simple approach provides a positive experience for your participants, setting a hospitable approach from start to finish.

## CREATING A WARM CLASSROOM ENVIRONMENT

As we've learned, hospitality begins the moment you walk in the door; saying hello to people on your way to class may help draw people into your class. But it doesn't end there. Once the class begins, you'll need to shift from one-on-one communication to addressing the group as a whole.

Begin by introducing yourself to the students, and describe the class and your cueing style. Explain where

---

## Ask the Pro

# What's in a name?

**CAROL MURPHY**
*Owner and Fitness Director*
*FitLife*
*Rochester, New York*
*2010 IDEA Instructor of the Year*

1. Remember your students' names and use them the next time you see them. Nothing sets someone at more at ease then being greeted by name. The ability to build rapport readily and easily and help participants connect with each other is one of the greatest skills an instructor can have. It all starts with an authentic smile, learning their name and taking a genuine interest in them. Although it's easy to feel overwhelmed at the task of building relationships with so many people, it is important to help people belong. Begin by making a conscious decision to remember people's names. Here are a few tips:

2. Repetition, Repetition, Repetition! Repeat their name during conversation and several times in your head. "Hi, Lindsey! Welcome to class. Lindsey, tell me a little about yourself. What are you hoping this workout will be like? Lindsey, it's important to do what feels right for your body. I am so glad you are here, Lindsey. Let me introduce you to Allie" — she'll help you get set up.

3. Associate their name with the person they are with. For example, if Stacie brought Kathleen to class, you can associate their friendship with their names. And if all else fails, you can discreetly ask Stacie to remind you of Kathleen's name.

4. Link their name to a characteristic. It's easier to remember a name when you know something unique about the person. For example: if you know someone named Mary who likes to run marathons, you might think of her as "Marathon Mary" or if Lori has a vulnerable knee, you might think of her as "Low Impact Lori."

5. Write it down. Provide opportunities for participants to communicate and learn more about your classes and fitness and wellness tips by visiting your company Web site or social networking page (*e.g.*, Facebook). These written additions to your "optional" mailing list are another way to help you recall their names and continue to inspire them beyond the classroom walls.

6. If you've forgotten someone's name, ask again. You might say, "I totally remember you, but for some reason, can't remember your name. Please remind me what your name is."

any equipment for the class can be found and address any environmental concerns, such as space (see Box 7.3). For example, if your classroom looks to be near capacity, members may assume there is no space to join. If you know there is room, take control and ask participants to kindly make space. Develop some language that you can use in these situations: "Would you kindly make room for those arriving? Next time it may be you arriving at this time, so be please be helpful. Thank you." Or "More students = more energy! Please make space for those coming in!" Turning members away from class when room is available will not serve either of you well.

Your environment will also change during the class. People may arrive late; others might leave early. In addition to teaching exercise fundamentals, you need to pay attention to changes in the room's environment and manage them throughout the class. In the case of a late arrival, welcome them and provide a few quick messages telling them what they need and what is coming next in the format. If the classroom is nearly full, help them find a spot by saying "Let's make some room for…." Use the student's name if you know it to make them feel welcome (see the Ask the Pro box, "What's in a Name?"). You might also set up one or two spaces ahead of time so latecomers can easily slip in.

## BOX 7.3    Avoiding Conflict around Space and Equipment

You will likely teach in many types of settings over the course of your group fitness career — and each one has a unique culture, as well as space limitations and equipment options. In addition to room size, you will find variance in the quality, type, and availability of equipment. For example, the number of bands, bars, and dumbbells (and the weight denominations of each) available for your class will vary depending on the club. Unfortunately, you will quickly see that equipment is one of the most frequent causes of conflict in a group classroom. You can avoid conflict by practicing the following skills:

- Evaluate the size and shape of the room. Each class format requires a different amount of space for each participant. According to ACSM guidelines, the recommended space is 40–60 square feet per expected member (3). Sometimes the participants will require a lot of room for lateral movement, but not as much for forward and back movement. Other classes may have different requirements. The point is that you should have an idea of how each of your classes will best fit into the room and then take a leadership role as participants come in. Tell them how and where to set up, if they need to be closer to their "neighbor" so that you can accommodate the most people. Hearing that instruction from you is much less likely to create conflict than if they have to ask one and another, for instance, "Can you believe that new guy told me to move over?" If your class is regularly crowded, you may want to designate spaces by setting up the room ahead of time to allow maximum participation.

- Inspect the equipment before class: If you are going to start teaching at a new club, it's a good idea to visit prior to your first class to evaluate the equipment they have available. If your class format typically includes a lot of dumbbell work and you see only a few pairs, you will need to make adjustments. If there are multiple studios, be sure that another class doesn't use the same equipment as your class. In both of these instances, consider how you might modify your class. Are there more resistance bands than dumbbells? Can you offer the bands or body bars or some other equipment as an alternative to the dumbbells?

- Encourage your students to share: A key way to help avoid conflict by instructing your students on how to share effectively. For example, in a toning or strength class, it is common for students to select a variety of weights to keep with them for use during different parts of the class. When this happens, you'll find that one particular type of equipment is fully claimed first (red bands, ten-pound dumbbells, etc.). However, one of your students may have a particular type of equipment that he or she is not using for a particular set or exercise that another student could use for that same set or exercise. To avoid negative feelings and conflict, provide instruction at the beginning of the class as to how to share: Advise your students that, if they need a particular piece of equipment that is not being used by someone else and they would like to use it, it is okay to ask for it as long as they return it after that set. This puts forth the expectation that sharing is expected and encouraged. It also eliminates your students' fear of asking for something they need, curbs resentment when someone has something they want, and dispels negative feelings about having to share "their" equipment. Another idea is to divide the class in half and have each side of the room use one piece of equipment for an exercise while the other uses another type of equipment, then having the sides switch. For example, have the left half of room use bands for biceps curl, while the right side uses dumbbells.

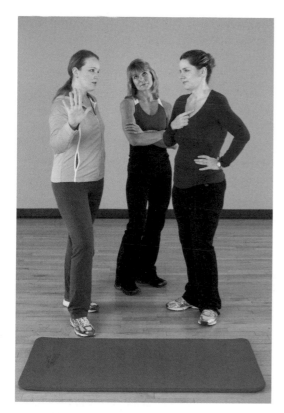

■ **FIGURE 7.1** Conflict can erupt quickly.

Late arrivals to your classroom can pose a safety risk to themselves or to others in the class, especially if the classroom is crowded. You should politely encourage habitual latecomers (see the Ask the Pro box, "Handling Latecomers") or newcomers who arrive late to make an effort to be on time. To avoid embarrassing or angering someone, address late arrivals in a general reminder to the entire class. Or, you may choose to speak to the individual one-on-one after class. The important thing is not to single anyone out in front of the group.

## DEALING WITH CONFLICT

So far, we have focused on strategies for avoiding conflict, and with good reason. As Benjamin Franklin once said,

"An ounce of prevention is worth a pound of cure" (6). However, even if you diligently and consistently apply the aforementioned techniques, it is almost certain that you will still find conflict in your classroom at some point in time. What do you do when that happens?

Conflict can erupt quickly (see Box 7.4 and Fig. 7.1). You should always be on the lookout for a potential or real problem as it is best managed when addressed early (see Box 7.3). Think of a soda bottle. Shake it a little, then stop. Nothing happens. Continue to shake it, and it eventually bursts, affecting you and everyone near you. Noticing and addressing conflict early is the key to managing it and keeping your environment safe.

## SAFE STRATEGIES FOR RESOLVING CONFLICT (*SEE, ASSESS, FACILITATE, ESCALATE*)

### SEE

If you are paying attention, it will be easy to see conflicts as they arise. If you are not focused on this aspect of your responsibilities, conflicts could get out of hand quickly and be difficult to manage. Observe body language. Highly animated use of hands while in conversation, facial expressions denoting emotional distress, vocal tones and yelling, or students moving quickly in or out of an area all signal potential problems.

### ASSESS

Assess the situation. Can you tell what the conflict is about? Can you think of a solution that would dissolve it or calm it until the end of class? Does it have the potential to interfere with members' safety by distracting them from their focus on you or their workout? Can you handle the situation alone? Do you need assistance from management? Most importantly, is it a physical altercation or do you fear that it may become physical?

### FACILITATE

Assessment is an important step because it will tell you how quickly you need to act and what your involvement

---

**BOX 7.4**    *Common Sources of Classroom Conflicts*

- That's my spot! Occurs when a new student sets up in a veteran student's favorite spot.
- You're too close! Occurs when classrooms are full and space is limited. Students (especially new ones) may set up too closely to others.
- I can't get in! Occurs when class size is limited due to space or equipment (number of bikes, steps, etc.) and you need to turn someone away.
- I can't hear! Occurs when cell phones and ongoing conversations disrupt the flow of class.

These distract both the instructor and the participants. (See "SAFE Strategies for Resolving Conflict" above.)

should be. But don't spend too much time assessing since the conflict could get worse in the interim. Below are two ways you can facilitate the resolution.

1. Look for a quick fix to "pause the conflict" and get through the class:
   - Is it a conflict over space? Try to help the participants solve this by suggesting alternate positioning.
   - Is there room to ask both participants to a different spot to separate them for the remainder of the class?
2. Follow through and complete your facilitation efforts after the class. Even if you managed to "pause" the conflict during the class, it doesn't mean it is resolved. If you don't follow through, there's a strong likelihood that the conflict will flare up again the next time the class participants are together again. Follow through by engaging all involved individually.

## ESCALATE

If the conflict is physical, or appears as though it could become physical, *you must escalate immediately*. In other words, you must decide whether or not to defer the situation to a manager. However, other conflicts may require escalation based on your club's policies, practices, culture, etc. You need to ensure you are familiar with what you need to report and to whom in your club *before a conflict occurs*. As a means of mitigating risk, ACSM recommends the following information should be included in managing and documenting an incident (4):

- Day, date, and time of incident
- Location of the incident
- Persons involved in the incident
- Witnesses to the incident
- Staff responding to the incident
- Actions taken by staff in responding to the incident
- Outcomes from these actions

Finally, always escalate if you feel uncomfortable, feel threatened, or feel that you need another teammate's help in resolving the conflict.

## DEALING WITH CONFLICT IN NONCLUB ENVIRONMENTS

While much of this chapter deals with working in a health club environment, many group fitness instructors work on their own and/or in other environments such as community centers and private residences. Though most of these techniques will work in settings such as boot camps, some environments may require you to adapt your hospitality and conflict prevention approaches accordingly. It's best to give it this some thought ahead of time. You don't want to be making the decisions as to how to adapt these approaches once conflicts arise.

Also, you won't have club management or club policies to guide you on how to report conflict. You may want to confer with your insurance providers to see if they can offer you any advice on conflict resolution or if they have specific reporting requirements.

## MORE TECHNIQUES TO FACILITATE CONFLICT RESOLUTION

### NEVER ASSUME

A common error in resolving conflict is to assume you know what the conflict is about. Sometimes these assumptions are based upon preestablished perceptions of the people involved (Bonnie is nice and Sue is sarcastic, so Sue must be wrong). But, remember that kind individuals (even if they're your friends) can be wrong in a particular situation.

### ACTIVELY LISTEN

Once you've dropped your assumptions, you need to actively listen, which means listening for meaning. Let the individuals know you value their participation in the class and want to solve the issue. Ask what happened and really listen; understand and try to imagine yourself in each participant's shoes, and, most important, reserve judgment.

### EMPATHIZE

Let people know you understand their frustrations, but remind them we are all here for a common goal. People will be much more likely to respond to your efforts if they feel they have been heard and understood.

### MIRROR

Make sure you really understand what you are hearing by mirroring (or reflecting) the information you receive back to the participant. In other words, rephrase what you believe you heard in your own words and ask if you have clearly understood what the participant has said. "Let me make sure I understand. What happened was…" or "I understand that this is what happened…. How did this make you feel?" "Is there more about this that I need to know?"

### ENGAGE THE PARTICIPANTS IN THE SOLUTION

Ask the involved parties what they think they can do differently the next time the same situation occurs to avoid conflict. You'll be surprised at how asking people to solve their own conflicts can sometimes be effective. And, if the resolution is their own, participants will be much more likely to follow through with it.

## SUGGEST A SOLUTION

Sometimes, people become so emotionally involved that it is difficult for them to see a solution on their own. You may need to suggest steps for resolution to each participant. Be sensitive to everyone's needs and feelings, but, above all, make sure you believe the resolution identified will actually work.

## GAIN COMMITMENT

Before finishing your conversation with each participant, reiterate the resolution and gain their commitment to following through with it. "So, we have established that it just isn't going to work for you and Mary to be next to each other during this class, and we have agreed that you will not set up near one and another. Do I have your commitment that you will set up somewhere else?"

## ANTICIPATE OBSTACLES

Anticipating obstacles that may occur and planning for them may assist in avoiding further conflict. Using the example in the previous point, I might follow up by asking, "What if Mary arrives before you and sets up in your usual spot? Do I have your commitment that you will set up in a different spot under those circumstances?"

## BE FAIR

Let each person know you will be asking the other for the same commitment to the solution. That will ensure everyone feels as though they have been treated fairly and that no one "is losing."

## RECOGNIZE PATTERNS

If you find, over time, that every conflict involves the same person and that they are really "the problem," discuss the matter with club management. It is management's prerogative and responsibility to maintain the club environment for the benefit of all. If you repeatedly encounter problems with the same individual, management should address that member appropriately.

---

### Ask the Pro

# Handling Latecomers

**CAROL MURPHY**
*Owner and Fitness Director*
*FitLife*
*Rochester, New York*
*2010 IDEA Fitness Instructor of the Year*

I handle latecomers by having an attitude and general spirit of respect for individual perspectives and care for others. How we talk to people makes a difference. If we focus on building strong relationships with our members, we will strengthen their desire to belong and become part of the solution. A few strategies for handling students who arrive late to class are as follows:

1. Place the class in a holding pattern of a move they are familiar with, while gladly welcoming the new participant and quickly assisting them with equipment set up.
2. Try to put yourself in their shoes. Life is busy. They are likely under stress as they rush to get to class. Place them at ease. Let them know you are genuinely happy they could squeeze class into their schedule. If they missed the warm-up, suggest that they gradually build intensity for their own safety.
3. For larger equipment-based classes, a second instructor or fitness center staff member could be used to assist the instructor before, during, and after class to handle situations like late arrivals and maintain a safe and effective workout environment.
4. Additional assistance may also be provided by a class participant. Regular students make terrific mentors to new participants.
5. Use these experiences to guide your teaching. In a future class, teach why the warm-up is so important. On the flip, for those students who skip out on the stretch, help them realize how recovery, relaxation, and mobility are essential to optimal functioning. Education is motivation. When we understand how it will help us, we are more likely to do it.
6. For a program in which it is not appropriate to enter late, professionally worded signage on the door is helpful to avoid member embarrassment.

## CONFLICTS AMONG STAFF

Conflict isn't limited to the students in your classroom. You may encounter friction with other instructors in your club. Conflicts among instructors may arise over a variety of issues — who has the "prime time" slots for classes, competitiveness over who can deliver a more popular workout, and even when instructors habitually end classes late and interfere with the start time of the next class. Perhaps the best practice you can use to avoid these types of conflict is to formulate an understanding that each instructor is part of a team who shares a common goal — to deliver safe, challenging, enjoyable, and effective workouts to the members of your club.

### RECOGNIZE THE TALENTS AND SKILLS OF OTHERS

There are many different instructors with many different styles. If a club's instructors work harmoniously, everyone can learn from each other and perhaps even incorporate some techniques of other instructors into their own classes. In these environments, where learning is continuous and informal, instructors can grow to reach their full potential.

### DON'T FALL INTO THE "PRIME-TIME" TRAP

A common conflict that brews between instructors is over the "prime time" class slots on the club's schedule. (While what is considered "prime time" will vary by club, usually the time periods immediately following the workday during the week and early on Saturday mornings will be the most desirable.) While it is important for everyone to lead well-attended, well-liked classes, some instructors create conflict over who has the "prime-time" classes on the schedule — especially if they believe their lower class attendance is a result of them being stuck in a less desirable class slot.

Don't fall into this trap. While a 6:00 p.m. class on a Thursday may have more potential attendees than a 2:00 p.m. class on a Friday, you will likely have little control over where you are placed on the schedule. What's important, and sometimes quite difficult to overcome, are the feelings of resentment you may have towards other instructors who have the "prime-time" slots. These feelings are bound to create conflict, and this is exactly what you want to avoid. You will have your time to shine in those "prime-time" slots — you just need to put in your time and learn that the number of participants in a class often has little or nothing to do with the time slot, but everything to do with the instructor and type of class that is offered in it.

### TEACH TO *YOUR* AUDIENCE

Since you can't control when your classes will fall on the schedule, tailor the type of class you are offering to the type of members that you see in the club at the time your class is offered. For example, if you find a larger number of senior citizens in the club on Friday at 2:00 p.m. and you teach a poorly attended class at that time, offer a class that is likely to appeal to that group. Maybe your current class is too difficult for that group, or too easy. Perhaps it is something as simple as your music style is not appreciated by the group or that your music is too loud or too quiet. Try to learn from other instructors who have taught in that time slot before. If each instructor strives to offer the best, most appropriate class for the time slot they teach in, everyone's class attendance can be strong, and schedule-related conflict can be limited or eliminated.

### LEARN FROM THE GROUP

Group fitness departments in clubs can easily feel like high school popularity contests. You need to make a sincere effort to avoid resentment of surrounding instructors' class attendance, style, and appeal to members. If you hear someone's spin or sculpt class is "better" than yours, don't sulk; use it as a learning experience. Talk with the other instructor. You may start this conversation by simply saying "Wow, I see you really draw a large crowd and they really seem to love you. What is your technique for keeping class attendance high?" Better yet, take the instructor's class. Listen to what other members say; look at, listen to, and learn from everything the instructor does. There is nothing that can compare to first-hand experience.

### ADDRESS TARDINESS ISSUES

When an instructor habitually ends his or her class late, it can interfere with the ability to start *your* class on time. This can be very frustrating. In this situation, it is best if you can gently discuss the matter with the "late" instructor, explaining the impact it has on your class. You may try saying something such as "I know people really enjoy your class and they never want it to end, but if possible, do you think you can try ending a few minutes sooner so you give us ample time to gather the equipment we need to begin?" You may also add something such as "sometimes I have a specific series of exercises, movements, etc., and it is so hard to fit them into an hour. If I start late, it is really difficult, and members complain that we can't get to everything." You may find this conversation to be very effective, but not everyone will respond well to this approach. If, after you address the matter with the other instructor, their class continues to run overtime, you will need to escalate this to management as it is simply not fair to you or your class participants. Sometimes the person who creates the schedule may need to place a 5-minute gap between classes to allow for the changeover.

## A WORD FOR THE GROUP EXERCISE DIRECTOR OR MANAGER

Most fitness professionals, regardless of their roles, enter the industry because they want to help others. They are "people people." They tend to like people, they enjoy working with people, and they innately put the needs of others ahead of their own. The Four Seasons organization, a global leader in the hospitality industry, takes this unique personality trait very seriously, hiring their employees based more on attitude as opposed to aptitude. Isadore Sharp, Founder, Chairman, and CEO, Four Seasons Hotels and Resorts, has observed, "We can't precheck service or sample it — production and consumption are simultaneous. Those few moments of service delivery are a company's make-or-break point, when reputation is either confirmed or denied... Most companies hire for experience and appearance, how the applicants fit the company image. We hire for attitude. We want people who like other people and are, therefore, more motivated to serve them. Competence we can teach. Attitude is ingrained" (2). Take it from hospitality experts at The Four Seasons, it is important to carefully select your group exercise instructors. A professional accredited certification is only one aspect of selecting the right employee. Audition your group exercise instructor candidates. Look for more than just how the candidate executes a grapevine or a squat. Engage the candidate to bring out personality traits that translate to leadership in the classroom.

## SUMMARY

*Despite all of the above, you will find your career as a group exercise instructor to be an enjoyable and rewarding one — especially if you are prepared for conflicts before they arise. It's important to set up a warm and friendly classroom environment as a preventative measure to control conflict. It is also important to have strategies to deal with conflict should they arise. The most important piece of information to take away is to NEVER let a conflict get out of control by leaving it unaddressed. Always confront the conflict sooner, rather than later. You, the other instructors and all the club's employees are there to serve members and provide them with a safe, challenging, and fun atmosphere. Unaddressed conflicts that are allowed to fester will make this goal difficult if not impossible to achieve.*

## References

1. Entertainment Cruises, Our Service System [Internet] http://www.entertainmentcruises.com/entertainment-cruises/our-service-system
2. Talbott BM. The Power of Personal Service, Industry Perspectives. The Center for Hospitality Research, School of Hotel Administration, Cornell University. CHR Industry Perspectives, No 1, September 2006.
3. Tharrett S, Peterson J, editors. *ACSM's Health/Fitness Facility Standards and Guidelines*. 3rd ed. Champaign, IL Human Kinetics; 2005. p. 35.
4. Tharrett S, Peterson J, editors. *ACSM's Health/Fitness Facility Standards and Guidelines*. 3rd ed. Champaign, IL Human Kinetics; 2007. p. 23.
5. The Ritz-Carlton Hotel Company, L.L.C. "Gold Standards", *Careers*, The Ritz-Carlton Hotel Company, L.L.C., 2011; [cited January 9, 2011]. Available from: http://corporate.ritzcarlton.com/en/About/GoldStandards.htm
6. US History.org, The Quotable Ben Franklin in the Electric Ben Franklin. Independence Hall Association, 1999–2010; [cited October 27, 2010]. Available from: http://www.ushistory.org/franklin/quotable/quote67.htm
7. www.dalecarnegie.com. Dale Carnegie's Golden Book. Dale Carnegie Training. [Internet] Dale Carnegie and Associates, Inc. 2006; [cited November 15, 2010].

# 8 Guidelines for Special Conditions

### NANCY J. BELLI

*objectives*

After completing this chapter, the reader shall be able to:
- Identify some of the more common physical conditions commonly seen in group exercise settings
- Understand if and how to make modifications in exercise leadership, class design, and exercise selection based on class participant's physical conditions

The variety of participants in group exercise classes over the past decade has expanded to include more males and more participants who have a variety of conditions. As the baby boomers age, those who have utilized group classes as their main mode of conditioning will most likely continue with this form of exercise but will also likely develop conditions that need to be monitored. Pregnancy is a commonly seen health condition that may require some "special care" in a group exercise setting. Hypertension, cardiovascular disease, diabetes, arthritis, and musculoskeletal issues are some of the most prevalent conditions that may be controlled through medication, diet, and exercise and that may also require special attention from a group exercise instructor (GEI). With an active generation of fitness participants living longer, there will be a greater demand for specialty classes geared toward common ailments that occur with aging, such as loss of balance, low back pain, and general loss of function.

As we age, there are numerous physiological and musculoskeletal changes that occur. Body systems do not function as well they did when we were younger. The documented loss of muscular strength during the decades of 50 through 70 years of age is significant (15% per decade) and can greatly impact one's functional ability, flexibility, and balance. Many research studies have reported that regular physical activity can mitigate the aging process and thereby help to keep us from becoming physically frail, dependent, or even disabled.

There are many conditions that participants in a group exercise class can present to an Instructor. Being prepared to make modifications and/or adjustments is a necessity for the GEI to create an atmosphere of confidence, competence, and safety. Having a basic knowledge of common medical conditions and their contraindications is just the start. There are specific knowledge and skills required to meet the standard of care threshold necessary

for competency. The GEI must also know the implications of omitting modifications for those individuals with medical conditions. The conditions discussed in this chapter are the most common but are by no means a complete list that a GEI may encounter. It is the duty and obligation of the GEI to be aware of the latest guidelines and recommendations for exercise for people with medical conditions, both chronic and acute.

## PREGNANCY

CLIP 8.1 Pregnancy temporarily alters a woman's physiology, anatomy, kinesiology, and biomechanics. These changes may be hormonal, physiologic, and musculoskeletal. Each trimester brings various challenges to the pregnant participant that may interfere with consistent physical activity. Exercise is contraindicated for women who experience specific complications with pregnancy, including specific forms of heart and lung diseases, cervical pain/ injury, a multiple pregnancy (twins/triplets) that is at risk for premature birth, vaginal bleeding, a history of preterm labor, premature rupture of membranes, and high blood pressure (2).

The many benefits of regular exercise that apply to all other healthy individuals also apply to pregnant women who do not have any complications that would limit their activity. Additional benefits for pregnant women who exercise consistently include a lower risk of developing pregnancy-specific conditions such as gestational diabetes mellitus, as well as some of the normal associated symptoms such as backaches, constipation, and bloating (26). Most healthy women can continue to exercise throughout their pregnancy with minor modifications as their pregnancy progresses and physiological changes occur.

Several governing agencies such as the American College of Obstetricians and Gynecologists (ACOG) and the American College of Sports Medicine (ACSM) recommend that a pregnant woman receive physician clearance prior to participating in an exercise program. The most widely used form, PARmed X for Pregnancy (refer to Figure 8.1 in *ACSM's Guidelines for Exercise Testing and Prescription*, 8th edition), was designed by the Canadian Exercise Physiology Society to screen pregnant participants for exercise. A thorough physical is needed to rule out any absolute and/or relative contraindications to exercise. (Refer to Box 8.1 in *ACSM's Guidelines for Exercise Testing and Prescription*,

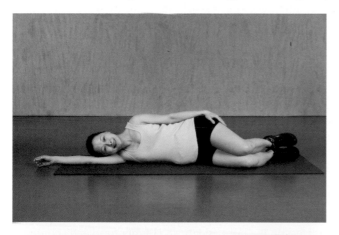

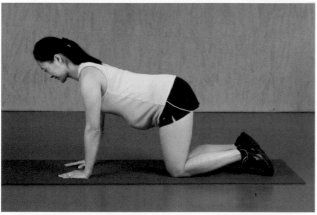

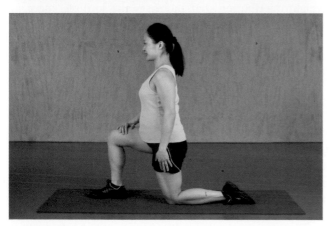

**■ FIGURE 8.1** Advise pregnant clients to transition slowly from the floor to standing.

8th edition.) It is especially important for pregnant women with specific medical conditions such as hypertension, gestational diabetes mellitus, and morbid obesity to see their physician prior to beginning an exercise program. Exercise intensity and programming will need to be adjusted according to the functional capacity, fitness level, symptoms, and daily energy fluctuations of the participant (28).

The increased blood volume and decreased venous return associated with pregnancy can compromise the cardiovascular system, so some precautions need to be followed in relation to intensity and volume of aerobic activity. Aerobic activity is important for keeping the heart and lungs strong, increasing circulation, and otherwise enhancing a woman's overall energy level. Moderate intensity should be safe for most participants, especially in the early stages of pregnancy. Ratings of perceived exertion (rating of perceived exertion [RPE] 12–14 on a 6–20 scale) and the "talk test" are good methods for monitoring exercise intensity. Heart rate ranges developed for pregnant women based on age by the Society of Obstetricians and Gynecologists of Canada in 2003 may also be useful for monitoring intensity. Activities such as low-impact aerobics, water aerobics, swimming, walking, and cycling for up to 30 minutes per day are all recommended for pregnant women of all fitness levels. Both continuous training and cross training are preferred over interval training to maintain fitness and decrease the risk of overuse injuries. The recommended frequency for aerobic exercise is a minimum of three times per week, and can be daily for those already participating in a program when they become pregnant. ACSM recommends that previously sedentary individuals begin with a shorter duration (between 5 and 15 minutes) 3 days per week and gradually lengthen their workouts (building up to 30 minutes) 4–5 days per week as they become more accustomed to regular exercise (28). 2002 ACOG guidelines indicate that most women can continue with their normal exercise routines until symptoms, discomfort, or decreasing capability indicate otherwise. Usually women will feel the need to decrease intensity, duration, or frequency as pregnancy progresses, especially in the second and third trimesters (26). There are, however, some situations when exercise should be terminated and the participant needs to contact her doctor (see the Take Caution! box, "Warning Signs to Stop Exercise").

The goal of resistance training is to maintain one's strength throughout pregnancy. Strength training may prevent some of the common aches and pains associated with this pregnancy. It is extremely important to build the stabilizing muscles of the upper back and shoulder for two reasons: first to counterbalance the increased weight of the breasts and, second, to be able to hold the newborn for extended periods of time without experiencing neck and shoulder pain. ACSM recommends multiple repetitions of moderate-intensity exercises such as rows, pull-downs, and reverse flies (12–15 repetitions), avoiding isometric exercises (28).

## Take Caution

### WARNING SIGNS TO STOP EXERCISE

The ACOG recommends that exercise should be terminated and the participant should contact her physician if any of the following occurs (2):

· Vaginal bleeding
· Dyspnea before exercise or increased shortness of breath
· Uneven or rapid heartbeat
· Dizziness or faintness
· Headache
· Chest pain
· Trouble walking or muscular weakness
· Calf pain or swelling (need to rule out thrombophlebitis)
· Uterine contractions that continue after rest
· Decreased fetal movement
· Fluid leaking or gushing from the vagina

While exercises such as squats and lunges are beneficial, deep knee bends should be avoided. Maintaining lower body strength and flexibility is important for being able to move the newborn both into and out of the cradle. The Valsalva maneuver should be avoided, as the increase in maternal blood pressure can be harmful to the fetus. Bearing down should be avoided, as it may stretch the pelvic floor. Encourage proper breathing techniques during exercise, *e.g.*, inhaling on the easy portion of the exercise and exhaling on the harder portion.

The pelvic floor is a series of muscles that provide the inferior support of the uterus, analogous to a hammock or the bottom of a grocery bag. Kegel exercises were designed to tone these pelvic floor muscles that play an important role in controlling bladder leaks and tightening the vaginal muscles that get stretched from delivering the baby. Although these exercises are important, and not normally done in class, some of the principles behind the exercises can be incorporated into general cues to be used in class, such as "drawing the pelvic floor up and in." The most common Kegel exercise is pretending to stop the flow of urine by squeezing the muscles for up to 10 seconds. This simple exercise can be done multiple times a day (up to 10–20 per set), but should not be performed when urinating since pregnant women have a higher risk of bladder infections.

Hormonal changes in the body require some modifications and precautions for exercise. Progesterone causes a reduction in smooth muscle tone that impacts the digestive and circulatory systems. This hormone causes vasodilation, creating a decrease in blood pressure, which slows the return of blood to the heart. Therefore, changing position quickly (like going from sitting to standing) and standing motionless over time can cause light-headedness.

Participants should be encouraged to move slowly from lying on the floor to sitting, to high kneeling, then to standing instead doing it in one movement (see Fig. 8.1). Also encouraging the woman to walk around between sets as well as after exercise will enhance circulation and venous return, mitigating the effect of this hypotensive response.

The hormone relaxin greatly increases over the course of pregnancy, with up to 10 times prepregnancy concentration levels occurring within the first trimester. This hormone allows the ligaments and connective tissue to stretch, which is vital during the delivery process. Since hormones do not target one area, all connective tissues surrounding joints have the ability to stretch beyond their normal length, thereby compromising joint integrity and overall stability. Certain movements need to be performed with caution, such as turns, quick changes of direction, high-impact exercises, exercises that place weight on the wrist while in extension, and exercises that work the lower back. Finally, end ranges should be avoided during stretching so as to not permanently stretch out the supporting structures of the involved joints.

A special condition that should be noted as it relates to the hormone relaxin is diastasis recti, which is a separation of the rectus abdominis due to the enlarged uterus pushing through the softened connective tissue. To test for diastasis recti, have the participant lie face up with her legs bent and feet on the floor. Ask her to lift her head and shoulders off the floor as if doing a crunch. Ask her to use her fingertips to feel for a ridge or separation about one inch above or below the bellybutton. A separation that is wider than two fingers indicates diastasis recti. These participants should avoid twisting and spinal flexion movements.

A pregnant woman can gain 25–35 lb during her pregnancy. During the third trimester, she will gain the greatest amount of weight, which will alter her center of gravity, and affect her balance. The distribution of this excess weight is mainly anterior, which can make it difficult for her to see her feet. Therefore, activities that challenge her balance should be avoided. Low back pain can often result from the altered center of gravity, and the anterior weight distribution that increases the lordotic curve of the spine, and stretches some of the lumbar ligaments.

Performing exercises such as the cat-cow (Fig. 8.2), bird dogs (Fig. 8.3), planks (Fig. 8.4), and side (lateral) bridges (both ways; Fig. 8.5) can build endurance in the core musculature, which may help to combat some of these structural and biomechanical changes.

As the fetus grows larger, especially during the second and third trimesters, exercises in the supine position should be avoided. The weight and position of the fetus can occlude the inferior vena cava, thereby diminishing the woman's venous return. This can be relieved by having the woman turn onto her left side (2). Pivarnik (26) suggests that supine exercises may be modified to a side-lying position or a semireclined position, as long as the head is higher than feet (Fig. 8.6).

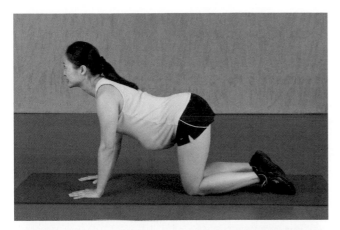

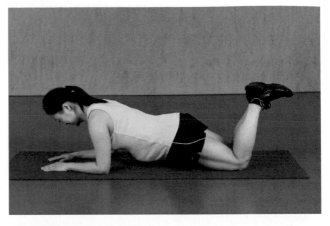

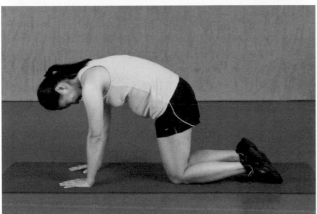

**■ FIGURE 8.4** Plank (modified).

**■ FIGURE 8.2** Cat-cow.

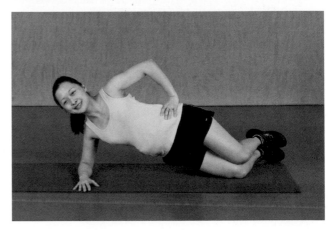

**■ FIGURE 8.5** Side bridge (modified).

Pregnant women should avoid contact sports and activities that may increase the risk of trauma to the abdominal area or present a high risk of falling, either of which may cause harm to the mother or fetus. Common sports that have an inherent risk of contact and/or trauma include racquet sports, soccer, basketball, skiing (water and snow), horseback riding, hockey, martial arts and kickboxing (2). Scuba diving presents an additional challenge to the fetus, since the fetus is unable to eliminate nitrogen from its system upon returning to the surface. This leaves the fetus unprotected from decompression sickness or gas embolisms and should therefore be avoided.

A woman's thermoregulatory system is compromised during pregnancy, increasing the risk of overheating. Since a woman's body temperature remains elevated throughout pregnancy, exercising in cool and well-ventilated environments can assist in the prevention of overheating. Wearing

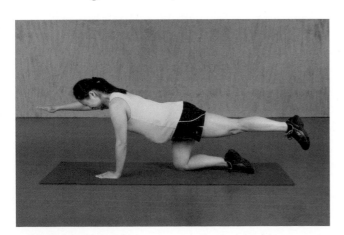

**■ FIGURE 8.3** Bird dog.

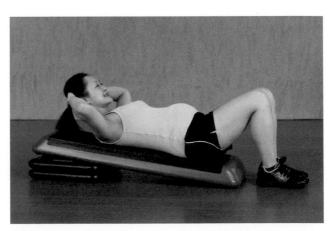

**■ FIGURE 8.6** Modify supine exercises to a semireclining position during pregnancy.

loose-fitting clothes and staying hydrated can also decrease the likelihood of overheating (26). Exercising in hot and/or humid environments as well as extremely intense or long-duration exercise should be avoided in order to not overtax the thermoregulatory system (5).

Adequate oxygen and fuel is required for a nonpregnant participant, but the added increased metabolic demand (resting energy expenditure can increase 5%–7% by the second trimester) of pregnancy requires a woman to ingest an additional 300 calories per day (28). Therefore, encourage pregnant participants to have a snack before exercise to ensure that adequate fuel is available.

During the postpartum period, exercise can be resumed gradually, usually within 4–6 weeks after delivery, provided there are no complications. ACOG postpartum guidelines for exercise state only that exercise may be resumed as soon as it is "physically and medically safe" (2). It is important that the postpartum participant remembers that it took 9 months to have a child and may take 9 months to return to prepregnancy exercise levels. Gradual progressions are recommended to enhance the new mother's physical and mental well-being.

> ✔ **RECOMMENDED RESOURCES:** *ACOG has a multitude of patient pamphlets concerning exercise and pregnancy-related conditions: www.acog.org/publications/patient_education*
> *They have also launched a separate Web site specifically dedicated to pregnancy and childbirth topics: www.yourpregnancyandchildbirth.com*

## DIABETES MELLITUS

According to the Centers for Disease Control and Prevention, the No. 6 cause of death in 2006 was diabetes mellitus, and the number of cases for this disease is on the rise. Research indicates that there is a correlation between the rise of obesity and the rise of diabetes, which can decrease the average life span by approximately 12 years and quality of life by 20 years (4). Diabetes mellitus is characterized as the inability to produce or use insulin properly. Without proper glucose regulation in the body, this condition eventually wears down many organs and creates multiple problems that fitness professionals need to address through modifications in their classes.

## Ask the Pro

# What are the three most important things to be aware of when dealing with a pregnant client in a large group setting?

**ANNETTE LANG**
*Owner*
*Annette Lang Education Systems LLC*
*New York, New York*

The three most important things to watch for when dealing with pregnant clients are as follows:

1. Keep feet moving when doing upper body exercises, especially when doing multiple sets in a row. ACOG recommends avoiding motionless standing as much as possible. This is because of the relaxation in the smooth muscles, making it easier to pass out when standing still.
2. Be aware of diastasis recti: separation of the rectus abdominis muscles. If a participant has difficulty getting up from a supine position due to belly size and/or you can see protrusion coming from her midsection as she exerts herself (it looks like an abnormal protrusion), she should be given regressions to avoid that movement/exercise. She needs to be taught deep abdominal stabilizer exercises, proper breathing patterns, and how to do that in her daily life outside of the gym.
3. Abnormal joint laxity due to relaxin and other hormones: ask participants to be aware of what their "normal" range of motion was and not to exceed that due to pregnancy, as they don't have the strength/stability and neural feedback to support this range. Fitness professionals need to be aware of what normal ranges of motion should be for participants.

The two most common forms of diabetes mellitus are type 1 and type 2. Type 1 diabetes is most often caused by destruction of the beta cells in the pancreas that produce insulin. Without insulin, the body's ability to regulate glucose is impaired, putting a person at risk for uncontrolled increases of blood glucose. Type 1 diabetes is often treated with insulin through either the conventional manner of injections or a self-regulated pump.

Ninety percent of diabetics have type 2 diabetes. Type 2 occurs when the body's ability to utilize the insulin becomes impaired. This resistance to insulin absorption and utilization produces elevated levels of insulin in the body which promotes fat storage and increase blood pressure. Exercise has an insulin-like effect and therefore promotes glucose utilization and can improve insulin sensitivity in people with both types of diabetes. Favorable changes in glucose tolerance and insulin sensitivity due to exercise usually deteriorate within 72 hours of the last exercise session, which is why regular exercise is imperative (4). For type 2 diabetics, exercise can also enhance fat loss and reduce other metabolic conditions, both of which can decrease the overall risk of cardiovascular disease (4,12).

The goal for people who have diabetes is glucose control while maintaining cardiovascular health and fitness (type 1) and weight loss (type 2). The first of these goals, glucose control, can be obtained by carefully balancing diet, exercise, and medications. The weight loss portion of the goal can be obtained in the same way, provided that the person is aware of how his or her body is reacting to each of the components. Moderate-intensity cardiovascular exercise (RPE range of 12–16 on a 6–20 scale) is recommended for 20–60 minutes at least 4 days per week. In addition, type 2 diabetics should expend approximately 2,000 calories per week. The role of consistent exercise in glucose regulation is so important that no more than 2 consecutive days of inactivity per week should be allowed. Certain modes of aerobic training are better suited for people with this condition, such as walking, non–weight-bearing machines (especially if neuropathy is present), and aquatic-based exercises (4).

Participants in your class have an obligation to come into your class prepared and ready to work, and this includes but is not limited to (28) the following:

- Wearing proper clothing and footwear
- Being properly hydrated before, during, and after exercise to ward off heat illness
- Ensuring adequate glucose levels prior to starting the class (glucose levels above 100 mg·dL$^{-1}$)
- Exercising when medication is not peaking so as not to increase the risk of hypoglycemia
- Avoiding muscles that will be used in exercise as injection sites; abdominal injection is recommended.

As the GEI, you need to be aware of and check in with these participants regularly to be sure they are responding in an appropriate manner to exercise and the intensity level they are using. In addition, if you intend to drastically change the intensity and/or exercises within a class format, it would be prudent to forewarn diabetic participants so they can properly prepare for these changes. Be mindful of and watch for signs of heat illness, as diabetes can compromise the thermoregulatory system.

Resistance training guidelines for diabetics are similar to those for a healthy population, provided that there are no contraindications: there is an absence of retinopathy, and no recent laser treatments have occurred (21,28). Moderate intensity (8–12 repetitions) of multiple sets of exercises for the major muscle groups is recommended two to three times per week. Circuit training is an effective method of resistance training, and multijoint exercises are most beneficial. Proper technique should be emphasized, and caution taken not to utilize isometrics, heavy weight lifting techniques, and exercises that involve sustained gripping or Valsalva maneuver, as these can cause an increase in blood pressure (10,28).

The most common problem that participants with diabetes may experience is hypoglycemia. As a fitness professional, you need to be aware of the common symptoms associated with hypoglycemia (see the Take Caution! box, "Hypoglycemia Symptoms") and how to respond when someone presents with these symptoms. Hypoglycemia is defined as a rapid drop in blood glucose and/or a blood glucose level of <70 mg/dL, and can occur several hours after exercise. Hypoglycemia may occur 4–6 hours after an exercise bout, so exercising late at night or before bedtime is not recommended. If late exercise is unavoidable, increasing carbohydrate consumption is recommended to minimize these effects (28).

## Take Caution

### HYPOGLYCEMIA SYMPTOMS

**Hypoglycemia (low blood glucose) is the most common problem that individuals with diabetes will experience. Recognizing the signs and symptoms hypoglycemia is vital to keeping participants exercising in a safe environment. Symptoms include**

- **Shakiness**
- **Weakness**
- **Tingling of the mouth and fingers**
- **Abnormal sweating**
- **Excessive hunger**
- **Anxiety**
- **Nervousness**

Hyperglycemia (or high blood glucose levels >300 mgdL$^{-1}$) is a common problem that can occur in type 1 diabetics who do not have good glucose control. Although moderate-intensity exercise is effective in obtaining glucose control, vigorous-intensity or extended activity may trigger an excessive release of adrenaline and other hormones, which could increase blood glucose levels (11). Common symptoms of hyperglycemia are

- Weakness
- Sweet, fruity breath odor (acetone breath)
- Increased thirst
- Fatigue
- Excessive urination

It should be noted that if fasting glucose levels are >250 mgdL$^{-1}$ with ketones or >300 mg/dL without ketones, exercise is contraindicated (28).

There are many complications that can develop as diabetes progresses. Peripheral neuropathy can impair the diabetic's ability to feel pressure and temperature changes. The implications associated with this are numerous. Balance is compromised due to the inability to sense pressure on the feet when stepping or moving. For this reason, sudden changes in position or quick steps may be a problematic for diabetics.

Proper foot care is critical for health and mobility of diabetics (see Box 8.1). Preventing blisters and keeping the feet dry and cushioned are important aspects to keeping diabetic participants active. If foot ulcers occur, it is imperative that the participant see his/her physician as soon as possible, since delay in treatment could cause major problems, up to and including amputation.

In autonomic neuropathy, diabetics lack the ability to sense changing pressures and temperature throughout their body, which can predispose them to experience blunted heart rate and blood pressure responses to exercise, and heat- or cold-related illnesses. Therefore, ratings of perceived exertion (or the RPE scale) should be used to assess exercise intensity for diabetics instead of heart rate (28).

Due to the excess stress and degenerative nature that diabetes places on the organs, additional complications will ensue. Hypertension is the most common of these

secondary conditions and affects approximately 60% of type 2 diabetics.

If a participant begins to experience these, it is imperative that she stop exercise, monitor blood glucose levels, and ingest rapid-acting carbohydrates such as juice, hard candy, soda, or glucose tablets (4,28).

> ✔ **RECOMMENDED RESOURCES:** *Additional information concerning diabetes can be found on the following Web sites, as well as ACSM resources listed:*
>
> · *American Diabetes Association: www.diabetes.org*
> · *Diabetes Exercise and Sport Association (DESA) Web site: www.diabetes-exercise.org*
> · *National Institute of Health Web site: www.niddk.nih.gov*
> · *Diabetes Network Web site: www.diabetesnet.com*
> · *Exercise is Medicine Web site: www.exerciseismedicine.org*

## HYPERTENSION

Hypertension is defined by a resting systolic blood pressure (SBP) that is ≥140 mm Hg and/or a resting diastolic blood pressure ≥90 mm Hg, or by taking antihypertensive medication. There are approximately 65 million people who are hypertensive, but only about a third of them have it under control and another third do not have it under control; the final third do not even know they are hypertensive, which is why hypertension is known as the silent killer. The high pressure on the arteries and blood vessels increase the risk of more serious cardiovascular diseases such as stroke, heart failure, and peripheral artery disease (17,18). Before the age of 45, men have a higher incidence

---

| BOX 8.1 | *Essential Foot Care* |
|---------|------------------------|

Peripheral neuropathy (inability to feel pressure or temperature in feet) can increase chances of getting sores on the feet, and poor circulation can decrease the healing process. Therefore, proper foot care is essential to prevent further medical complications. This includes the following:

**WASH FEET DAILY WITH WARM WATER.**
- Check feet daily for sores, blisters, redness, or calluses.
- If skin is dry, use lotion (not between toes).
- Smooth calluses and corns gently with a pumice stone.
- Cut toenails about once per week.
- Wear shoes and socks — be sure footwear fits properly.
- Protect feet from hot and cold.
- Keep blood flowing to feet: put them up when sitting.

Adapted from Prevent Diabetes Problems: Keep your Feet and Skin Healthy. NIH Publication. No. 08–4282 May 2008, National Diabetes Information Clearinghouse, 1 Information Way Bethesda, MD 20892–3560. Available at www.diabetes.niddk.nih.gov

of high blood pressure than women, but after the age of 64, women have a much higher incidence than men (15).

The National Heart Lung and Blood Institute (NHLBI) of the National Institute of Health (NIH) in conjunction with the National High Blood Pressure Education Program created a Joint National Committee (JNC) to extensively research the prevention, detection, evaluation, and treatment of high blood pressure. During the Seventh Report of the JNC in 2003, the classifications for blood pressure were redefined, and a new category of prehypertension (SBP of 120–139 mm Hg or diastolic blood pressure 80–89 mm Hg) was created as a warning that without changing certain lifestyle habits, a person would be at an increased risk of developing this condition. These lifestyle habits are the first line of defense for decreasing one's SBP (Table 8.1).

Exercise causes blood vessels to dilate, leading to a reduction in blood pressure (3,11). Aerobic exercise is an instrumental component to the control of hypertension because of the reduction in blood pressure (average reduction of 5–7 mm Hg in both systolic and diastolic pressures) that occurs after a single mild- to moderate-intensity exercise bout. This postexercise hypotension can persist for up to 13 hours after exercise (7). These results suggest that hypertensive people should participate in moderate-intensity activities for 30–60 minutes, daily. Exercise can be performed continuously or intermittently (10-minute bouts that accumulate to the total recommended time) and may include activities such as walking, jogging, swimming, and cycling. A long cool-down (5–10 minutes) is recommended to avoid abrupt postural change (3,9).

Resistance training in the form of circuit training is recommended for hypertensive people. There has been evidence to show that aerobic training plus circuit training has a greater effect of lowering blood pressure than resistance training alone (23). Resistance training of at least one set of 8–12 repetitions can be performed 2–3 days per week (28). Terminate a set when RPE is between "somewhat hard" and "hard" (RPE 13–15). It is important to refrain from gripping weights or handles tightly as this could increase blood pressure of the smaller vessels of the upper body. Participants must avoid heavy weight

lifting, isometrics, and the Valsalva maneuver, since all of these activities will increase the blood pressure of the participant, and since it is recommended that exercise SBP remains below 200 mm Hg (see the Take Caution! box, "Hypertensive Precautions") (3).

### Take Caution

### HYPERTENSIVE PRECAUTIONS (28)

- Participant should not exercise if resting SBP is >200 mm Hg and/or diastolic blood pressure is >110 mm Hg.
- During exercise, SBP should remain below 220 mm Hg and/or a diastolic blood pressure of <105 mm Hg.
- Exercise should be terminated if SBP is >250 mm Hg and/or the diastolic blood pressure is >115 mm Hg.

Most hypertensive individuals are prescribed one or more types of medications that are designed to slow the heart rate response, keep the blood vessels open (dilation), or decrease the volume of fluid within the body. Here are some suggestions to use while conducting a class to keep hypertensive participants safe from the side effects of antihypertension medications while exercising:

- Use ratings of perceived exertion (RPE scale) to monitor exercise intensity.
- Avoid changing posture/position quickly since certain medications can produce sudden decreases in blood pressure. Keep the classroom at a comfortable temperature and well ventilated.
- Have the participant stay hydrated — certain medications can affect the thermoregulatory system.
- Extend the cool-down period and monitor participants during cool-down since certain medications may produce sudden reductions in postexercise pressure.
- Watch participants for hypoglycemic signs and symptoms as some medications can increase the risk of this response.

| Table 8.1 | SUGGESTED LIFESTYLE MODIFICATIONS TO REDUCE BLOOD PRESSURE | |
| --- | --- | --- |
| **LIFESTYLE HABIT** | **DEFINED** | **APPROXIMATELY DECREASES SBP** |
| Maintain healthy weight | BMI of <25 | 5–20 mm Hg/10 kg weight loss |
| Decrease salt intake | No more than 2400 mg per day$^{-1}$ | 2–8 mm Hg |
| Stay physically active | 30 min of PA on most days | 4–9 mm Hg |
| Moderate alcohol intake | No more than 2/men and 1/women per day | 2–4 mm Hg |
| Adopt DASH eating plan | Foods rich in whole grains, poultry, fish, fruits, vegetables, and low fat dairy (protein and fiber). | 8–14 mm Hg |

SBP, systolic blood pressure.

aAdapted from Report The Seventh Report of the Joint National Committee on Prevention, Detection, Evaluation, and Treatment of High Blood Pressure (JNC 7), National Heart, Lung, and Blood Institute, National High Blood Pressure Education Program, Aram V. Chobanian, M.D., Chair. *JAMA*. 2003;289(19):2560–2571. Published online May 14, 2003 at: http://www.nhlbi.nih.gov/guidelines/hypertension/jnc7full.pdf.

✔ **RECOMMENDED RESOURCES:** *Additional information concerning hypertension can be found on the following Web sites, as well as ACSM resources listed:*

- *American Heart Association Web site: www. americanheart.org*
- *National Heart, Lung, and Blood Institute Web site: www.nhlbi.nih.gov JNC 7 Express Report and Facts about the DASH Eating Plan*
- *Your Guide to Lowering Blood Pressure Web site: www.nhlbi.nih.gov/hbp/index.html*

## MUSCULOSKELETAL CONDITIONS: SHOULDER, BACK, KNEE

In 2005, one in two people reported a chronic musculoskeletal condition, which is twice the rate of reported circulatory or respiratory conditions (21). A group fitness professional may need to modify exercises for participants with injuries to any of three major musculoskeletal areas. Movements involving sprains and strains are the most common injuries that will be presented. A sprain is an injury that occurs to a ligament that attaches bone to bone across a joint. Two of the most common areas where a sprain will occur are in the ankle and knee. Strains are injuries that occur to the muscle. The most common areas where strains occur are the low back and rotator

cuff muscles. The anatomical structure of the joints, improper lifting techniques, poor posture, and/or body mechanics can predispose a participant to injury. Knowledge of the joint structure, mechanics, and movements can assist the instructor in providing safe and appropriate modifications for participants in classes.

### SHOULDER

▶ CLIP 8.2    The American Academy of Orthopedic Surgeons reported that in 2006, approximately 7.5 million people went to the doctor's office for shoulder and upper arm sprains and strains. Of these 7.5 million visits, 4.1 million of these were rotator cuff–related injuries. Injuries to the rotator cuff can occur due to repetitive overhead movements associated with sports or everyday activities such as gardening (1).

The shoulder is one of the most complex joints of the body due to its lack of bony support coupled with its vast range of motion. Dr. Simon Kemp in the Sports Injury Bulletin for the Shoulder reports that "the shoulder can assume no <1,600 positions" (27). The shoulder is comprised of the shoulder girdle and the shoulder joint. The shoulder girdle consists of the scapula and its supportive musculature, while the shoulder joint is where the humerus articulates with the pear-shaped glenoid fossa (Fig. 8.7). In actuality, only about 30% of the humeral head articulates with the glenoid fossa, similar to a golf ball on a tee or a ball balancing on a seal's nose. This is why the shoulder relies on its surrounding musculature

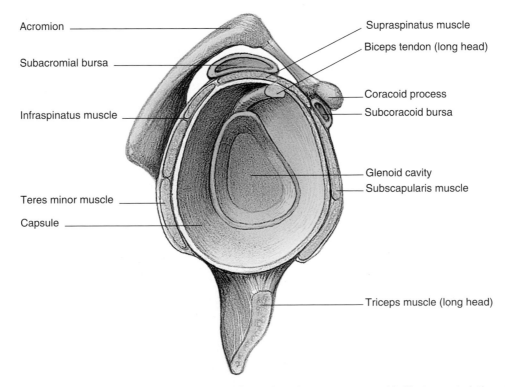

Acromion — Supraspinatus muscle
Subacromial bursa — Biceps tendon (long head)
Infraspinatus muscle — Coracoid process
Subcoracoid bursa
Glenoid cavity
Subscapularis muscle
Teres minor muscle —
Capsule —
Triceps muscle (long head)

■ **FIGURE 8.7** Shoulder joint socket showing glenoid fossa (glenoid cavity). (Asset provided by Anatomical Chart Co.)

for its stability, mobility, and strength. Smooth coordination between the shoulder girdle and the shoulder joint is therefore imperative for complete movement of the arm (16,27).

The scapula and its surrounding musculature provide a variety of movements. Because the scapula is not directly connected to the torso, it can slide along the posterior aspect of the thoracic area of the torso in an effort to put the arm and hand into a position to move. The scapula also provides the surface for the anchor of the rotator cuff muscles. When you shrug your shoulders, the scapula slides up and then down. These movements are known as elevation and depression. When the scapula slides toward the midline, then away from the spine, the movements are called retraction and protraction, or adduction and abduction, respectively. There is a certain amount of rotation that occurs with the scapula in coordination with the previously mentioned movements. Without these movements, your ability to wave "hello" would be severely limited.

The shoulder joint also has movements that are unique to it. When you swing your arm forward and then backward by your side, the movements are flexion and extension. When you make an angel in the snow, the movement as the arms go up by your head is abduction and the movement as the arms go down by your sides is adduction. When you place your hand over your heart, the movement at the shoulder joint is horizontal adduction, and when a football player "clothes-lines" another player, the movement is horizontal abduction. The movements of external and internal rotation are unique to the shoulder and hip. When you watch a baseball pitcher throw a pitch, you see the extremes of this movement. Some baseball pitchers can get their throwing forearm parallel to the ground during the windup phase of a pitch. This is an example of extreme external rotation. As the pitcher proceeds through his pitching motion and into the follow-through phase of the pitch, his arm will internally rotate. These movements are very important in all major sports, especially ones with a stick, bat, or racquet.

One of the most neglected areas of the shoulder joint is the rotator cuff. These four muscles (supraspinatus, infraspinatus, teres minor, and subscapularis) stabilize the humerus in the glenoid fossa. Every time the arm moves, these muscles are activated in some way. Most of the time, they contract to assist in moving or stabilizing the head of the humerus while the larger muscles contract to create larger arm movements, and yet, rarely are these muscles strengthened. This is the reason why approximately 55% of the total number of upper arm and shoulder sprains and strains reported in 2006 were rotator cuff related injuries as reported by the American Academy of Orthopedic Surgeons (1).

The shoulder joint is most vulnerable when the arm moves behind the plane of the head with applied pressure, especially in an externally rotated position. The other common position for many injuries is that of falling on an outstretched arm in an effort to mitigate a fall. Therefore, exercises and movements that mimic these positions should be avoided in class.

## Implications for Group Exercise Instructors

Incorporating scapular- and shoulder-specific exercises within class is recommended. Including exercises such as rows and lateral raises into a class format will help maintain scapular strength and stability. Rotator cuff–specific exercises such as external rotation at 0, 45, and 90 degrees of shoulder abduction utilizing bands or light weights will help these muscles continue to be strong and active. Scapular-specific exercises such as the row and pull-down will provide inferior and medial strength that is imperative for providing a stable base on which the arm can move. Body bars, bands, and dumbbells can all be utilized to strengthen these muscles. Reverse flies (Fig. 8.8) are also an important exercise to provide some stability to the posterior aspect of the shoulder that is important in slowing the forward motion of the arm.

Participants in class may already have injuries when they come to take class, and therefore modifications must be made so further injury does not occur. Always instruct the participants to work in a pain-free range of motion. Impingements and tendonitis are injuries that typically occur from repetitive overhead movements, which are sometimes caused by a muscular imbalance between weak external rotator muscles and the strong internal rotator muscles. Pain usually occurs when one is raising or lifting one's arm above the level of one's shoulder. The inflamed muscle gets pressed up against the superior border of the joint that elicits a pain response. Most of the time, avoiding overhead movements and/or keeping movements below shoulder height will keep the pain to a minimum. Externally rotating the arm prior to overhead movement can dissipate the pain due to the head of the humerus having better clearance of the superior aspect of the joint. Therefore, this is a preferred arm/shoulder

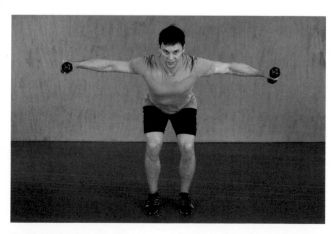

■ **FIGURE 8.8** Reverse fly.

position for shoulder flexion exercises. Ronai suggests modifying overhead movements by limiting motion to within pain-free ranges, and avoiding the 90/90 position (90 degrees of abduction and 90 degrees of external rotation) to decrease the shoulder pain that can occur with these movements (27).

Participants may present a rounded shoulder posture. Poor posture and alignment can exacerbate the anatomical predisposition to rounded shoulders. Tight pectoral and anterior deltoid muscles may also be contributing factors to this posture. Performing exercises that strengthen the shoulder girdle, such as reverse flies and rows, may provide some muscular balance to counteract the effects of the tight anterior muscles. Including upper body stretches for the chest and anterior shoulder (Fig 8.9), the latissimus dorsi (Fig. 8.10), and the triceps (Fig. 8.11) will keep the shoulder able to move through its full range of motion.

## LOW BACK

CLIP 8.3    Lower back pain is such a common condition that statistics show that 80% of Americans will be affected by it during their lifetime. The onset of pain, mechanism of injury, length of discomfort, and length of recovery can differ from person to person and from occurrence to occurrence. There are many muscular forces that impact the lower back area, which is why the specific cause pain is often difficult to determine (20). Some common causes for low back pain are poor mechanics while lifting objects, muscular weakness or poor coordination of the "core muscles," and herniated discs from repetitive lumbar flexion/ rotation (19). Postural issues such as excessive or insufficient lordosis, anterior or posterior pelvic tilt, and/or increased thoracic curvature can all impact the low back area. People who sit all day long can develop tight muscles in the back, legs, and hips. These postural habits and occupational challenges are difficult to correct within a 50-minute class structure.

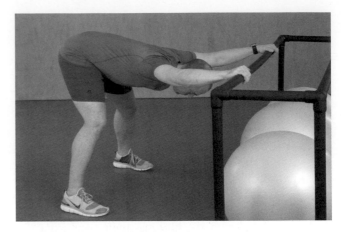

■ **FIGURE 8.10** Stretch for latissimus dorsi.

The back has multiple layers of muscles, some that attach to each vertebra, some that attach to multiple vertebrae, and some that attach to other bones and joint structures, which allow for multidirectional movement and to provide a conduit through which power generated from the hips can be transferred to the upper body. The spinal ligaments attach the vertebral bodies to each other to provide the stability to the spine. The discs separate the vertebral bodies to provide shock absorption for the spinal column. When the jelly-like substance that normally lies in the center of the disc protrudes through the more dense outer layer of the disc, this "herniation" can put pressure on the nerve root(s) that emanate from the spinal cord, causing localized pain or pain that radiates down one or both legs (1).

The overall goals for programming for low back pain are to reduce pain; to improve exercise tolerance,

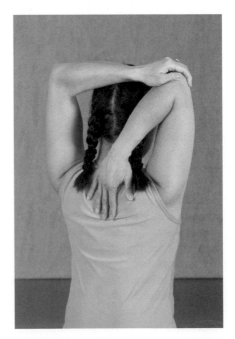

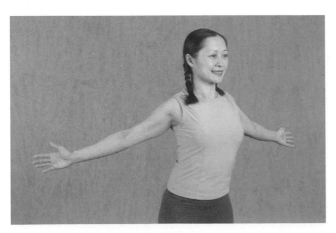

■ **FIGURE 8.9** Stretch for the chest and anterior shoulder.

■ **FIGURE 8.11** Stretch for triceps.

muscular endurance of the core, and flexibility of the back and hip musculature; and to improve gait and posture (20). All group fitness classes contain some element of core training, so selecting or modifying exercises that are appropriate for all populations is crucial. There are several categories of low-back conditions that will need your attention, such as chronic strains, postural imbalances, poor lifting techniques, and poor general mechanics. Alignment, impeccable form, and proper progressions for exercises are crucial for all participants. Dr. Stuart McGill suggests that building endurance through repetitions of static holds (no longer than 10 seconds) in core exercises is better than increasing the length of total time that a position is held because it provides better oxygen supply to the muscles (19).

A gentle dynamic warm-up of the spine is recommended prior to performing exercises. The cat stretch (unloaded flexion and extension of the spine) is an excellent means of increasing the circulation to the muscles and "flossing" the spinal nerve roots in preparation of exercise (6,18).

Specific low back exercises should begin with stability-type exercises. Exercises such as planks and bridges can typically be performed by all participants. Planks are an exercise that can train the rectus abdominis along with the "core" or spinal stabilizers, while sparing the spine from excessive load forces. Bridges are an excellent exercise because they recruit the gluteal muscles, and cocontract hamstrings and low back muscles in hip extension (19). Progressing through the following adaptations can increase the strength and stability of the surrounding musculature by coordinated cocontraction of the core muscles (Fig. 8.12). Begin with a short lever on a stable surface and gradually increase the repetitions with which the movements can be performed. As strength increases, lengthening the lever, in the case of the plank, (moving from bent knees to on the toes) will increase the difficulty of the exercise. In the case of bridges, moving to a shorter base (one foot from two feet) will accomplish the same purpose. The next set of progressions can include moving to an unstable surface, such as a BOSU or physioball, or placing balance pads under the feet. The final progression for stability is to move the limbs while keeping the torso still, in the plank and/or bridge. This progression provides multidirectional stresses to the core without any dynamic movement of the low back area.

Exercises that move the limbs while holding a stable core are next in the progression. McGill's research on back injuries shows that this goal can be obtained without increasing tremendous load to the intervertebral discs as occurred in traditional exercises like the prone "superman" (18). The "bird dog" exercise provides strength through the spinal musculature along a diagonal from the shoulder to the hip without excessively loading the discs. Making a fist to cocontract the arm and shoulder will enhance the upper erector spine contraction (19).

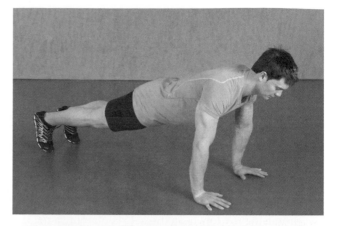

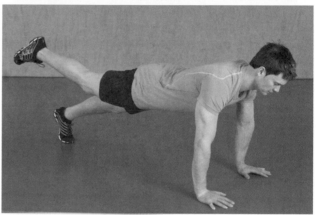

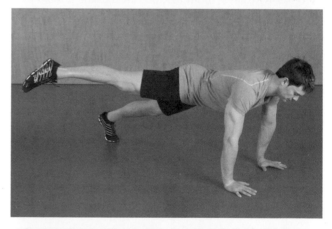

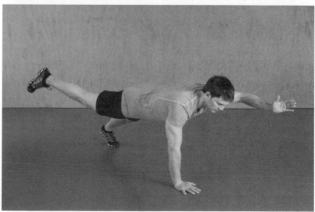

■ **FIGURE 8.12** Plank progression.

Side-lying hip abduction may be utilized to enhance the strength of the gluteus medius. Once stability and control are accomplished, then dynamic and functional exercises can safely be added.

Finally dynamic exercises are the ones with which we are most familiar. Abdominal curl-ups, back extensions (static hold), and other large superficial muscle exercises all fall into this category. Side bends and one-arm carries will provide strength to the quadratus lumborum that will provide some lateral strength and stability to the lumbar spine. The wood chop exercise (Fig. 8.13) is a wonderful example of training the core dynamically through a coordinated contraction of the core musculature without compromising the low back discs. (Maintaining a neutral spine and hinging at the hips throughout movements that involve lifting, carrying, pushing, pulling, and rotation afford a complete transfer of power from the hips through the upper body. McGill states that "bending the spine or bending at the waist during the transfer of power would cause a loss in power or an energy leak" (18). Additional progressions for athletes can be found in Recommended Resources by McGill (18–20).

One of the conditions that needs particular attention is disc injury. Most of the time, a herniated disc will protrude in a posterior and lateral direction. Exercises that include forward flexion, and especially forward flexion with rotation, will exacerbate this condition. Rotational exercises with or without flexion through the lumbar area should be restricted since they may irritate this condition. Most rotation should come from the thoracic area and hips through recruitment of muscles that power and stabilize the body (18). Planks in both the side and prone positions will maintain muscular strength and stability without irritating this condition.

Certain exercises should be avoided if one suffers from low back pain. High-impact aerobic activity can increase compression of the spine, thereby causing more pain. Lifting weights overhead or loading weight onto the shoulders or back (such as a bar) can also increase

spinal compression, and therefore should be avoided. As stated earlier, rotational movements, especially when the feet are planted, may exacerbate disc problems. Unsupported forward spinal flexion relies on the spinal ligaments for support instead of the muscles. Rapid flexion and extension, especially early in the morning, places an excessive load on the discs (18). Static holding with both legs extended while lying supine will also place excessive loads on the back.

## KNEE

CLIP 8.4

In 2003, knee injuries were the most common reason for visits to the orthopedic surgeon's office as reported by the American Association of Orthopedic Surgeons (1). The knee is composed of three joints that are held together by ligaments (Fig. 8.14). The tibiofemoral joint is a hinge joint and the largest joint in the body. The patellofemoral joint is a modified plane joint. Finally, the superior tibiofibular joint is a plane synovial joint between the proximal tibia and the head of the fibula. Movement at this joint occurs with any activity involving the ankle. Since the skeletal structure of the knee lends little or no support or stability to this joint, any movement can be a challenge (6). This joint also receives a tremendous load from both directions: bodyweight from the superior direction and ground forces from the inferior direction.

The majority of the support for the knee stems from four major ligaments: the anterior and posterior cruciate ligaments and the medial and lateral collateral ligaments. The collateral ligaments provide medial and lateral support and stability to the knee, while the cruciate ligaments help to control rotation and keep the tibia from

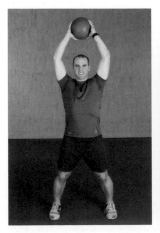
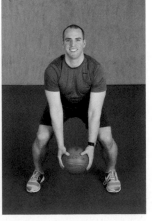

■ FIGURE 8.13 The wood chop.

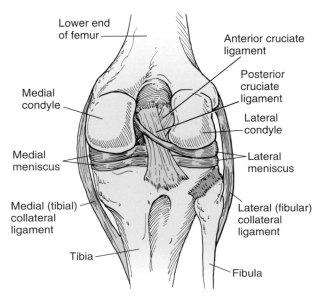

■ FIGURE 8.14 Bones, ligaments and the menisci of the knee region — posterior view — with the knee flexed and patella removed. (From Cipriano J. *Photographic Manual of Regional Orthopaedic and Neurological Tests.* 2nd ed. Baltimore (MD): Lippincott Williams & Wilkins; 1991.)

moving too far forward or too far backward in relation to the femur. The menisci are the thick pieces of cartilage that lie on the tibial plateau. The medial and lateral menisci help stabilize the joint and deepen the articular surface. Not only does this cartilage act as a shock absorber between the femur and the tibia, the menisci also provide some control for rotational movement at the knee.

The basic movements of the knee include flexion, extension, and some rotation; however, the alignment of these joints during movement is under the control of the surrounding musculature. Weakness or muscular imbalance in the hip and thigh, and/or instability at the ankle or even the foot can affect the proper mechanics of the knee. For example, you may notice that a participant who complains of knee pain, struggles to keep her knees from caving in medially during a squat. A pronated foot (foot that rolls toward the instep) can place the knee in a more medial deviated position. Similarly, weak gluteus muscles may not be effective in keeping the hips from internally rotating, which may also place excess stress on the knee joint. Closed chain activities (where the foot is fixed to the floor) can provide better control for the lower body and decreases the sheer forces on the joint ligaments. For these reasons, you may need to provide some participants with modifications on certain lower body exercises to limit range of motion at the knee, and encourage proper joint tracking (6).

### Implications for GEIs

Incorporating lower body exercises that strengthen all the lower body muscles in a variety of planes is recommended. It is important to watch the knee alignment of your participants to check for proper patellar tracking or provide modification if needed. Lunges performed in multiple directions (Fig. 8.15), carioca, backward and forward stepping, and sidestepping provided in a logical progression will work the lower body muscles globally to enhance balance and strength throughout the kinetic chain and aid in preventing injury.

Unilateral leg strength is important to quality functional movement. Incorporate one-legged exercises in multiple planes and directions (like hopping and skipping) to enhance balance and unilateral strength. Watch for proper landing technique that includes landing with the knee over the second toe and the chest over the knee while keeping a straight back and neutral spine position. The hips, knees, and ankles should all be flexed upon landing, as well as landing on the ball of your foot and sinking into the heel to properly absorb the impact.

A thorough stretching routine for the lower body is recommended for keeping the knees healthy; however, end ranges should be avoided if pain is present or a participant is recovering from an injury.

Participants with knee injuries may require modifications to some exercises. The most common injury to the knee joint is a sprain to one of the ligaments. Caution participants with knee sprains to use caution with the movements that change direction quickly, or otherwise place stress on either the lateral or medial aspect of the knee. Encourage these participants to perform exercise in a pain-free range of motion. There are a few additional modifications you may need to incorporate if someone has a meniscus injury. Participants with a meniscus injury should avoid high-impact exercises, quick starts and stops, and quick changes of direction. As with any injury, if the pain gets worse, or does not get better within a week of the onset, the participant should seek appropriate medical attention.

✔ **RECOMMENDED RESOURCES:** *For additional information on knee injuries, AAOS has a dedicated Web site that includes topics such as keeping knees healthy, exercise, common knee problems, injury prevention, and others. http://www.saveyourknees.org*

## ARTHRITIS

Arthritis is currently the most prevalent chronic condition and the leading cause of disability in the US, affecting about one-third of adults. The findings from the National Health Interview Survey (2003–2005) indicated that more than 46 million adults (one in five) had doctor-diagnosed arthritis, and 17.4 million had activity limitations that were attributed to arthritis. By the year 2030, an estimated 67 million or 25% of the projected total adult population aged 18 years and older will have diagnosed arthritis (22).

Although arthritis is a general term for a group of more than 100 inflammatory diseases that affect joints, it's not just an older adult disease. The prevalence of this disease does increase with age, but more than half of those (some estimate two-thirds) with arthritis are under the age of 65, and it affects more women than men by a ratio of 60%–40% (22). Although there is no cure, exercise, maintaining a healthy weight, and maintaining good muscular strength and balance may mitigate the impact that this disease has on the functional status of those afflicted with it.

Osteoarthritis is a degenerative disease in which articular cartilage deteriorates, leaving a joint's exposed bone surfaces to rub against each other, producing pain, stiffness, and swelling in the joints or supporting structures. Ultimately, this process leads to loss of function and movement. The pitting of articular cartilage also causes the underlying bone to thicken and form bony spurs (osteophytes) near the articular surfaces of the bone. The joint lining (synovium) becomes inflamed due to the cartilage breakdown. This inflammation introduces enzymes and proteins to the joint, which cause further damage to

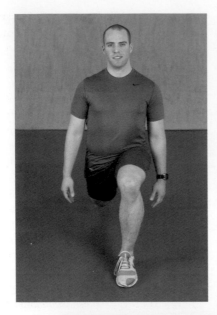
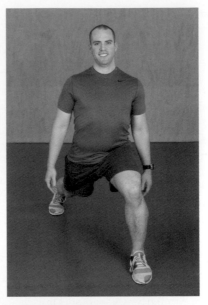
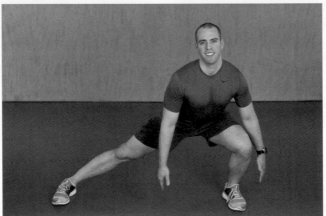
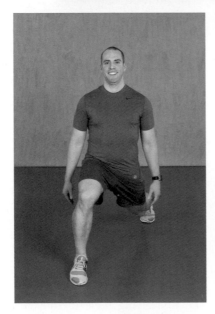
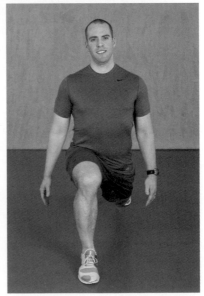

■ **FIGURE 8.15** Multidirectional lunges.

the cartilage. Although the cause of osteoarthritis is not completely known, there are some risk factors that may contribute to the onset of the disease such as age, obesity, injury, overuse, and genetics. Obese adults are up to four times more likely to develop knee osteoarthritis than normal-weight adults, and excess body weight is also associated with about 35% of adults who have been diagnosed with arthritis (14,15). Osteoarthritis most often affects the hands, lower spine, knees, and hips. There is no cure for this condition, and the progression of the disease is the leading cause of hip and knee replacements (13,24).

Exercise and weight loss have been used as therapeutic options for patients with osteoarthritis of the knee. Studies have shown that pain and disability improve with short-term exercise (3–6 months) and that lower-extremity training increases strength and improves function of the arthritic knee (14). Similarly, weight loss ranging from 7.5% to 11% of an obese person's bodyweight can significantly improve self-reported function due to the decreased stress to the joint structures. Weight loss of as little as 11 lb reduces the risk of developing osteoarthritis of the knee among obese women by 50% (8).

ACSM guidelines for aerobic activity are initially low intensity and short duration (5–10 minutes), gradually increasing the duration to 20–30 minutes per day, three to five times per week or 150 total minutes per week, emphasizing duration over intensity. Cross-training methods utilizing low-impact and/or non–weight-bearing activities (cycling) should decrease the impact and load on the affected joints. Nordic walking with poles has been successful in Finland for reducing the load on the hips and knees, while swimming and other aquatic exercise is recommended since working in multiple angles and planes helps joint integrity. Water, as a medium, may also reduce pain and stiffness and decrease the reliance on pain medication. Activities to avoid are running, jumping, high-impact aerobics, and tennis due to the high-impact nature of these activities and their affects on the joint (28).

Resistance training will increase the strength of the muscles surrounding the joint, thereby displacing the load and reducing the stress on the joint. Isometric exercises may be utilized if there is joint pain, with the goal of gradually building up (10% per week) to one or more sets of 10–15 repetitions, two to three times per week (28). Bands, dumbbells, and water can be used as the resistance once dynamic movement is tolerable. Circuit training can also be used as a type of resistance training due to the low-resistance exercise being performed during a prescribed time versus a specific number of repetitions (8). Progressing to functional patterns and activities such as rising from a chair and climbing stairs can be added on a daily basis as pain and symptoms tolerate to improve neuromuscular control and balance required by activities of daily living (28).

Flexibility exercises should be performed one to two times daily using a pain-free range of motion as an index

of intensity. Utilizing both active and passive motion is important to joint mobility and function, especially for the affected joints and surrounding areas. Holding static stretches for 30 seconds and repeating these stretches may provide some relief.

There may be many different modifications that a GEI needs to provide since the variety of symptoms and their severity can differ from participant to participant. As pain and swelling decrease, the person may be able to tolerate more, thereby making any progression symptom limited. It is imperative not to place excessive loads around the damaged joints and to provide appropriate warm-up and cool-down (~5–10 minutes of range of motion exercises). Avoiding strenuous exercise during flare-ups is recommended; however, gentle range of motion exercises can be performed since total inactivity should be avoided (28).

Exercise during the same time of day when medication is peaking and pain is least severe is recommended for maintaining adherence. Appropriate shoes that have good shock absorption and stability may decrease some of the load that is transferred to the joint. Although there may be some discomfort during and immediately following exercise, joint pain that lasts 2 hours after exercise and exceeds preexercise pain severity is a warning sign that the duration and intensity of exercise should be reduced in the future. Exercise should be terminated if there is unusual or persistent fatigue, increased weakness, decreased range of motion, and increased joint swelling or continuing pain (25,28).

> ✔ **RECOMMENDED RESOURCES:** *Additional information concerning osteoarthritis can be found on the following Web sites, as well as ACSM resources listed:*
>
> - *National Institute of Arthritis and Musculoskeletal and Skin Diseases Web site: www.niams.nih.gov*
> - *Arthritis Foundation: www.arthritis.org*
> - *American Association of Orthopedic Surgeons Web site: www.AAOS.org*

## LIABILITY/RISK MANAGEMENT

One of the best defenses against liability is to work within your scope of training and expertise. Your education, both formal and informal training, as well as your experience, all contribute to the standard of care that you are expected to deliver. Maintaining your certifications and staying abreast of the latest research in the industry through continuing education courses will help you provide the latest techniques that are safe for your participants to perform. You can apply your knowledge about these medical conditions to provide your members with a safe programming environment. It is also important to maintain a nationally recognized First Aid and Cardiopulmonary Resuscitation (CPR)/Automated External Defibrillation (AED) certifications. These certifications will keep your lifesaving and first aid skills sharp.

The primary sources for the latest research are trade journals which are produced by the nationally recognized certifying agencies. An additional resource to help you stay abreast of the latest research is the NIH Web site, which contains the most current research for many common conditions. There are approximately twenty-seven agencies within the NIH that house information about any condition from musculoskeletal (NIAMS) to heart, lung, and blood (NHLBI), to diabetes and digestive conditions (NIDDK). Within each of these agencies are links to other organizations that provide patient information for the general public about specific conditions. The fitness industry also offers seminars, conferences, and publications that contain the latest business and programming information. There are multiple venues and resources available to those who take the time and effort to utilize such reputable sources. The best defense against liability is being prepared for any situation that may come your way.

## SUMMARY

*This chapter has highlighted some of the most common medical conditions that you will encounter in your classes, and has provided a foundational knowledge and basic understanding of these conditions so that appropriate modifications can be utilized when needed. Due to the nature and progression of medical conditions, it is important to obtain a physician's clearance prior to participation. There are general recommendations that typically apply to all conditions, such as having an extended warm-up and cool-down (approximately 10 minutes) so the body can gradually acclimate to the class intensity and to avoid blood pooling or faintness after the work portion of class. Instruct participants to work in a pain-free range of motion, and to inform you of any changes in their medical condition they may be experiencing prior to beginning every class. (Refer to the discussion of the ACSM Quick Screen in Chapter 2.) Be watchful of the proper alignment of the joints and overall posture during exercises. Most medical conditions require a lower intensity and shorter duration due to a compromised system, so instruct participants to listen to their bodies and not push themselves to total fatigue. Be sure participants stay hydrated before, during, and after class (5,28), and be sure the classroom is well ventilated to mitigate the possibility of heat illness.*

*As the number of participants in group fitness classes increases, so does the possibility that multiple medical conditions will exist among them. It is important to have an understanding of common medical conditions and the implications that exercise and commonly associated medications can have on your participants. It is as vital to stay abreast of new guidelines for common medical conditions as it is to search out new program trends and opportunities. Providing a safe class for all of your participants is a minimum standard that is expected by the public, and is your responsibility as a group fitness instructor.*

# References

1. American Association of Orthopedic Surgeons Web site: AAOS Web site: http://orthoinfo.aaos.org—updated July 2009; accessed 6/5/10.
2. American College of Obstetricians and Gynecologists. Exercise during pregnancy and the postpartum period. ACOG Committee Opinion No. 267. *Obstet Gynecol*. 2002;99:171–3.
3. American College of Sports Medicine Position Stand. Exercise and hypertension. *Med Sci Sport Exer*. www.acsm-msse.org. 2004;533–53.
4. American College of Sports Medicine Position Stand. Exercise and type 2 diabetes. *Med Sci Sport Exer*. www.msse.org. 2004;1345–60.
5. American College of Sports Medicine Position Stand. Exercise and fluid replacement. *Med Sci Sport Exer*. 2007;39(2):377–90.
6. American College of Sports Medicine. Exercise programming for musculoskeletal disorders. *ACSM Certified News*. 2009;19(4):1–2.
7. Bibi KW, Niederpruem MG, editors. *ACSM's Certification Review*. 3rd ed. Lippincott Williams & Wilkins Baltinere, MD; 2010;39–40.
8. CDC: Targeting Arthritis: The Nation's Leading Cause of Disability, In: Centers for Disease Control and Prevention, Promising Practices in Chronic Disease Prevention and Control: A Public Health Framework for Action. Anonymous. Atlanta Department of Health and Human servises, 2003, p. 5–19.
9. Chen C-Y, Bodmam AC. *Postexercise hypotension: Central mechanism*. *Exerc Sport Sci Rev*. 2010;38:122–7.
10. Colberg SR. *The Diabetic Athlete: Prescriptions for Exercise and Sports*. Human Kinetics; 2001.
11. Durstine, JL, Moore, GE, editors. *ACSM's Exercise Management for Persons with Chronic Disease and Disabilities*. 2nd ed. Human Kinetics; Champaign, IL 2003. p. 217–21.
12. Exercising with type 2 diabetes Exercise is Medicine Web site: www.exerciseismedicine.org. Accessed June 2010.
13. Felson DT, Zhang Y. An update on the epidemiology of knee and hiposteoarthritis with a view to prevention. *Arthritis Rheum*. 1998;41:1343–55.
14. Felson DT, Zhang Y, Anthony JM, Naimark A, Anderson JJ. Weight loss reduces the risk for symptomatic knee osteoarthritis in women. *Ann Inter Med*. 1992;116:535–9.
15. Hootman J, Bolen J, Helmick C, Langmaid G. Prevalence of doctor-diagnosed arthritis and arthritis-attributable activity limitation—United States, 2003–2005. CDC, MMWR 2006;55:1089–92.
16. Jonathan A Pye. An Introduction to Shoulder Injuries: prevention and treatment. Sports Injury Bulletin. www.sportsinjurybulletin.com/shoulder. Accessed June 2010.
17. Lloyd-Jones D. Adams R, Carnethon M, et al. Heart disease and stroke statistics—2009 Update: A report from the American Heart Association Statistics Committee and Stroke Statistics Subcommittee. *Circulation*. 2009;119:e87–90.

18. McGill, S. Core training: Evidence translating to better performance and injury prevention. *Strength Cond J*. 2010;32:33–46.

19. McGill, S. *Low Back Disorders: Evidence Based Prevention and Rehabilitation*. Human Kinetics Champaign, IL; 2002.

20. McGill, S. The painful lumbar spine. *IDEA Fit J*. January 2010;7:30–7.

21. Messier SP. *ACSM's Resource Manual for Guidelines for Exercise Testing and Prescription*. 5th ed. Baltimore (MD): Lippincott Williams & Wilkins; 2006.

22. CDC, National Center for Health Statistics, National Health Interview Survey, 2005 CDC, MMWR 54(19):484–488.

23. National Heart, Lung, and Blood Institute and National High Blood Pressure Education Program. "Seventh Report of the Joint National Committee on Prevention, Detection, Evaluation, and Treatment of High Blood Pressure Express" (JNC 7). Aram Chobanian, M.D., Chair.

24. National Institute of Health: National Institute of Arthritis and Musculoskeletal Diseases Web site. Health Topics: Osteoarthritis. July 2002.

25. National Institutes of Health: NIH Web site: www.nih.gov. Accessed June 2010.

26. Pivarnik JM, Mudd L. Oh baby! Exercise during pregnancy and the postpartum period. *ACSM's Health Fit J*. 2009;13:8–13.

27. Ronai P. Shoulder stability exercise training. *ACSM Certified News*. 2002;12:1–3.

28. Thompson WR, editor. *ACSM's Guidelines for Exercise Testing and Prescription*. 8th ed. Lippincott Williams & Wilkins; 2010.

# Specialty Classes

### KAREN A. KENT

*Objectives*

**At the end of this chapter, you will be able to:**
- Explain the different types of class styles
- Identify the guidelines for popular class styles
- Describe the components of class design (warm up, stimulus, cool down)
- Design a basic group exercise class

Specialty classes have become increasingly popular in group exercise programs. This chapter is devoted to four common varieties often seen in mainstream group exercise programs: indoor cycling, aquatic exercise, Pilates, and yoga. There are other specialties including the ever-growing popular trend called "fusion," which is the blend of any two or more styles of exercise to create a new form of exercise. Blending yoga and Pilates styles together to create Yogilates (27) is one example. While the list and combinations of fusion classes and new trends in group exercise offerings continues to grow, the specialties highlighted are considered staples in group exercise programs today.

## Take Caution

### GO FOR THE GOLD STANDARD

**Earning an NCCA-accredited group exercise instructor certification like the ACSM Certified Group Exercise Instructor credential, is a smart start to a GEI's career. Additional training and practice of specialty programs is often recommended and sometimes required. While certifications are offered in many specialties, these should be earned in addition to an NCCA-accredited "generalist" certification in order for you to meet the highest and most rigorous and processional industry standards. Keep in mind that safety and effectiveness are the foundations of any workout or class.**

## STATIONARY INDOOR CYCLING CLASS

 **CLIP 9.1** Stationary indoor cycling classes are a popular group fitness modality. These classes are usually conducted in a dedicated room, complete with specialized indoor bikes, sound system, and microphone. This class is about the ride or "journey" itself

so that individuals can work at their own fitness level, regardless of their experience or physical work capacity. It is important that you instruct students on the various methods of measuring exercise intensity. The use of heart rate monitors is popular and can be beneficial if students are educated on their training heart rate and the proper use of the monitor. Also, students who take medications that alter their heart rates will require more information and education on using HR monitors. For these reasons, the use of RPE is often the easiest tool to use. The recommended RPE ranges used in this chapter are based on the 0-10 scale (see Appendix C).

Indoor cycling classes are an ideal mode of training for cardiovascular fitness, burning an average of 475 kcal per 40-minute ride excluding the warm-up and cool-down portion (17). Ideally, participants should have at least a moderate level of cardiovascular conditioning prior to engaging. The use of heart rate monitors (60% of heart rate reserve [HRR]) or more detailed instruction of the rating of perceived exertion (RPE) (Borg) scale is highly recommended for the novice as reported by John and Schuler (29). Research on indoor cycling class has reported that the standing, climbing, high-resistance settings and jumping maneuvers elicited the highest heart rates, RPE, oxygen consumption, and caloric expenditure (11,18,19,53). That said, the prescreening of participants is a safety concern and is recommended whenever feasible (see ACSM Quick Screen, discussed in Chapter 2). Starting with several introductory beginner class sessions is a good strategy to ensure adequate progression and understanding of safety and technique concerns for the participant. Introductory class format is comprised of 20–30 minutes to teach the basic bike setup and seat and hand positions, along with an understanding of the ratings of perceived exertions derived by the resistance, body positions, and speed variables created by the tempo of the music or cadence of the workload on the muscles of the lower body and cardiovascular system.

BOX 9.1     *Bike Setup and Alignment*

1. Seat post height is the key for healthy knees.
   - Adjusting a cyclist's bike seat height is a simple way to improve the comfort and safety of the ride.
   - To determine the right height, the cyclist places his or her feet in the toe cages or clips into the pedals and rotates the pedals until one leg reaches the bottom of the pedal stroke. That leg should have a 25- to 35-degree bend in the knee.
2. Fore/aft seat position
   - The seat also adjusts forward and backward, so that cyclists' knees will be properly aligned relative to their feet.
   - To set the seat position, cyclists sit on the saddle in riding position, with their hands on the handlebars and the balls of their feet over the center of the pedals.
   - They then position the pedals so they're level with each other.
   - Using their forward leg for the alignment check, they picture an imaginary line (or have someone hold a plumb line) from the front of their kneecap straight down.
   - The seat is in the right position when the cyclist's kneecap is directly above the center of the pedal.
3. Handlebar height
   - Is dependent on the cyclist's ability to maintain a neutral spine, flexibility in the hamstrings and hips, arm length, and his/her experience level.
   - Adjust the handlebars to a position that is comfortable and limits unnecessary strain on your neck and back.
4. Pedal concerns/safety
   - If toe cages and straps are used, be sure to align the ball of your foot over the center of the pedal. This is the firmest, widest part of your foot and therefore the most efficient and comfortable foot position.
   - If clipless pedals are used, make sure that your cleats are aligned properly on your shoes so that the ball of your foot is positioned on the center of the pedal. Encourage stiff-soled shoes, to remain rigid over the pedals and to have shoelaces tucked in.
   - Use clips or baskets with straps for efficiency.
   - Encourage the rider to keep feet on pedals while in motion.
   - Use the emergency brake if feet come out of the pedals and keep feet clear of crank arm.
5. Riders should maintain a neutral spine and pelvis with upper body inclined forward about 45 degrees from upright, both scapula slightly depressed and retracted (Fig. 9.1).
   - Avoid pelvic tilt and hyperextension of the neck.

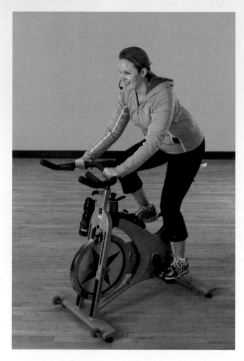

■ **FIGURE 9.1** Proper seated bike alignment. Note the neutral spine position while maintaining a forward incline of the torso-about 45 degrees from upright seated position.

*Source*: Spinner® Bike Setup, Spinning Training Tips. *Mad Dogg Athletics*. 2010.

| BOX 9.2 | Teaching Essentials: Warm-up Segment |
|---------|--------------------------------------|

- Sit upright with neutral spine, easy pedaling, provide overview of planned ride
- Warm up with dynamic movement for 5–10 minutes to increase heart rate gradually
- Rehearse the various positions, explaining proper alignment and cycling techniques
- Give clear cues, verbal directions, and intensity information or guidelines
- Use music of moderate tempo, *e.g.*, 120 bpm equals 60 rpm for the cadence

| BOX 9.3 | Teaching Essentials: Cardiovascular Training Segment |
|---------|------------------------------------------------------|

- Increase the intensity gradually
- Vary the cycling techniques
- Do not use one technique for a prolonged period of time
- Encourage fun interaction between participants
- Use good form and alignment, give clear verbal cues and directions
- Match the volume and tempo of music appropriately. Use a gradual tapering of the intensity for cool-down (1)

## INJURY PREVENTION

Improper bike setup may cause injury or unnecessary muscle soreness for the cyclist. Before starting class, ask if there are any new students or if anyone needs special assistance with their bike setup. Scan the room to ensure that all students are correctly positioned and that all questions have been addressed.

## SAFETY

### Hand Positions

The three hand positions used in indoor cycling were developed with safety and comfort in mind.

1. Hand position 1 (Fig. 9.2) is the basic hand position used in the seated position. Note that the heels of the hands are resting on the straight bar and the fingers are touching on the curved section of the bar.
2. Hand position 2 (Fig. 9.3) is commonly used for seated climbing, running, jumping, and sprinting. This position assists in maintaining an upright posture with no restrictions on breathing and is a more stable hand position when performing certain advanced movements out of the saddle.
3. Hand position 3 (Fig. 9.4) is used solely for standing climbing. The hands are over the ends of the handlebar extensions. The palms are turned inward, knuckles face outward with the fingers wrapped around the bar.

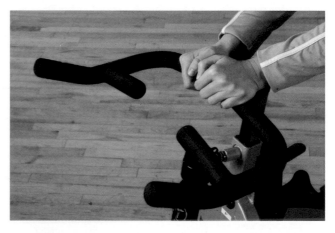

■ **FIGURE 9.2** Hand position 1.

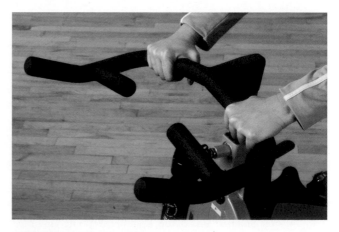

■ **FIGURE 9.3** Hand position 2.

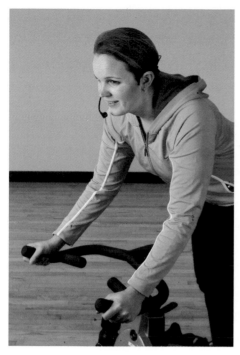

**FIGURE 9.4** Hand position 3.

### Out-of-the-Saddle Movements

For more advanced movements such as standing and jumping, caution your class to have the proper amount of resistance, typically an RPE of 6 or higher. This will ensure that they will be able to stay in control. Running out of the saddle is an advanced move and is not for the beginner. Instruct your class to follow these guidelines:

- The body should be positioned over the center of the bike with bodyweight applied to the pedals.
- Hands should be in position 2 with very light amount of pressure on the handlebar.
- The shoulders should be relaxed with slightly bent elbows.
- The tip of the saddle should lightly touch the back of the thighs.
- Always use moderate resistance of at least an RPE of 6.

**Take Caution**

**BRAKE ADJUSTMENT**

- It is imperative to teach your students how to use the brake knob that works with a uniformly weighted flywheel.
- In the event of an emergency, they should activate the brake adjustment knob and keep their feet away from the moving pedals.

### Stretching

An important part of the cool-down is stretching. Upper body stretches on the bike are safe. Have your students dismount the bike to perform lower body stretches, using the frame of the bike to assist with positions as needed.

**Take Caution**

**NO STRETCHING ON THE BIKE**

Incorporating flexibility training into an indoor cycling class doesn't take a lot of time, and the benefits are immeasurable. The safest type of stretch for flexibility training is a static, sustained stretch. Cyclists should always stretch gradually, to the point of mild discomfort, and hold each stretch for at least 30 seconds. Bouncing or ballistic stretching should be avoided, and stretching should always be done off the bike!

When it Comes to Stretching – Don't Skimp, Spinning Training Tips. *Mad Dogg Athletics*. 2010.

### Intensity

The indoor cycling program should be simple, fun and easy to do, but intensity involves some coaching. Please encourage your students to follow these guidelines:

- There is no competition in this class; encourage your students to train at a level they feel most comfortable.
- Familiarize your students at a moderate pace before increasing the speed. Your student should always have some resistance on the flywheel, except during warm-up or cool-down.
- Remind your students to stay in control, making smooth transitions with good form.
- If a student is having any type of problem, immediately dismount your bike and offer assistance.
- Use RPE and encourage the students to stay within their target heart rate range.

## BASIC MOVES

Your goal is to simulate an outdoor ride or "journey." Use your favorite music for specific goal-intensity segments using seated flats, seated and standing climbs, jumps, and sprints, which are the basic moves or segments of class using an interval format.

### Seated Flat

A basic cycling technique is the seated flat. Using various levels of speed on a flat road will help the cyclist to warm up, creating the cardio stimulus and the cool-down. The cadences will vary from 80 to 110 rpm. (see Fig. 9.1).

### Seated and Standing Hill Climbs

Increasing the resistance on the bike creates seated and standing hill climbs (Fig. 9.5). The body weight is shifted to the back of the seat to protect the knees and gain more

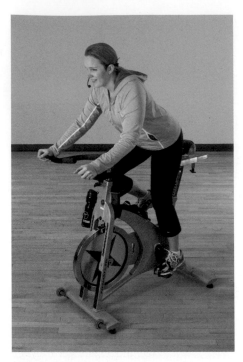

■ **FIGURE 9.5** Standing position.

power from the gluteus. A slower cadence is required, 60–80 rpm, and can be very strenuous.

### Standing Flat Run or Jog

For endurance segments, the resistance is moderate and the cadence is 80–95 rpm. Keeping the spine neutral with slightly bent hips is important, and light touch on the handlebars is encouraged.

### The Downhill or Flushing Segment

Perform the downhill or flushing segment in the seated position with lighter resistance or RPE of 5. This is used after a heavy hill climb, for recovery of breathing and heart rate to moderate levels.

### Rebounds, Jump, or Lifts

Advanced moves used to increase intensity are rebounds, jumps, or lifts. These are usually done with eight counts up out of the saddle and eight counts back in the saddle. Jumps can be hard on the knees; therefore, we recommend limiting or avoiding jumps in most cycling classes.

### Sprints

Sprints, also known as spin-outs, fast hammers, and power drills, could be performed in a seated (see Fig. 9.1) or standing position (see Fig. 9.5). The cadence will change to a very fast pace of 100–120 rpm with light to moderate resistance. Watch for bounding hips, and cue participants to increase the amount of resistance for more effective training when necessary.

### Cool-down and Stretching

Be sure to conclude the cycling class by directing your students to decrease tension on the flyer wheel progressively for about 5 minutes, also reducing the cadence for at least a minute of class before dismounting the bike. Make sure you stretch the major muscle groups using the bike for balance.

> ✔ **RECOMMENDED RESOURCES:**
> *Trademarked by names such as Spinning are specialized organizations which provide certifications.*
> **Mad Dogg Athletics, Inc.**
> *2111 Narcissus Ct.*
> *Venice, CA 90291*
> *800-847-SPIN*
> *www.spinning.com*
> *Keiser*
> *800-888-7009*
> *www.keiser.com/m3/mtraining.html*

## WATER EXERCISE CLASS

Over the last 20 years, water exercise has grown in popularity. Water exercise provides a forgiving cross-training modality for competitive athletes with the cushioning effects of water, and for individuals with potential risk to impact stress from weight-bearing exercise, such as the elderly, obese, individuals with a soft tissue injury, or those with an orthopedic disorder, who may also find water to be the most desirable environment for exercise (35). A great advantage of water exercise is the ability to utilize total-body functional and sport-specific movement through optimal ranges of motion while minimizing joint stress (5,47,50).

Water exercise is a perfect medium for providing cardiovascular and resistance training stimuli. Although it is important to discuss the heart rate response to the aquatic medium, the scientific-based evidence shows that while standing in water at chest level, there are marked increases in central venous pressure, stroke volume, and cardiac output, which results in a decrease in heart rate. The combined influence of water temperature and hydrostatic pressure help to explain why, at a given $VO_2$, heart rate has been shown to be up to 20 bpm lower in water than on land (40). Results conclude that the heart rate is lower when participating in the water exercise as compared to land-based exercise because of the hydrostatic effects of water causing a shift of blood volume from the periphery of the body to the thorax (2). It has been shown that the heart rate response in water depends considerably on water temperature (3). Consequently, RPE is a preferred indicator of work intensity in water-based fitness classes.

BOX 9.4

## Unique Qualities of Water Exercise

- When one walks at chest height in the water, the buoyant force of water results in a 90% reduction in body weight and strengthens abdominals (30).
- Water is capable of providing a full-body multiplanar resistive force through which the extremities can move.
- The density of water is approximately 800 times that of air, which is an important contribution to the energy cost of water exercise (16).
- The water environment allows for high levels of energy expenditure, while reducing or eliminating next day soreness (often referred to as Delayed Onset Muscle Soreness or DOMS) by emphasizing concentric resistance (7).

## WARM-UP

Warm-up in the water is different than a typical land-based class. The water-based class requires a vigorous warm-up of dynamic movements to promote thermo-regulation of the body in the cooler water temperature, typically at 82°F–86°F. Additionally, the warm-up should increase ranges of motion (ROM) and then gradually increase speed and lever length to progress the exercise at the prescribed cardiovascular training zone.

Deep and shallow water have fundamental differences of how the human body is affected by buoyancy. Provide an orientation in the shallow water using basic movements, and then progress using buoyancy equipment teaching the awareness of center of buoyancy over center of gravity, how to recover when alignment is lost, and then progressing into the deep water after mastery of recovery drills are achieved.

Water safety and progression plays a large role in the psychological and physical adjustment to the buoyant environment. Progression should begin with familiar land-based movements, with appropriate buoyancy equipment rehearsed in the shallow area of the pool, and then proceed to the suspension movements or deeper water (39). The kinesthetic awareness of body parts and alignment in vertical movement, especially in the deep water is a new learning experience and must be properly cued, demonstrated, and reinforced in a variety of approaches.

BOX 9.5

## Essential Teaching Skills

Warm-up Segment

- Use full ROM, multidirectional dynamic movements
- Provide rehearsal of simple moves before adding more complex combinations
- Stretch major muscle groups with appropriate instruction
- Give clear cues and verbal direction
- Use music to match the movement

Cardiovascular Segment

- Increase the intensity gradually
- Use a variety of longer and shorter lever techniques
- Change water technique routinely, but not too often
- Transition to slower water movements to cool down
- Provide clear cueing, as well as demonstrating good alignment and form

Progressive Resistance

- Increasing speed results in more resistance
- Increasing the surface area results in more resistance
- Traveling against a current creates additional overload
- Using drag equipment will increase resistance

## TECHNIQUE AND SAFETY

- For safety purposes, be sure to explain any physical concerns about the pool area.
- Have a lifeguard present on deck.
- Be sure to inquire about the water temperature comfort.
- Move at "water speed" when demonstrating on-deck.
- Emphasize full ROM, engaging of specific muscles, and alignment.
- When using total-body movements, bring participants' attention to engaging the core.
- Use multidirectional movement planes and vary lever length to change workload.
- Encourage participants to work at their own level and modify where necessary.
- Instruct from the water only when the class understands the movement, moving out on deck to demonstrate as necessary.
- Name your movements with fun, descriptive names.
- Group the movements in a series, (e.g., jumping jacks (JJ) for lower extremities, then pyramid press for upper extremities), so routine and familiarity is learned to ease the auditory concerns in the pool area.

## BENEFITS OF INTERVALS

Allows the participants to perform at intense workloads with periods of recovery (34).
- Workload changes are physically demanding, yet fun (20).
- As a higher state of conditioning occurs, increasing the length of the work bout and decreasing the recovery time allows for a higher metabolic response or the calories expended (above resting values) after an exercise bout. This is referred to as "excess post-exercise oxygen consumption (EPOC)" (52).

## USING EQUIPMENT

After 6–8 weeks, the initial adaptation to the water exercise has occurred, and more overload is required (36).
- Surface area or drag equipment is good in both deep and shallow water.
- This equipment uses concentric muscle contraction; otherwise know a positive resistance working both antagonist and agonists muscle group.
- Buoyancy equipment offers aide in safety for deep water exercise or an injured lower extremity.

 **RECOMMENDED RESOURCES:** *Below are Web sites that relate to water exercise.*

www.hydrotone.com
www.aquatherapeutics.com
www.aeawave.com
www.poolates.com
www.waterfit.com
www.aquajogger.com

## PILATES

This type of exercise class is considered a "mind-body" program, which means that the participants should be mentally focused and introspective as they perform the exercises. The Pilates method of body conditioning is a unique system of stretching and strengthening exercises developed over 100 years ago by Joseph H. Pilates. The Pilates method originated with a small group of dancers and elite athletes in New York City and became popular in the 1990s in other areas of the world. Since then, the 2007 IDEA Health and Fitness Association Program and Equipment Survey found that 68% of program directors at fitness facilities offered Pilates mat classes as a staple on their group fitness schedule (45). The Pilates system was developed to create a healthy body, a healthy mind, and a healthy way of life with a message of balance. Pilates basic principles include concentration, centering, breathing, controlling (including strength), precision, flowing movement, isolation (including flexibility), and routine with the focus being that the quality of the movement is superior to the quantity.

Contrology develops the body uniformly, corrects wrong postures, restores physical vitality, invigorates the mind, and elevates the spirit, centered on the basic principles, as stated above.

- Centering relates to the "powerhouse" of strength (pelvis, spine, neck, and shoulder girdle), from which all movements emanate.
- It is the control through the abdominals that provide fluidity of movement from the center, not just strength.
- The Abdominal Hollowing or B-line is an age-old approach to abdominal control by drawing the transverse abdominal wall into the spine from the navel to stabilize the spine (25).
- Imprinting of the spine into the mat entails flattening of the lumbar curve, a posterior tilted pelvis by contracting the rectus abdominis.
- Control is essential to preventing injuries, as in a prone plank position, inhale on the leg lift. This braces or engages the powerhouse and protects weaker muscles.
- Precision requires thought, mental feedback, and controlled action, without which the movement becomes sloppy or aesthetically unappealing. The work is performed slowly so the stronger muscles do not over power the weaker ones.
- Flowing movement is conscious muscular control through all ranges of movement preventing stiff, jerky movements.
- Isolation aids in the flexibility of the limb, lever, and joints when you are able to contract the muscle independently. As the weaker muscles become stronger, they move independently of other body parts.
- Routine practice of 1¼ hours should be established — at least 2–3 days a week is recommended (38).

General breath rules to follow and cue when moving include the following:

- In a supine position, exhale as appendages move vertically away, and inhale on the return to center.
- Inhale when appendages move laterally from midline, and exhale on return to center.
- In a prone position or lying on the side, engage abdominals B-line, (B-Line is a Pilates term which means: "behind the line of the hip bones" and refers to abdominal muscles being as close as possible to the spine) exhale as you lift and inhale as you lower appendages.
- In a quadruped position, inhale as you elongate and exhale moving toward the center.
- Exhale when contracting (curling forward) or rotating the torso.

## THE NEUTRAL SPINE

**CLIP 9.2** A neutral spine is a keystone of the modern Pilates practice (Fig. 9.6). Muscle imbalances are generally the major causes of poor posture. Inherited conditions, habits from occupational or repetitive movements, and disease can also alter the correct body alignment of the skeletal structure. To bring the body back into balance, one has to stretch the tighter, overworked muscles and strengthen the weaker muscles. Establishing and maintaining the correct position of the limbs, pelvis, or torso is crucial to the final outcome. Most experts maintain that a neutral spine distributes the stress, shock, and impactful forces in the safest way possible (41,12,37).

## WARM-UP

The Pilates mat class is basically practiced on the floor as the warm-up prepares the mind to focus on key concepts as follows: proper breathing, neutral spine, spinal mobility, abdominal hollowing, imprinting, lengthening, control, precision, and mindfulness are introduced. Below is a sample warm-up:

- Seated breathing practice with 3–5 breaths
- Round and release. Exhale while rounding and flexing spine to a posterior tilt with abdominal hollowing. Inhale while lifting spine up, pelvis to neutral sitting up on sits bones (ischial tuberosities) for 3–5 breaths.
- Spinal imprinting and release
- Spinal articulated bridge
- Spine rib cage placement
- Quadruped cat-cow tilts

## VERBAL CUES AND MUSIC

Be sure to offer a variety of verbal cues to provide a full understanding of how to articulate the movement with the breath for all segments of the exercise. If you notice a participant experiencing discomfort or pain, give cueing to reduce the range of motion, to change the pressure on the

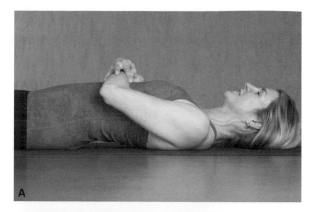

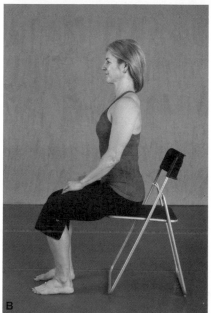

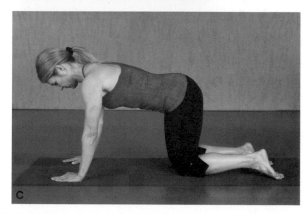

**■ FIGURE 9.6** The neutral spine in the (**A**) supine, (**B**) seated, and (**C**) quadruped positions.

joint, or offer a pillow/prop to facilitate comfort and safety. The choice of music should be soft, soothing background music to elicit calmness and relaxation for the mind.

## TECHNIQUE AND SAFETY

Pilates exercises can be very basic to quite extreme and lead to potential injury. The task of teaching at

| BOX 9.6 | Benefits of Pilates |
|---|---|

- Improved posture
- Stronger abdominals and back musculature
- Improved pelvic control
- Improved muscular endurance
- Body Awareness
- Better coordination and sense of balance
- Reduction in back pain and potential injury
- Increased muscle flexibility
- Improved ability to correctly contract the transverse abdominus
- Increased spine mobility

*Source*: Pilates Method Alliance. PMA position statement: On Pilates. Miami (FL): Pilates Method Alliance; 2006:2.

multiple levels is very important. As Siler (46) states, some of the more advanced exercises may not be best suited to your particular body, and that is okay. As an instructor, you should be aware of the potential injury to the joints or spine such as with unsupported spinal flexion, unsupported spinal flexion with rotation, unsupported lateral flexion, extreme lumbar hyperextension, long-lever traction, and weight bearing on the cervical spine; therefore, seek further training and certification.

## BASIC MOVES

These are some of the basic movements: the hundred, roll up, rolling like a ball, single-leg stretch, double-leg stretch, single-leg circle, breast stroke, side-lying, spine stretch forward, seated spine twist, plank, and the leg pull front.

### The Hundred

1. Lying in a supine position with the knees pulled into your chest. Inhale deeply, and then exhale while allowing the belly to sink.
2. Fold forward from your back; tilt your chin to look at your belly.
3. Press your shoulder blades into the mat as you extend your arms by your sides.
4. Extend your legs to the ceiling,
5. Pump the extended arms up and down, as if you were slapping water.
6. Inhale for five counts and exhale for five counts, as you continue to reach.
7. Lower your legs to a 45-degree angle, as long as you maintain your lumbar spine pressed in the mat.
8. Continue for 10 sets to perform the 100 counts of breathing.

### Take Caution

**TECHNIQUE AND SAFETY CHECKLIST**

**To keep your class safe, remember to**

- **Provide the proper warm-up**
- **Teach progression with basic or modified exercises first**
- **Avoid high-risk exercises**
- **Cue for alignment and details in various ways for each exercise**
- **Give mindful breath instructions on each phase of the movement**

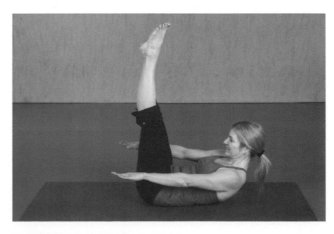

**■ FIGURE 9.7** The hundred.

9. Relax the head into the mat and pull the knees into the chest, and then lengthen out your arms and legs in preparation for the roll-up (Fig. 9.7).

## The Roll-Up

1. In a full extension of the torso, engage your buttocks and press the posterior aspect of your thigh into the mat.
2. Extend your arm over your chest.

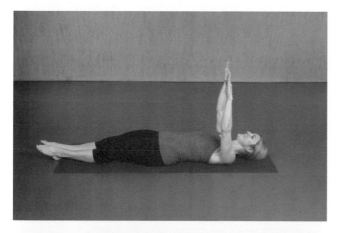

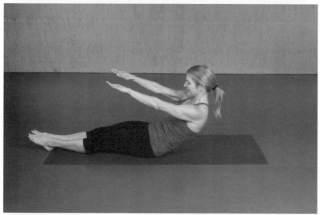

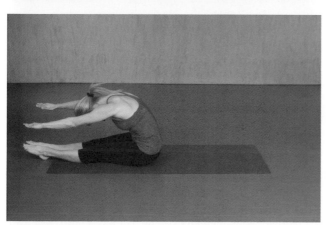

**■ FIGURE 9.8** Roll up.

3. Lengthen the back of the neck while performing a chin tilt to the chest and inhale as you articulate one vertebra at a time off the mat to roll up and forward.
4. Exhale as you stretch forward from your hips while keeping your navel pulled into the spine.
5. Exhale as you flex the spine lifting one vertebra at a time off the mat.
6. Complete three to five cycles (Fig. 9.8).

## Rolling Like a Ball

1. Sit toward the front of the mat with your knees bent into your chest as you grab your ankles.
2. Lift up your heels off the mat balancing on your tailbone with your chin tucked into your chest.
3. Engage your abdominal muscle toward the spine, and fall backward.
4. Inhale as you roll back, and exhale as you come forward.
5. Continue to roll like a ball for five or six times, and then sit back on the mat to prepare for single-leg stretch (Fig. 9.9).

## Single-Leg Stretch

1. Sit in the center of the mat with your knees bent. Pull your right knee into your chest by placing your left hand just below the knee and right hand on your

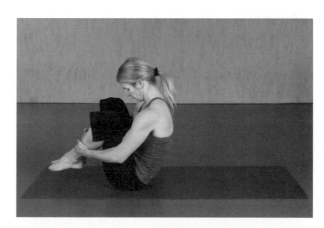

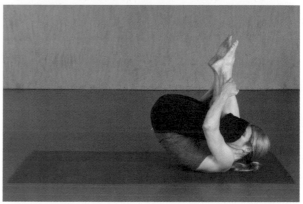

**■ FIGURE 9.9** Rolling like the ball.

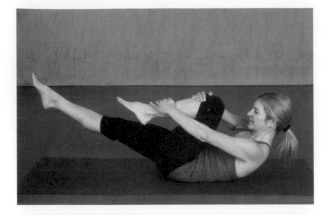

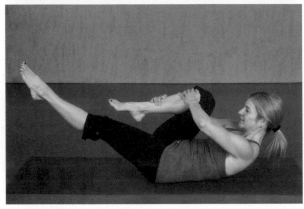

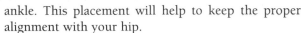

■ **FIGURE 9.10** Single-leg stretch.

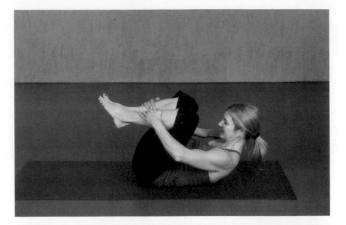

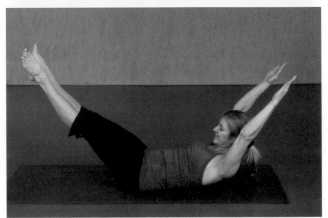

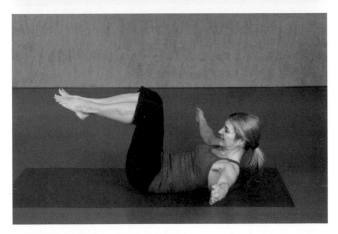

■ **FIGURE 9.11** Double-leg stretch.

ankle. This placement will help to keep the proper alignment with your hip.

2. Roll your back down on the mat, maintain the knee to chest position.
3. Extend your left leg out in front of you just above the mat to allow the spine to be supported.
4. With your arms extended and your chin lifted toward your chest, inhale and engage your abdominals toward the spine.
5. Exhale and switch legs; bring the outside hand to the ankle and the inside hand below the knee. Stretch your extended leg out from your hip and to the center of the body.
6. Continues for 5–10 sets of the single stretch and then pull both knees into the chest for double-leg stretch (Fig. 9.10).

### Double-Leg Stretch

1. Lie on your back and pull both knees into your chest with arms extended, head lifted with chin tuck.
2. Inhale deeply while stretching your body long, reaching your arms back by your ears and with your legs extended in front of you at a 45-degree angle.
3. As you exhale, draw your knees back into your chest by circling your arms around to meet them.
4. Repeat the sequence 5–10 times, remaining still in your torso as you inhale to stretch and exhale to pull back to start position (Fig. 9.11).

### Single-Leg Circles

1. To prepare stretch by pulling one knee into your chest, then straighten the leg while holding the ankle or the calf.
2. Place your arms back down by your sides, and leave your leg reaching straight up to the ceiling at as close to a 90-degree angle as possible. Lengthen the back of your neck by pressing into the mat.
3. The opposite leg should be centered and reaching long in front of you for stability.
4. Stretch your leg across your body, then circle it down, around, and back up to its starting position with your

leg slightly turned out so that the posterior hip stays in contact with the mat.

5. Continue three to five repetitions, inhaling as you begin the movement and exhaling as you complete it. Reverse the direction of the circles, and complete three to five repetitions, making sure you remain stabilized in your hips at all times.

6. Change legs to repeat the stretch and leg circles with the other leg (Fig. 9.12).

## BEFORE TEACHING A PILATES CLASS

As with any exercise program, there is risk for injuries, so prescreening and if necessary medical clearance is required. Seek out additional training and certification in Pilates.

## YOGA

### PHILOSOPHY

This type of exercise class is considered a "mind-body" program, which means the participants should be mentally focused and introspective as they perform the exercises. The yoga practice is an ideal way to improve the quality of life, as it enhances both the physical and psychological well-being. The yogi believes that yoga is a complete system of living. The word yoga means to "yoke" or unite. The practice of yoga integrates every aspect of a human being from the innermost to the external. Hatha, one of many forms of yoga, provides a comprehensive system of stretches designed for physical health, emotional balance, mental clarity, and spiritual health development, including breath work. The breath work, meditation, positive thinking, healthy diet, and

 **RECOMMENDED RESOURCES:** *Below are some helpful Pilates resources.*

**Books**
- *Menezes A. The Complete Guide to Joseph H. Pilates Techniques of Physical Conditioning. Alameda, CA: Hunter House; 2000.*
- *Lessen D. The PMA Pilates certification exam study guide. Miami, FL: Pilates Method Alliance; 2005.*
- *Siler B. The Pilates Body. New York: Broadway Books; 2000.*

**Web sites**
- *Balanced Body, www.Pilates.com*
- *Physical mind Institute, www.themethodpilates.com*
- *Pilates Method Alliance (PMA), www.pilatesmethodalliance.org*
- *Stott Pilates, www.stottpilates.com*

services to others of the mind are key components of this discipline of conscious living. The purpose of yoga is to enhance and maintain the health of the physical body while creating calmness in the mind, which uses the breath as the link. This is accomplished through the mobility of the torso and joints along with the stability of the spine. Typically the sequencing is organized in a complementary manner-with a principle pose and then a counter pose. Practitioners believe that all of the internal systems such as circulatory, respiratory, glandular, nervous, and digestive systems are fine-tuned in practice (8). The technical terms of Yoga are in Sanskrit, the classical language of India. Most yoga instructors have translated the Sanskrit names into common usage names.

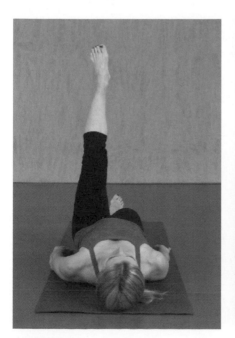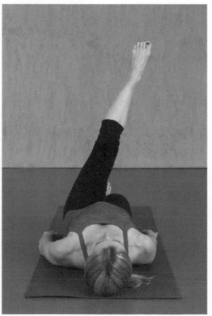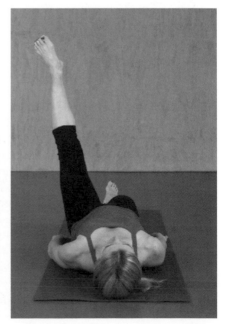

■ **FIGURE 9.12** Single-leg circles.

The American College of Sports Medicine exercise guidelines recommend that we should be engaging in cardiovascular activity on most days of the week, 2–3 days of resistance training and 2–3 days per week of flexibility. The following studies have validated yoga as a viable means in satisfying the ACSM's fitness guidelines. ACE commissioned a study, finding 50 minutes of power yoga burned approximately 237 cal and elevated the participant's heart rate 62% of $HR_{max}$ along with increased flexibility, balance, and strength and endurance in the abdominal and chest areas (43). Adelphi University found that the metabolic demand of Ashtanga yoga was similar to that of moderate-intensity aerobic dance or walking (9). Another study found improvements in muscle strength, endurance, flexibility, cardiorespiratory fitness, body composition, and lung function after an 8-week training program in which subjects participated in yoga class 2 days per week (51).

## THE NEED FOR ADDITIONAL EDUCATIONAL TRAINING AND CERTIFICATION

Since yoga is a unique and comprehensive philosophy, its complex system of physical movements differs from the systems of movements of traditional physical fitness. It is highly recommended that you seek out additional training and certification before you lead yoga classes. For more information on training and certifications, see the list of yoga Web sites.

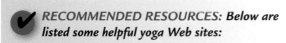

**✔ RECOMMENDED RESOURCES:** *Below are listed some helpful yoga Web sites:*

*www.yogajournal.com*
*www.yogafit.com*
*www.yogaalliance.com*

## TYPICAL YOGA CLASS STRUCTURE

There are many styles of yoga, from gentle and therapeutic to the very vigorous forms which are well known, such as hot yoga or power yoga. People at any fitness level can find and explore the right kind of yoga for them. Raja (royal) yoga uses moral discipline and meditation. Karma yoga seeks transcendence and spiritual freedom. Jnana yoga practices of discernment, wisdom, and the path of the sage. Tantra yoga is a ceremonial form of yoga. Bhakti, the yoga of devotion, is said to be having an open heart and Hatha yoga, the physical postures, including Iyengar, Bikram, Viniyoga, Jivamukti, Kripaula, Sivananda, and Anusara. In the fitness setting, however Hatha Yoga is the most common style of yoga offered.

### How to Begin a Yoga Class

- Start with breath work or "Basic Abdominal Breathing" by focusing attention on taking a breath deep into the belly as the diaphragm contracts downward and the abdomen is pushed out during inhalation, and the diaphragm relaxes back up as the abdominal muscles engage during exhalation.
- Pranayamas are techniques used to control or harness one's breath that prepare or brace the body for the movement into poses or asanas.
- Centering oneself means being mindful of the breath and its powerful way of staying present in the moment and letting go of the business of the day.
- During practice, the mind stays connected to the body through the breath, exploring the sensations in the body and calming the mind.

### Warm-up

Bringing yourself into the moment with the warm-up and breathing exercises, the cat pose or cat/cow tilts is an exercise bringing awareness and flexibility to the entire length of the spine. Coupled with the breath, cat and cow pose's (Fig. 9.13) key is the awareness through the slow movement.

1. Use a quadruped position with the hands just ahead of the shoulders and the hips over the knees
2. Inhale deeply into the spine as you drop your belly toward the mat. Move your breastbone forward and up as your tailbone extends upward. Keep the back of your neck long as you gaze upward.

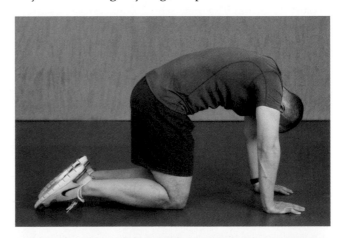

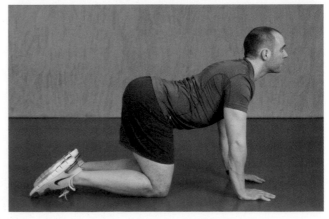

■ **FIGURE 9.13** Cat/cow tilts.

3. As you exhale, round your back. Your upper back arches naturally in this way, so place particular awareness in the movement of the lower back as it follows this new curve upward as you tuck your pelvis under. Observe how the shoulder blades spread apart. As you finish your exhalation, move your chin toward your breastbone.

4. Repeat up to 10 more rounds, arching and rounding deepening with your breath as you increase your awareness in the moment.

### Yoga Class Structured Warm-up

Other limbering moves on the hands and knees include

- Child pose
- Downward dog and or standing forward bend
- Sun salutations

Modified warm-up flow (beginners and/or participants with special concerns):

- Sit in cross-legged pose or modified sitting position for breath and or meditation.
- Swing arms up and down for three sun breaths.
- Side stretching alternating sides for three cycles.
- Spinal Rotation, exhale with straight spine to the right and inhale to return to center and repeat to the left.
- Extend legs out in front, circle feet clockwise three times and reverse. Move into dorsiflexion and plantar flexion of the ankles.
- Transition into a quadruped position for cat/cow tilt, exhale into cat stretch as the spine rounds and the head and tail point down, and inhale as the spine lengthens and the head and tail point up.
- Maintaining quadraped position and neutral spine, engage abdominals and laterally flex the spine from side to side (wag your tail slowly). Exhale as you flex to the right; inhale as you flex to the left.

- Transition to circling the pelvis, allowing the spine and head to move as it feels comfortable.
- Transition to pressing the right heel into the floor, switch to the left heel and finally press both heels back moving into a downward dog position.

### Sun Salutation

CLIP 9.3 Sun salutation is a flow of postures (Table 9.1 offers variations for various poses). This graceful flow is intended to be performed without stopping. The directional cue of inhaling and exhaling is given with each posture and used in meditation. Yogic breathing exercises have improved asthma symptoms in study subjects (14).

## VERBAL CUEING AND MUSIC

There are various types of cues that could be used in teaching yoga. Typically, yoga instructors speak in soft, calm tones and offer suggestions on how you may want to participate.

The music can vary depending on the style or segment of a class. During the beginning or end of class, a selection of soft introspective music is suitable, whereas during a rigorous, repetitive power type of class, a stronger drumming background is often selected. The volume is lower than in other type of group fitness classes.

## MODERN USAGE OF YOGA

An increasing numbers of medical doctors, chiropractors, back specialists, and therapists are recommending yoga practice for their patients. Yoga is being prescribed as a preventive and remedial measure for the spine and stress reduction (4). Yoga has been found to be an effective modality for relieving low back pain (22,24,28,48,54,55).

| Table 9.1 | SUN SALUTATION VARIATIONS | |
|---|---|---|
| STEP | SUN SALUTATION 1 | SUN SALUTATION 2 |
| 1 | Mountain pose, prayer position — Exhale | Mountain pose, arms overhead — Inhale |
| 2 | Mountain pose, arms overhead — Inhale | Forward bend — Exhale |
| 3 | Forward bend — Exhale | Monkey pose, head up—Inhale |
| 4 | Lunge, right foot back, head up — Inhale | Forward bend — Exhale |
| 5 | Plank position — Hold breath | Plank — Inhale |
| 6 | Chaturanga dandasana — Exhale | Chaturanga dandasana — Exhale |
| 7 | Upward-facing dog — Inhale | Upward-facing dog — Inhale |
| 8 | Downward facing dog — Exhale | Downward facing dog — Exhale |
| 9 | Lunge left foot back — Inhale | Monkey pose, head up — Inhale |
| 10 | Forward bend — Exhale | Forward bend — Exhale |
| 11 | Mountain pose, arms overhead — Inhale | Mountain pose, arms overhead — Inhale |
| 12 | Mountain pose, arms at sides — Exhale | Mountain pose, arms at sides — Exhale |

Kennedy C, Yoke M. Methods of Group Exercise Instruction. Champaign, (IL): Human Kinetics, 2009; 269–288.

| BOX 9.7 | Yoga Class Preparation Guidelines |
|---|---|

- Warm-up of simple poses, which allow the body to prepare for movement.
- Proceed into the selected group of poses for the day.
- End with relaxing poses that allow the work done to be assimilated in the body.
- Repetition of postures such as standing poses, sitting poses, and twisting poses is recommended with special care in selection relative to the fitness level of class participants.
- Progression in the length of time postures are held is also contingent to the fitness level.
- Breathing in the postures: do upward movements with an inhalation and downward movements with an exhalation, so that one cycle of breath is completed within the posture. Never hold the breath while in a posture. The instructor should cue the class on the transitions.
- Select appropriate form of music.

| BOX 9.8 | Examples of Yoga Cues |
|---|---|

- Alignment Cue
  "Lengthen up through your crown, root down into your sits bones." (ishical tuberosities)

- Breathing Cue
  "As you inhale, notice how your ribs elevate, expand, and then fall with each breath."

- Informative Cue
  "As you allow your head to hang downward, you are making space in your spine with the traction created by the weight of your head."

- Injury Prevention Cue
  Using a yoga block will ensure that you do not overstretch, and it will give you more stability, and help you maintain proper alignment."

- Imaging Cue
  "Before coming into a pose, close your eyes and visualize yourself clearly in a strong, stable, steady pose."

- Affirming Cues
  "I am breathing into my spine, making space; I am letting go."

- Inward Cues
  "Be clear of your intent, but begin each practice with an open mind."

The application of yoga for a group fitness instructor would be highly recommended and beneficial for your students. Yoga postures can be blended or fused into the traditional exercises to facilitate muscular balance between strength intervals or as a restorative cool-down. This type of class is referred to as a fusion style class.

## SUMMARY

*Chapter 9 discusses specialty group exercise classes. Among the recommendations made in this chapter is that such specialty classes require special training and education on the part of the instructor. Specific study beyond earning an accredited group exercise instructor certification is recommended and will help facilitate a safe, comprehensive, and effective program.*

*This chapter provided a broad overview of four of the more common specialty classes found in mainstream fitness today. These include indoor stationary cycling classes, aquatics classes, Pilates, and yoga.*
*We reviewed the basics of indoor cycling, including the bike setup, proper positioning on the bike, and safety issues. We also covered the proper warm-up, basic moves, different class formats, intensity rating, cueing for the class, and cool-down of the indoor cycling class. Use your creativity in music selection and formatting of class and then take a journey on every ride. Teaching this type of class is fun and can create a lot of camaraderie for your clientele.*

*We discussed the benefits of water exercise, including how it provides an accommodating modality that adapts to all fitness levels and ages. It offers a nonimpact environment, and whether the participant is an neophyte or a competitive athlete, they all gain from the multiplanar resistance and buoyant effects of the water in either the shallow or deep area of the pool. Safety is first in the aquatic environment, as it is in every class mode. Teach from the deck initially and then in and out of the water to coach your class with visual, verbal, and directional cueing. Adding drag resistance or buoyancy devises will continually challenge your students and keep things interesting.*

*The Pilates methods of exercise are very popular in group fitness classes, small-group training, and one-on-one training. This chapter has covered the benefits and the basic principles of Pilates exercises. We provided a sampling of the basic exercises in hopes this may encourage you to seek further education and certification in Pilates.*

*Yoga has emerged from its ancient Indian origins as a discipline for living; to take a place in the modern fitness industry. This holistic practice unites body, mind, and spirit. We covered some basic yoga philosophy, styles and types of yoga, fundamentals of breath work, research findings, verbal cues, music, warm-up, and the basic sun salutation. Today, medical professionals are referring individuals to yoga for its therapeutic and stress-reducing benefits. It is beneficial to fitness instructors to become educated and certified to broaden their class structure to include fusion of yoga into their basic classes as a stretching and restorative modality. Namaste!*

## References

1. Aerobics and Fitness Association of America. *Indoor Cycling Workshop Manual*. Sherman Oaks (CA): Aerobic Fitness Association of America; 2005.
2. Arborelius M Jr, et al. Hemodynamic changes in man during immersion with the head above water. *Aerospace Med*. 1972;43:592–98.
3. Avellini BA, Shapiro Y, Pandolf KB. Cardio-respiratory physical training in water and on land. *Eur J Appl Physiol Occup Physiol*. 1983;50:255–63.
4. Bijlani RL, et al. A brief but comprehensive lifestyle education program based on yoga reduces risk factors for cardiovascular disease and diabetes mellitus. *J Altern Complement Med*. 2005;11(2):267–74.
5. Bravo G, et al. A weight bearing, water-based exercises program for orthopedic women: its impact on bone, functional fitness, and well being. *Arch Phys Med Rehabil*. 1997;78(12):1375–80.
6. Brown C. *The book of Yoga*. UK: Parragon Publishing, HE; 2002.
7. Byrnes W. Muscle soreness following resistance exercise with and without eccentric contractions. *Res Q Exerc Sport*. 1985;56:283.
8. Carrico M. The philosophy of yoga. *IDEA Today*. 1992:26–8.
9. Carroll J, et al. The metabolic requirements of Vinyasa yoga. *Med Sci Sports Exerc*. 2003;35(5):S155.
10. Chapman A, et al. Do muscle recruitment patterns differ between trained and novice cyclist? *Med Sci Sports Exerc*. 2004;36(5):S169.
11. Chinsky A, et al. A comparison of two types of spin classes. Abstract. *Med Sci Sports Exerc*. 1998;30(5):S954.
12. Cholewicki J, Panjabi MM, Khachatryan A. Stabilizing function of flexor-extensor muscles around a neutral spine posture. *Spine*. 1997;22(19):2207–12
13. Cochrane T, Davey RC, Matthes Edward SM. Randomized controlled trial of the cost-effectiveness of water-based therapy for lower limb osteoarthritis. *Health Technol Assess*. 2005;9:iii–76.
14. Cooper S, et al. Effects of two breathing exercises (Buteyko and pranayama) in asthma, a randomized control trail. *Thorax*. 2003;58:674–9.
15. Crews L. Mind-body exercise: yoga and Pilates. *ACSM Fit Society Page*. 2005;Spring.
16. Di Prampero PE. The energy cost of human locomotion on land and in water. *Int J Sports Med*. 1986;7:55–72.
17. Falsetti HS, et al. Heart rate response and caloric expenditure during a Spinning class. In: Goldberg J, editor. *Spinning Instructor Manual B2.1–B2.4*. Venice (CA): Johnny Goldberg Productions; 1995.
18. Flanagan K, et al. The metabolic and cardiovascular response to selected positions and resistance during spinning exercise. Abstract. *Med Sci Sports Exerc*. 1998;30(5):S944.
19. Francis PR, Witucki AS, Buono MJ. Physiological response to a typical studio cycling session. *ACSM Health Fitness J*. 1999;3(1):30–6.
20. Frangolia D, Rhodes E, Taunton J. The effects of deep water running on maximal oxygen consumption. *J Strength Cond Res*. 1996;210(4):215–9.
21. Frangolia D, Rhodes E. Maximal and ventilatory threshold responses to treadmill and water immersion running. *Med Sci Sports Exerc*. 1995;27(2):1007–13.
22. Galantino et al. The impact of modified hatha yoga on chronic low back pain: a pilot study. *Altern Ther Health Med*. 2004;10:56–9.
23. Gehring M, Keller B. Water running with and without a floatation vest in competive and recreation runners. *Med Sci Sports Exerc*. 1997;29(10):1374–8.
24. Herman. Comparing yoga, exercise, and a self-care book for chronic low back pain. *Ann Intern Med*. 2005;143(12):849–56.
25. Hodges P, Richardson C, Jull G. Evaluations of the relationship between laboratory and clinical tests of transverse abdominis function. *Physiother Res Int* 1996;1(4):269.
26. Hoeger W, Warner J, Fahalson G. Physiologic response to self-paced water aerobics and treadmill running. Abstract. *Med Sci Sports Exerc*. 1995;27(5):83.
27. IHRSA 2010 Global Report. *International Health, Racquet & Sportsclub Association*. Boston (MA); 2010.
28. Jacobs BP, et al. Feasibility of conducting a clinical trial on hatha yoga for chronic low back pain: methodological lesson. *Altern Ther Health Med*. 2004;10:80–3.
29. John DH, Schuler P. Accuracy of using RPE to monitor intensity of group indoor stationary cycling. Abstract. *Med Sci Sports Exerc*. 1999;31(5):S643.
30. Kennedy C, Sanders M. Strength training gets wet. *IDEA Today*. 1995;May:25–30.
31. Kennedy C, Yoke M. Methods of group exercise instruction. *Human Kinetics*. 2009:215–26.
32. Kennedy C, Yoke M. Methods of group exercise instruction. *Human Kinetics*. 2009:227–45.
33. Kennedy C, Yoke M. Methods of group exercise instruction. *Human Kinetics*. 2009:269–88.
34. Kravitz L. The effects of music on exercise. *IDEA Today*. 1994;October:56–61.

35. Kravitz L, Mayo JJ. *The Physiological Effects of Aquatic Exercise: A Brief Review*. Nokomis (FL): Aquatic Exercise Association; 1997.

36. Mayo J. Practical guidelines for the use of deep water running. *J Strength Cond Res*. 2000;22(1):26–9.

37. McGill, S. *Low back disorders*. Champaign, IL: Human Kinetics; 2002.

38. Menezes A. *The Complete Guide to Joseph H. Pilates' Techniques of Physical Conditioning*. Alameda (CA): Hunter House; 2000.

39. Michaud D, et al. Aquarunning and gains in cardiorespiratory fitness. *J Strength Cond Res*. 1995;9(2):78–84.

40. Mougios V, Deligiannis A. Effect of water temperature on performance, lactate production and heart rate at swimming of maximal and submaximal intensity. *J Sports Med Phys Fitness*. 1993;33, 27–33.

41. Norris CM. *Back Stability*. Champaign (IL): Human Kinetics; 2000.

42. Pilates Method Alliance. *PMA position statement: On Pilates*. Miami (FL): Pilates Method Alliance; 2006:2.

43. Porcari, Boehde. Does yoga really do the body good? *ACE Fitness Matters*. 2005;9–10:7–9.

44. Sander M, Lawson D. Use water's accommodation properties to help clients recovering from knee injuries return to sports. *IDEA Fitness J*. 2006;September:40–7.

45. Schroder J, Friesen K. Programs and equipment survey. *IDEA Fitness J*. 2007;July:7–12.

46. Siler B. *The Pilates body*. New York: Broadway books; 2000:25–7.

47. Simmons V, et al. Effectiveness of water exercise on the elderly: an experimental study on balance enhancement. *J Gerontol Med Sci* 1996;51A(5):M233–8.

48. Sherman KJ, et al. Comparing yoga, exercise, and a self-care book for chronic low back pain. *Ann Intern Med*. 2005;143(12):849–56.

49. Spinner® Bike Setup, Spinning Training Tips. *Mad Dogg Athletics*. 2010.

50. Suomi R, et al. Postural sway characteristics in women with lower extremities arthritis before and after and aquatic exercise intervention. *Arch Phys Med Rehabil*. 2000;8(6):780–5.

51. Tran MD, et al. Effects of yoga practice on the health-related aspects of physical fitness. *Prev Cardiol* 2001;4(4):165–70.

52. Vella CA, Kravitz L. Exercise after-burn: a research update. *IDEA Fitness J*. 2004;1(5):42–7.

53. Williford HN, et al. Maximal cycle ergometry and group exercise: a comparison of physiological responses. Abstract. *Med Sci Sports Exerc*. 1999;31(5):S423.

54. Williams, et al. Therapeutic application of Iyengar yoga for healing chronic low back pain. *Int J Yoga Ther*. 2003;13:55–67.

55. Williams, et al. Effect of Iyengar yoga therapy for chronic low back pain. *Pain*. 2005;115:107–17.

56. Yogilates was created in 1997 by certified Pilates instructor and personal trainer Jonathan Urla. *http://www.webmd.com/fitness-exercise/guide/yogalates-blend-of-exercises*

57. When it Comes to Stretching – Don't Skimp, Spinning Training Tips. *Mad Dogg Athletics*. 2010.

# Legal Issues and Responsibilities for Group Exercise Instructor

SHIRLEY ARCHER

**After completing this chapter you will be able to:**
· Understand the primary areas of potential liability
· Understand the role of industry standards and guidelines
· Learn practical strategies to manage risk

*objectives*

As a group exercise instructor (GEI), you must understand legal issues and responsibilities before assuming leadership of any exercise classes. Regardless of whether you are an employee or an independent contractor, you need to know what areas of potential liability affect your job performance, what industry standards and guidelines direct these areas, and what measures you can take to manage risk effectively. All physical activity involves risk of injury; accidents can and will happen. To maintain professionalism and to protect the longevity of your health and fitness career, you need to proactively anticipate risk areas and manage them with common sense. This knowledge of, and commitment to, safety and injury prevention not only minimizes the likelihood of professional liability but also improves service quality and may save lives.

This chapter discusses liability specifically related to group exercise instruction (1) and does not expand into broader issues such as type of business organization, copyright, or trademark issues that are more appropriately covered in other chapters and books devoted specifically to business practices. Local rules and regulations, definitions of standards of care, and the acceptability of informed consent forms and waivers of liability vary from state to state, county to county, and even city to city. This chapter is not intended to be legal advice and should not be considered a substitute for legal counsel on specific liability issues pertaining to individual situations.

## TERMINOLOGY AND CONCEPTS

### DEFINITION OF LIABILITY FOR THE GEI

Before discussing liability issues, all GEIs must understand the concept of liability. Liability exists as a public policy to encourage responsible behavior and to protect the public. Legal liability simply means that one has a legal responsibility for one's acts or omissions, or in other words, the failure to act. This liability is based on one's duty or standard of care. A professional GEI's responsibility is to lead safe, effective group exercise programs that meet standards and guidelines set by professional organizations and other relevant codes, laws, and regulations.

The legal liability of a GEI can be understood without becoming overly technical. A person is considered legally liable if he or she fails to meet or, in other words, "breaches" the standard of care. As an exercise professional, if you fail to meet certain expectations of professional conduct, you will be held legally accountable. The best way to protect yourself from exposure to liability, therefore, is to know the standards of care that are expected of you and to proactively take steps to always conduct yourself professionally. Additional measures to further reduce liability risk include using legal forms such as waivers and releases, maintaining your GEI certification, and obtaining liability insurance. See Box 10.1 for a list of key terms such as "duty of care" and "negligence."

## POTENTIAL AREAS OF PROFESSIONAL LIABILITY

Legal considerations affect many aspects of the exercise training experience. Areas of potential exposure for liability include the physical setting where program activities occur; the equipment used; the nature and quality of exercise instructional techniques, advice, and services rendered; the degree of emergency preparedness and responsiveness; and the method of keeping and protecting records. While legal principles affect the training environment, as a practical matter most cases today are settled out of court and therefore never actually create case law.

| BOX 10.1 | *Key Terms* |

*Contract law:* Body of law that regulates the rights and obligations of parties who enter into a contract. A contract is an agreement between two or more parties that creates an obligation to do, or not to do, something that creates a legal relationship. If the agreement is broken, the parties have the right to pursue legal remedies. A contract can be written or verbal. The important elements of a contract include an offer and an acceptance, also referred to as a "meeting of the minds" and the exchange of something of value.

*Duty of care:* Refers to the level of responsibility that one has to protect another from harm. In general, the legal standard is reasonable care under the circumstances, which is based on an examination of factual details.

*Informed consent:* A process that entails conveying complete understanding to a client or patient about his or her option to choose to participate in a procedure, test, service, or program.

*Negligence:* A failure to conform one's conduct to a generally accepted standard or duty that results in harm.

*Release or waiver:* An agreement by a client before beginning participation, to give up, relinquish, or waive the participant's rights to a legal remedy (damages) in the event of injury, even when such injury arises as a result of the service provider's negligence.

*Risk management:* A process whereby a service or program is delivered in a manner that fully conforms to the most relevant standards of practice and that uses operational strategies to ensure day-to-day fulfillment, ensure optimum achievement of desired client outcomes, and minimize risk of harm to or dissatisfaction with clients.

*Standard of care:* The degree of care — attention, prudence, caution — that one needs to exercise in order to meet the duty of care. If you have a duty of care and you fail to meet the standard of care, then you may be found negligent.

*Tort law:* A body of law that regulates civil wrongdoing.

From Herbert DL, Herbert WG, Herbert TG. *Legal Aspects of Preventive, Rehabilitative and Recreational Exercise Programs.* 4th ed. Canton (OH): PRC Publishing; 2002; Koeberle BE. *Legal Aspects of Personal Fitness Training.* 2nd ed. Canton (OH): PRC Publishing; 1994; American College of Sports Medicine. *ACSM's Resource Manual for Guidelines for Exercise Testing and Prescription.* 6th ed. Baltimore (MD): Lippincott Williams & Wilkins, 2010; and Cotten DJ, Cotton MB. *Legal Aspects of Waivers in Sport, Recreation and Fitness Activities.* Canton (OH): PRC Publishing; 1997.

To help you as a GEI to understand the practical issues, this chapter is organized according to the most common types of incidents likely to occur during day-to-day business. The application of legal concepts such as negligence to these particular circumstances is then examined, and the role of professional standards, guidelines, position statements, and recommendations from professional organizations is considered. Exercise training is a business/invitee relationship. In these types of relationships, the ante for invitee responsibilities is raised.

## SAFE PREMISES

Although most GEIs focus on learning the latest training techniques and class formatting, in reality, GEIs are most vulnerable to professional liability for incidents that result from conditions of the physical setting where program activities occur. In general (12), any business owner who allows people to enter upon land or into a building is required to provide a reasonably safe environment under theories of tort law (see Box 10.1). The area of tort law that regulates these issues is termed "premises liability." Box 10.2 lists 21 standards identified by the ACSM to which facilities must

adhere (3). Because GEIs offer services in a variety of locations, including health and fitness facilities, the outdoors, or offsite at hotels, corporations, or churches, before you begin teaching any program, you should take basic precautions to ensure that every training setting is safe.

### Slip and Fall

The number one claim against fitness facilities and professionals is for injuries related to falls on the training premises, according to many insurance providers (7). Courts have consistently held that clients are entitled to "safe" conditions. As a GEI, you can foster safe conditions by observing a regular practice of inspection for, and correction and warning of, any hazards in the workout and access areas to the workout location (8). These are typically commonsense situations. For example, if items are on the floor that may cause a fall, you should clear these away before beginning a session. If floor surfaces are wet and incapable of correction before the session occurs, you should move or reschedule the session. If safety conditions require, it is always better to be conservative and reschedule a class rather than to continue training in the

## BOX 10.2 Standards for Health/Fitness Facilities

1. All facilities offering exercise equipment or services must offer a general preactivity cardiovascular risk screening, *e.g.*, Physical Activity Readiness Questionnaire and/or a specific preactivity screening tool, *e.g.*, Health Risk Appraisal, Health History Questionnaire, to all new members and prospective users.

2. All specific preactivity screening tools (*e.g.*, Health Risk Appraisal, Health History Questionnaire) must be interpreted by qualified staff, and the results of the screening must be documented.

3. If a facility becomes aware that a member or user has known cardiovascular, metabolic, or pulmonary disease, or two or more major cardiovascular risk factors, or any other major self-disclosed medical concern, as a result of a preactivity screening, that person must be advised to consult with a qualified health care provider before beginning a physical activity program.

4. All facilities with qualified staff must offer each new member a general orientation to the facility, including identification of resources available for personal assistance with developing a suitable physical activity program and the proper use of any exercise equipment to be used in that program.

5. Facilities must have in place a written system for sharing information with users and employees or independent contractors regarding the handling of potentially hazardous materials, including the handling of bodily fluids by the facility staff in accordance with the Occupational Safety and Health Administration.

6. Facilities must have written emergency response policies and procedures, which must be reviewed and rehearsed regularly, as well as documented. These policies must enable staff to handle basic first-aid situations and emergency cardiac events.

7. Facilities must have as part of their written emergency response system a public access defibrillation program.

8. The fitness and health care professionals who have supervisory responsibility for the physical activity programs (supervise and oversee members, users, staff, and independent contractors) of the facility must have an appropriate level of education, work experience, and/or certification.

9. The fitness and health care professionals who serve in counseling, instructional, and physical activity supervision roles for the facility must have an appropriate level of professional education, work experience, and/or certification.

10. Fitness and health care professionals engaged in preactivity screening, instructing, monitoring, or supervising of physical activity programs for facility members or users must have current automated external defibrillation and cardiopulmonary resuscitation (AED and CPR) certification from an organization qualified to provide such certification.

11. Facilities, to the extent required by law, must adhere to the building design standards that relate to the designing, building, expanding, or renovating of space as presented by the Americans with Disabilities Act.

12. Facilities must be in compliance with all federal, state, and local building codes.

13. The aquatic and pool facilities must provide the proper safety equipment and signage according to state and local codes and regulations.

14. Facilities must have a system in operation that monitors the entry to and usage of the facility by all individuals, including members and users.

15. Facilities that offer a sauna, steam room, or whirlpool must ensure that these areas are maintained at the proper temperature and that the appropriate warning systems are in place to notify members and users of any unacceptable risks and changes in temperature.

16. Facilities that offer members and users access to a pool or whirlpool must ensure that the pool water chemistry is maintained in accordance with state and local codes.

17. A facility that offers youth services or programs must provide appropriate supervision.

18. Facilities must post the appropriate caution, danger, and warning signage in conspicuous locations where existing conditions and situations warrant such signage.

19. Facilities must post the appropriate emergency and safety signage pertaining to fire and related emergency situations, as required by federal, state, and local codes.

20. Facilities must post all required Americans with Disabilities Act and Occupational Safety and Health Administration signage.

21. All cautionary, danger, and warning signage must have the required signal icon, signal word, signal color, and layout, as specified by the American National Standards Institute and reflected in the American Society of Testing and Materials standards for fitness equipment and fitness facility safety signage and labels.

From American College of Sports Medicine. *ACSM's Health/Fitness Facility Standards and Guidelines.* 3rd ed. Champaign (IL): Human Kinetics; 2007. p. 1–2.

presence of known dangers. If you teach in an aquatics facility, you need to be particularly vigilant about deck conditions and pool access areas, as wet surfaces increase the likelihood of a slip-and-fall incident.

In addition to routinely inspecting locations before and during exercise sessions, all GEIs should follow a procedure of proper equipment storage when equipment is not in use (7). Whether in a dedicated group exercise studio, gym, or community room used for group exercise, encourage designating specific storage places for equipment so items are not left where people can trip over them. Different types of equipment require different types of storage. Make sure to use storage practices that not only store equipment effectively out of people's way under conditions as advised by the manufacturer but also secure equipment from being used for inappropriate purposes. For example, many types of exercise training equipment are attractive to young children and may be best stored in locked cabinets if children potentially can access the training room where they are kept.

### Footwear and Protective Gear

GEIs should educate clients about appropriate clothing and footwear to prevent injury and to enhance training. Clothing should be comfortable, breathable, and allow movement. In particular, you need to check the footwear of class participants and not allow clients to train with inadequate shoes. Factors such as poor fit, excess wear, and unsuitability to the activity all increase the risk of injury. An awareness of foot care issues is also important if you work with clients who have certain types of diabetes. GEIs who work with people who are new to exercise may ask their supervisor to provide a client handout that outlines appropriate exercise apparel and other exercise safety issues. If you train clients in a setting in which protective gear is necessary, such as pads for inline skating, you should make sure that you, as a role model, *and* all the class participants wear all recommended protective equipment (8).

### Environmental Concerns

Environmental conditions such as air quality, temperature, humidity levels, and other related matters also impact safety, but have not resulted in a significant number of claims against fitness professionals. Whether leading group exercise classes indoors or outdoors, you should insure that class participants are not exposed to conditions that may hamper health and should judge safety as it impacts the most vulnerable participants, *e.g.*, older adults, prenatal or postnatal women, or children. If conditions cannot be corrected to be suitable for these individuals, class should be rescheduled.

Four additional environmental considerations include space, wall surfaces, lighting, and noise levels. Since fitness activities involve movement, each participant requires enough space to move freely without risk of colliding into others, into equipment or into any other dangerous surfaces. Class size limits need to be respected. On a related note, before you teach a class, you should scan the exercise environments and check whether wall surfaces are protected or if any other hazards present sharp edges. If activities require rapid movements or tossing of balls, you need to be particularly careful to provide safety cues and to keep activities within the skill level of participants. You also need to ensure that lighting conditions are adequate for planned activities; if any essential lighting fixtures need repair, consider offering class alternatives.

Noise from accompanying class music or any distracting background noise may also impact safety. Background music volume should be motivating, but not so loud as to interfere with the ability to hear class cues. If talking by some class participants distracts others and makes it difficult to hear class instructional and safety cues, you need to develop methods to manage this situation. Some suggestions for managing "class talkers" include providing specific opportunities for classmates to interact and mingle within the class period or announcing reasons to the entire class regarding why talking is disruptive without pointing out individual participants. Often, people are unaware that they are disturbing others, and only a very gentle reminder is required.

## EQUIPMENT USE

Pay attention whenever using equipment, because the second leading reason for claims against GEIs according to insurance providers is injury resulting from equipment use (8). These cases are based on legal theories from tort law that a GEI's duty or standard of care (see Box 10.1) is to exercise reasonable care that a client does not suffer injury. A GEI who fails to take reasonable precautions, which is determined based on an evaluation of facts surrounding an incident, could be deemed to be negligent and therefore liable or responsible for injuries from equipment use.

Professional organizations such as the ACSM and National Strength and Conditioning Association offer industry standards and guidelines relating to matters of facility and equipment setup, inspection, maintenance, repair, and signage. Although these standards and guidelines do not have the force of law, they can be introduced as evidence of the GEI's duty or standard of care. See Box 10.3 for an explanation of the difference between standards and guidelines.

Keep in mind that the law does not envision that accidents never happen; laws exist to encourage proactive safe behavior to avoid preventable accidents. What this means as a practical matter is the following. If an accident happens, but the fitness professional has taken every reasonable step to prevent this accident, the accident will not be considered to be the professional's fault. In other words, the accident does not result from any failure to perform professional responsibilities.

| BOX 10.3 | *Standards Versus Guidelines* |
|---|---|

In the context of the ACSM's Health/Fitness Facility Standards and Guidelines publication, editors offered the following definitions to help understand the differences between standards and guidelines.

*Standards* are base performance criteria or minimum requirements that ACSM believes each health/fitness facility must meet to satisfy a facility's obligations to provide a relatively safe environment in which every physical activity or program is conducted in an appropriate manner.

These standards are not intended to give rise to duty of care or to establish a standard of care; rather, they are performance criteria derived from a consensus of ACSM leaders. The standards are not intended to be restrictive or to supersede national, regional, or local laws and regulations and are qualitative in nature. Finally, as base performance criteria, these standards are steps designed to promote quality and to accommodate reasonable variations, based on local conditions and circumstances.

*Guidelines* are recommendations that ACSM believes health and fitness operators should consider using to improve the quality of the service they provide to users. Such guidelines are not standards, nor are they applicable in every situation or circumstance; rather, they are illustrative tools that ACSM believes should be considered by health and fitness operators.

From American College of Sports Medicine. *ACSM's Health/Fitness Facility Standards and Guidelines*. 3rd ed. Champaign (IL): Human Kinetics; 2007. p. 4–5.

Therefore, when it comes to using equipment safely, the question then becomes what steps can you, as a GEI, take to prevent foreseeable accidents? In other words, you should always use safe, reliable, and appropriate equipment and always use equipment for its intended purposes according to manufacturer guidelines (13). The reason that this is important is that equipment manufacturers are only responsible for a piece of equipment's safety and performance when it is used as intended.

Whenever you direct class participants to use equipment, you need to provide proper instruction and supervision. In addition, policies and procedures for routine safety inspections, maintenance, and repair should be in place and observed systematically. Supervisors of GEIs or facility managers should keep written records to demonstrate compliance with these policies and procedures. All of these steps taken together are likely to minimize the risk of an accident. And, if an accident occurs and everything has been done to prevent it, then it is likely to be considered the type of accident that could not have been prevented by taking reasonable precautions.

### Fitness Tools of the Trade

For a concrete example of potential liability for client injury from equipment use, consider this common scenario that involves an experienced personal trainer supervising an apparently healthy client who is performing a squat or similar exercise with free weights. The trainer encourages the client to use a heavier weight and to perform more repetitions even though the client complains

of fatigue. The client suffers a debilitating back injury and sues the personal trainer and fitness facility. While most of the case law involves personal trainers, a GEI could theoretically also be held responsible in a similar group training situation.

Under theories of negligence, a GEI owes this participant a duty to exercise reasonable care to prevent injury. Reasonable steps that you can take to avoid this type of incident include encouraging open communications with class members to encourage feedback and listening when any individual states that he or she is reaching fatigue. In addition, as the class leader, you should know how to spot signs of fatigue, be proactive to recommend that people *not* push themselves beyond their limits, and be conservative when implementing program progressions. In other words, only advanced students should do advanced moves. In every setting, if you have a variety of ability levels, progressions must be provided, and you, as the class leader and role model, after demonstrating modifications, should do the exercise at the lowest intensity relevant for class participants.

One of the most important points that you must remember as the GEI is that your purpose is to train class participants safely and effectively. This theme cannot be overemphasized. The group exercise class is *not* an opportunity for you to work at your personal level to achieve personal fitness gains. You are there for your class members. Your role is to lead, motivate, and instruct participants and to be particularly attentive to those class members who may be most vulnerable to injury. Personal training goals must be pursued on personal time, not while leading clients in the exercise classroom.

## Machines: Cycles, Pilates Reformers, Suspension Devices, etc.

The topic of product liability is complex and outside the scope of this chapter. However, the GEI should be aware that equipment product managers are now pursuing clubs *and* GEIs for improper installation and maintenance in cases that the manufacturers may lose a claim to an injured participant under product liability. What that means is that the injured individual may be successful in winning a claim against an equipment manufacturer. In turn, the manufacturer will then go after the individual instructor, the instructor's supervisor, and the facility to recover the claim by arguing that either the instructor did not provide appropriate instruction or the equipment was not properly used or was not properly maintained.

Instances where this situation can occur to GEIs include classes that are conducted primarily on equipment such as indoor cycling, small group equipment-based Pilates (*e.g.*, reformer), or suspension devices. In every class, as the instructor, you must provide safety information. In ideal circumstances, a facility will hold introductory workshops for those new to these class formats in which thorough equipment orientation and safety education is provided. When teaching an equipment-based class, however, you should never assume that any new class participant has undertaken this equipment education. At the beginning of every class, new individuals need to be identified and oriented.

A consistent practice of regular inspections and correction of any known hazards is an additional way in which a GEI can exercise reasonable care to ensure that participants do not suffer avoidable injuries. Potential hazards to look out for include either worn or faultily maintained equipment. Any time that you notice machines that you think require service or repair, provide notice to your supervisor, and do not use the equipment in question. While clients may be upset by a last-minute need to reduce class size or to require more people to share individual equipment items, it is far better to err on the side of safety (8).

When working with mechanical equipment such as indoor cycles, Pilates machines, or suspension devices, the GEI can develop a procedure of instruction and supervision for each class that includes an equipment and body scan to check for proper equipment setup and body alignment. Creating this type of instructional technique so that inspection becomes a routine part of each and every group exercise session can go a long way toward preventing accidents. In this manner, you can also invite participants to assist in the safety checking process and learn how to take more responsibility for their own well-being.

Factors that courts have looked at in equipment-related cases include whether or not the equipment has been maintained appropriately and used for its intended purpose per specific manufacturer guidelines. In particular, courts examined whether or not parts had been replaced in a timely manner and whether or not facility owners had ensured that routine inspections and maintenance were conducted and documented (7). Regardless of the setting, a GEI should be proactive in learning about equipment safety inspections, maintenance, and record-keeping policies as well as the procedures for reporting the need for repairs. Before putting a participant on any piece of equipment, the GEI should have first-hand knowledge of its readiness for use (8).

Keep in mind that courts also examine appropriateness of use. In one case, hotel management had placed equipment in a hotel gym that was intended for private home use. The court found the hotel liable for injuries suffered by the client. A training facility should provide commercial equipment; manufacturers do not design home equipment to withstand the wear and tear of frequent use by multiple users. A GEI should use professional equipment that is designed for the club or studio setting when leading group exercise classes. And you should provide personalized progressions for individual ability levels, cueing, and role modeling to ensure people work at the appropriate intensity.

None of these points should discourage any GEI from using equipment to condition participants. Equipment is an essential part of creating effective training programs and is largely responsible for continuing enthusiasm in group exercise programs. These tips simply underscore that whenever equipment is being used, you must remain alert to the special risks presented and take proactive steps to manage and minimize these risks (13). In other words, have fun and be responsible.

## SCOPE OF PRACTICE

Another important area of potential liability for the GEI pertains to scope of practice. As fitness professionals work more closely together with health care providers to deliver a continuum of care to individuals, it is important to define respective roles. According to ACSM's Code of Ethics for Certified and Registered Professionals, "[ACSMCPs] practice within the scope of their knowledge, skills, and abilities. [Group exercise instructors] will not provide services that are limited by state law to provision by another healthcare professional only" (4). See Box 10.4 for ACSM's Code of Ethics. This is particularly true of GEIs with advanced academic degrees or training and when working with clients who may have special exercise considerations. Both criminal and civil actions are possible for practicing without a license.

### Principles and Standards

#### Responsibility to the Public

ACSM's GEIs shall be dedicated to providing competent and legally permissible services within the scope of the Knowledge and Skills (KSs) of their respective credential. These services shall be provided with integrity,

## BOX 10.4 Code of Ethics for ACSM Certified and Registered Professionals

### PURPOSE

This Code of Ethics is intended to aid all certified and registered ACSM credentialed professionals (to establish and maintain a high level of ethical conduct, as defined by standards by which ACSM GEIs may determine the appropriateness of their conduct. Any existing professional, licensure, or certification affiliations that ACSM GEIs have with governmental, local, state, or national agencies or organizations will take precedence relative to any disciplinary matters that pertain to practice or professional conduct. This Code applies to all ACSM GEIs, regardless of ACSM membership status (to include members and nonmembers). Any cases in violation of this Code will be referred to the ACSM Committee on Certification and Registry Boards (CCRB).

competence, diligence, and compassion. ACSM GEIs provide exercise information in a manner that is consistent with evidence-based practice.

- ACSM's GEIs should respect the rights of clients, colleagues, and health care professionals, and shall safeguard client confidences within the boundaries of the law.
- Information relating to the ACSM GEI-client relationship is confidential and may not be communicated to a third party not involved in that client's care without the prior written consent of the client or as required by law.
- ACSM's GEIs should be truthful about their qualifications and the limitations of their expertise and provide services consistent with their competencies.

#### Responsibility to the Profession

- ACSM's certified professionals maintain high professional standards. As such, an ACSM-certified professional should never represent himself or herself, either directly or indirectly, as anything other than an ACSM-certified professional unless he or she holds other license/certification that allows him or her to do so.
- ACSM GEIs practice within the scope of their KSs and in accordance with state law.
- An ACSM-certified professional must remain in good standing relative to governmental requirements as a condition of continued credentialing.
- ACSM GEIs take credit, including authorship, only for work they have actually performed and give credit to the contributions of others as warranted. Consistent with the requirements of their certification or registration, ACSM GEIs must complete approved, additional educational course (continuing education) work aimed at maintaining and advancing their KSs.

### Principles and Standards for Candidates of ACSM Certification Examinations

Candidates applying for a credentialing examination must comply with candidacy requirements and, to the best of their abilities, accurately complete the application process.

### Public Disclosure of Affiliation

- Any ACSMCP may disclose his or her affiliation with ACSM credentialing in any context, oral or documented, provided it is currently accurate. In doing so, no ACSMCP may imply college endorsement of whatever is associated in context with the disclosure, unless expressly authorized by the college. Disclosure of affiliation in connection with a commercial venture may be made provided the disclosure is made in a professionally dignified manner; is not false, misleading, or deceptive; and does not imply licensure or the attainment of specialty or diploma status.
- ACSM GEIs may disclose their credential status.
- ACSM GEIs may list their affiliation with ACSM credentialing on their business cards without prior authorization.
- ACSM GEIs and the institutions employing an ACSMCP may inform the public of an affiliation as a matter of public discourse or presentation.

### Discipline

Any ACSMCP may be disciplined or lose his or her certification or registry for conduct that, in the opinion of the Executive Council of the ACSM CCRB goes against the principles set forth in this Code. Such cases will be reviewed by the ACSM CCRB Ethics Subcommittee, which will include a liaison from the ACSM CCRB executive council, as appointed by the CCRB chair. The ACSM CCRB Ethics Subcommittee will make an action recommendation to the executive council of the ACSM CCRB for final review and approval.

✔ **RECOMMENDED RESOURCES: ACSM Code of Ethics for ACSM Certified and Registered Professionals is available on the Internet at http:// www.acsm.org/AM/Template.cfm?Section=Home_ Page&TEMPLATE=/CM/HTMLDisplay. cfm&CONTENTID=2385**

The contemporary delivery of health care services itself is in a state of flux because of high costs and attempts to reduce costs by expanding the roles of paraprofessionals in the medical context. As a result, states vary widely on what constitutes the practice of medicine and what is appropriate behavior for a nurse, physician assistant, or other paraprofessional.

As a GEI, you need to become familiar with the relevant guidelines for scope of practice that are established at your affiliated organizations and institutions. If you operate your own business, it would be wise to seek the advice of local counsel and to take all other steps to manage risk effectively, such as maintaining certifications, obtaining releases and waivers or consents as applicable, and carrying liability insurance.

## Supplements

Claims related to violations of scope of practice occur most frequently in the area of supplements and involve personal trainers, not GEIs. A high-profile case brought against a personal trainer and a large fitness chain involved a scenario in which a personal trainer sold supplements, including one that contained ephedra, to a client. The client, who had hypertension, died. Survivors filed a suit. In another example, a personal trainer sold steroids to a client, who later suffered adverse consequences and filed a claim against the personal trainer (7).

In another incident, an exercise training company combined supplement sales with its fitness packages to increase revenue. The company eventually had a client who was allergic to an ingredient in the supplement. The problem was compounded when the client assumed that if she took more than the recommended dosage, she would see more results. She ended up in the hospital, and even though she had been a loyal client for some time, she sued the personal trainer and the business. The case was settled out of court, and the personal trainer lost his business. The problem was not that the personal trainer had sold the client the products, but that he had given her a written plan specifying what to eat and when to take the supplements. The fact that the client overdid it did not matter (7).

According to insurers, the problem with supplements is worsened by the fact that most supplement manufacturers do not carry any insurance coverage. Therefore, the people selling the supplements do not have any product liability coverage. Furthermore, most of the insurance policies for fitness professionals do not include protection for product liability. These case examples would serve as precedents if the facts involved a GEI. The principles and logical reasoning regarding why liability is relevant would apply to any fitness professional who sold supplements.

In today's market, no one, even professional registered dietitians, can be certain about the ingredients in many supplements because they are not subject to government regulation. In addition, one can never be certain regarding who may have severe allergic reactions, including the risk of death, to any particular ingredient. To proactively protect client safety and to minimize the risk of professional liability, you should avoid selling supplements.

### Medical or Dietary Advice

No cases have yet been litigated to conclusion that involved a client suing a GEI for faulty medical or dietary advice, except in the case of supplements. However, remember that health care is a highly regulated area. The consequences of stepping over the line into the protected area of a licensed health care practitioner — such as a medical doctor, physical therapist, registered dietitian, or chiropractor — vary by state. You are exposed to potential liability for acting outside the scope of practice if your "advice" could be interpreted as the unauthorized practice of medicine and if this advice results in a client injury. The best practice is to develop a comprehensive network of allied professionals and actively refer clients who request or require specialized services to the appropriate health care provider (6).

## SEXUAL HARASSMENT

Sexual harassment claims represent the third area of potential exposure to liability that is seeing growth in the number of claims against personal trainers, but not GEIs, according to insurance providers (7). Because the exercise training relationship can seem "intimate," it lends itself to creating more opportunity for abusive conduct on the part of the trainer or for a misinterpretation of actions on the part of the client. Numerous cases involve a male personal trainer and a female client. The female client believes inappropriate touching has occurred and that she has been violated. Or a personal relationship develops between the personal trainer and the client that then raises questions about the legitimacy of the business services rendered. The client believes undue influence was used to create an exploitive situation.

Sexual harassment is difficult to prove and often rests on credibility. Even though most reported incidents involve personal trainers, it does not mean that GEIs are not vulnerable to this type of claim. As an instructor, therefore, you should act professionally at all times. One strategy to protect against a claim of inappropriate touching is to always ask a client for permission to use tactile spotting, and to avoid it unless absolutely necessary. Some GEIs do not touch clients directly, but spot them through the use of another prop, such as a ball. Also, avoid any situation with a member behind closed doors where no one else is present. If a personal relationship develops with a class participant, discontinue the professional relationship and suggest that the participant take classes with another instructor unless and until the relationship becomes more defined. Check with your employer to determine what, if any, is the organization's policy on dating. Some organizations frown on it, while others suggest discretion.

## PROPER QUALIFICATIONS

Although no specific case on the books has held that GEIs have a higher standard of care based on their specific training in individual assessment, program design, and supervision, clients have filed claims after injuring themselves, based on the fact that a GEI did not have the qualifications represented in a facility's advertising literature. This claim was based on a theory of breach of contract since the facility failed to provide GEI with the level of qualification that it had promised (6). The takeaway lesson from this case is that you should never falsify any of your qualifications or imply that you have any specialized training that you have not undertaken.

The best evidence that you can show as an instructor that your training services meets professional standards is to maintain your certification and to conduct business according to the KSs that are expected as minimum competencies by the certifying organization. The ACSM certified GEI's job is defined as "works in a group exercise setting with apparently healthy individuals and those with health challenges who are able to exercise independently to enhance quality of life, improve health-related physical fitness, manage health risk, and promote lasting health behavior change. The GEI leads safe and effective exercise programs using a variety of leadership techniques to foster group camaraderie, support, and motivation to enhance muscular strength and endurance, flexibility, cardiovascular fitness, body composition, and any of the motor skills related to the domains of health-related physical fitness" (11).

The issue of a GEI's responsibility for advising appropriate levels of training intensity is even more critical as more people with special needs attend group exercise programming. If your services are advertised to targeted clientele such as older adults or people with arthritis, and you claim that you are trained to serve these niche markets, you need to be sure that you are sufficiently prepared to serve these clients' needs. Evidence of sufficient preparation would include additional training and experience in working with people with particular needs. All GEIs should therefore keep written records of all certifications, continuing education, and work-related experience.

An important precaution to ensure that you deliver services that are appropriate to the client is the prescreening health and medical history. As a GEI, you should be fully informed of the policies in place at the facility where you work. If you are an independent contractor, some process must be in place to ensure that prescreening is conducted. In addition, the ACSM has developed

the Quick Screen (see Chapter 2). As a GEI, you need to be able to assess risk and determine when a medical clearance is necessary. The Quick Screen is a secondary screen used in the classroom. The prescreen should happen with the Physical Activity Readiness Questionnaire or other health assessments as directed by your organization. The Quick Screen gives you an opportunity to meet newcomers and determine any modifications that may be required. It also quickly assesses if the class style is appropriate for the student. After all these precautionary steps are taken, you need to be able to determine the recommended level of training that will be safe and effective for any particular participant (2).

The risk of exposure to liability for a GEI may be even greater when training services are delivered in a medical setting. In a 2003 Indiana case, a court held that even though a personal trainer was employed by a hospital and the fitness facility was owned by the hospital, the personal trainer was not a health care provider. The case, therefore, did not qualify as a medical malpractice case. The significance of this case, however, is that the client did try to sue both the fitness club and the hospital on the basis of injuries sustained while engaged in the exercise training program, and the court did examine the fact that the training occurred in a setting with a close connection to a hospital. Another court might have found that this type of training did need to meet the standards of health care practitioners (7,12).

## EMERGENCY RESPONSE

As yet, no specific case has involved a claim against a GEI for wrongful death in a situation in which a client has had a heart attack or other medical emergency and died while under the supervision of an instructor. However, as most GEI certifications require that GEIs have CPR training (and many require first aid training and AED training), it is possible that a claim could be filed against a GEI who failed to provide an emergency response if that failure led to a death that could have otherwise been avoided.

The ACSM and the American Heart Association (AHA) published a joint position stand in 1998 with recommendations for health/fitness facilities regarding screening of clients for the presence of cardiovascular disease, appropriate staffing, emergency policies, equipment, and procedures relative to the client base of a given facility (5). In 2002, the ACSM and the AHA published a joint position stand to supplement the 1998 recommendations regarding the purchase and use of AEDs in health/fitness facilities (9,10). These organizations agree that a comprehensive written emergency plan is essential to promote safe and effective physical activity.

The AHA, the ACSM, and the International Health, Racquet and Sportsclub Association recommend that all fitness facilities have written emergency policies and procedures, including the use of automated defibrillators, which are reviewed and practiced regularly (see Fig. 10.1). Staff who have responsibility for working directly with program participants and provide instruction and leadership in specific modes of exercise must be trained in CPR. These staff should know and practice regularly the facility's

emergency plan and be able to readily handle emergencies. In addition, these organizations encourage health and fitness facilities to use AEDs (9).

As evidence of professional competency and to remain in readiness in case of a true emergency, GEIs should

---

### *Form 26*
## Emergency Procedures Sheet

In the event that an emergency should occur and no medical personnel are present, the following guidelines should be followed:

1. A staff person should identify him or herself as a professional rescuer trained in emergency care. This helps to reassure the victim and bystanders. If the victim is conscious, legally we must ask permission to assist the victim. (The law assumes that an unconscious person would give consent.) A senior staff person should stay with the individual at all times. He or she should attempt to reassure the person and protect the individual from personal bodily harm. Senior staff person will assume control of the situation and issue further orders as needed.

2. A second staff member will call 911 and give the following information:

   A. Phone number of location

   B. Title of location (building name, address, specific suite or room number)

   C. Site-specific entrance instructions for ambulance driver

   D. Brief description of the problem. If it is a definite cardiac event (i.e., respiratory arrest) and CPR is in progress, an Advanced Life Support unit will be sent. If it is nonlife-threatening (i.e., seizures), a Basic Life Support unit will be sent.

   E. After 911 has been called, a staff member will notify building security (list phone #: _____), put elevator on hold (if applicable), and wait in the lobby to meet the ambulance at the main entrance to escort them to the emergency.

3. The individual should be monitored at all times. This will include:

   A. Checking heart rate, noting the regularity and strength of each heart beat.

   B. Monitoring and recording blood pressure.

   C. Observing skin color and breathing pattern.

   D. Maintaining open airway.

   E. Establishing unresponsiveness and initiating CPR when appropriate.

   F. Before the individual is transported (if unconscious), give the EMTs as much information as possible regarding individual's name, age, medical considerations (folder, if possible), and home phone emergency numbers. The attending physician and the hospital will make the call to the family.

4. Once the individual is transported, the senior staff person in charge should:

   A. Notify the individual's emergency contact.

   B. Assume responsibility for personal belongings and valuables. Please remember that it is important to respect the individual's privacy. Be as brief as possible when disclosing the information pertinent to the event.

   C. Fill out an accident report and file one copy in the member's folder and one copy with the Center Director.

---

■ **FIGURE 10.1** Sample emergency procedures sheet. (Adapted from American College of Sports Medicine. *ACSM's Health/Fitness Facility Standards and Guidelines.* 3rd ed. Champaign (IL): Human Kinetics; 2007.)

keep CPR, first aid, and AED certifications current. Wherever you work, you should proactively familiarize yourself with your organization's emergency plan and be ready to implement the plan's procedures in case of emergency. If you operate your own business, creating an emergency plan should be a top priority. GEIs who provide training services outdoors or in any alternative setting to a traditional institutional facility should also have written emergency policies and procedures.

In addition to having an emergency plan, you also need to document any accident or incident immediately, using an Incident Report Form (see Fig. 10.2). When

---

### *Form 20*
## Incident Report Form

Date of accident _____ Time of accident _____

Member's name _____ Member number _____

Address _____

Home phone _____ Business phone _____

Location of accident _____

Staff attending _____ _____

_____ _____

Witnesses (nonstaff) _____ _____

_____ _____

Details of accident _____

_____

_____

_____

Action taken by staff _____

_____

_____

_____

Staff reporting _____ Date _____

Department head's signature _____ Date _____

_____
*Note.* The law varies from state to state. No form should be adopted or used by any program without individualized legal advice.

■ **FIGURE 10.2** Incident report form.

completing any form, only include the facts surrounding the incident and do not offer any opinions regarding what may or may not have caused the incident. Names and contact information of witnesses also should be included. And the person who experienced the incident should sign the form. Insurers will provide incident reporting forms, and as a professional GEI, you should always carry one when providing professional services (3,13).

Keep in mind that completing incident forms and documenting what happened at the time of an incident is only the beginning of a matter. It is also important to follow up and to determine the final outcome of a situation. One can express concern without admitting any fault. Maintaining good relationships is also a positive method to avoid an incident from escalating into a legal issue.

## CLIENT CONFIDENTIALITY

The failure to protect client confidentiality is another emerging area of potential liability for fitness professionals. This is rooted in the concept of preventing potential harm to a participant's reputation. If you gather any personal information or if you read any participant's fitness assessment or health history, please follow carefully your employer's guidelines. The ACSM's guidelines for the fitness testing, health promotion, and wellness area state, "a facility should ensure that its fitness testing, health promotion, and wellness area has a system that provides for and protects the complete confidentiality of all user records and meetings. User records should be released only with an individual's signed authorization" (3).

In general, as a GEI, you are not required to disclose any personal information. If, however, you want to use personal information for marketing purposes, such as a member testimonial or "before and after" photos, it's a good idea to get and store a signed release form from the member. A law passed by the U.S. Congress requires health care professionals to have strict policies regarding the safety and security of private records (the Health Insurance Portability & Accountability Act of 1996, Public Law 104-191, which amends the Internal Revenue Service Code of 1986, also known as the Kennedy-Kassebaum Act) and came into effect on April 14, 2003. While it is still unclear if the Health Insurance Portability & Accountability Act extends to GEIs, it is wise to become familiar with this law and how it may affect the release of any personal information to a third party.

## RISK MANAGEMENT STRATEGIES

By now, you realize that GEIs should manage risk exposure with a multilayered approach that incorporates a number of important strategies. We have already reviewed many proactive steps that you can take to protect yourself that are grounded in common sense. These include checking your environment, equipment, and

participants; always keeping safety concerns first and foremost; providing appropriate instructions, modeling, and progressions as needed; and holding yourself out to the public in a way that accurately reflects your true training, knowledge, and experience. In addition to these commonsense approaches, you can further manage your professional risk by using any of several legal instruments described below, by maintaining a liability insurance policy, by keeping your certifications and training current, by creating protective legal business structures, and by always conducting yourself in a positive, professional manner.

## WRITTEN POLICIES, PROCEDURES, AND FORMS

As the first line of defense, all GEIs should learn about and closely observe all written policies, procedures, and forms that meet industry standards and guidelines that are used by their employers (2,3,6,7,8,12,13). If you work as an independent contractor, then you may need to hire a local attorney to prepare relevant written policies, procedures, and forms. This strategy of observing written policies and procedures minimizes the likelihood that you would fail to demonstrate that you exercised reasonable care under the circumstances. In other words, you need to proactively make every effort to not be negligent.

In addition, if a GEI has his or her own business or provides services as an independent contractor to an organization that does not have preactivity screening procedures or a written emergency plan, then the GEI will also need to have those documents.

## INFORMED CONSENT, RELEASE, OR WAIVER

The second strategy involves using a release or waiver (Fig. 10.3) or informed consent (Fig. 10.4), depending on which legal document is recognized under the laws of the place where you provide services (14). See Box 10.5 for descriptions of each of these documents. The purpose of these documents is either (a) to demonstrate that the facility or the GEI, as the case may be depending on the business status of the GEI, fully informed the client of all of the potential risks of physical activity and the client decided to undertake the activity and waive the GEI's responsibility or (b) to demonstrate that the client knowingly waived his or her right to file a claim against the GEI even if the GEI is negligent. In most institutional settings, the facility will have the participant sign this form and store it with member records. If the GEI is working as an independent contractor, then the GEI should provide the relevant waiver or informed consent to class participants, obtain signatures, and keep these records indefinitely and in a safe place. Consent forms are not infinity contracts, so provisions should also be made for an annual signing of these important documents.

## Form 6

## Agreement and Release of Liability Form

1. In consideration of gaining membership or being allowed to participate in the activities and programs of _____ and to use its facilities, equipment, and machinery in addition to the payment of any fee or charge, I do hereby waive, release and forever discharge _____ and its officers, agents, employees, representatives, executors, and all others from any and all responsibilities or liability for injuries or damages resulting from my participation in any activities or my use of equipment or machinery in the above-mentioned facilities or arising out of my participation in any activities at said facility. I do also hereby release all of those mentioned and any others acting upon their behalf from any responsibility or liability for any injury or damage to myself, including those caused by the negligent act or omission of any of those mentioned or others acting on their behalf or in any way arising out of or connected with my participation in any activities of _____ or the use of any equipment at _____ . (**Please initial** _____)

2. I understand and am aware that strength, flexibility, and aerobic exercise, including the use of equipment, is a potentially hazardous activity. I also understand that fitness activities involve a risk of injury and even death and that I am voluntarily participating in these activities and using equipment and machinery with knowledge of the dangers involved. I hereby agree to expressly assume and accept any and all risks of injury or death. (**Please initial** _____)

3. I do hereby further declare myself to be physically sound and suffering from no condition, impairment, disease, infirmity, or other illness that would prevent my participation in any of the activities and programs of _____ or use of equipment or machinery except as hereinafter stated. I do hereby acknowledge that I have been informed of the need for a physician's approval for my participation in an exercise/fitness activity or in the use of exercise equipment and machinery. I also acknowledge that it has been recommended that I have a yearly or more frequent physical examination and consultation with my physician as to physical activity, exercise, and use of exercise and training equipment so that I might have recommendations concerning these fitness activities and equipment use. I acknowledge that I have either had a physical examination and have been given a physician's permission to participate, or that I have decided to participate in activity and/or use of equipment and machinery without the approval of my physician and do hereby assume all responsibility for my participation and activities, and utilization of equipment and machinery in my activities. (**Please initial** _____)

Date _____          Signature _____

*Note.* The law varies from state to state. No form should be adopted or used by any program without individualized legal advice.

Reprinted, by permission from D Herbert, 1989, "Avoiding allegations of misrepresentation/fraud in program documents," *The Exercise Standards and Malpractice Reporter* 3(2):30-31.

■ **FIGURE 10.3** Agreement and release of liability form.

In numerous states, courts are holding up waivers more and more as valid means of protection against litigation. In 2001, a California case was dismissed after a court held that the waiver form signed by a facility member when she joined protected the facility and its owners from liability when the member filed a lawsuit claiming that she slipped and injured herself. This case is consistent with other California cases (7).

## *Form 7*

# Informed Consent Agreement

Thank you for choosing to use the facilities, services, or programs of _____. We request your understanding and cooperation in maintaining both your and our safety and health by reading and signing the following informed consent agreement.

I, _____, declare that I intend to use some or all of the activities, facilities, programs, and services offered by _____ and I understand that each person, myself included, has a different capacity for participating in such activities, facilities, programs, and services. I am aware that all activities, services, and programs offered are either educational, recreational, or self-directed in nature. I assume full responsibility, during and after my participation, for my choices to use or apply, at my own risk, any portion of the information or instruction I receive.

I understand that part of the risk involved in undertaking any activity or program is relative to my own state of fitness or health (physical, mental, or emotional) and to the awareness, care, and skill with which I conduct myself in that activity or program. I acknowledge that my choice to participate in any activity, service, and program of _____ brings with it my assumption of those risks or results stemming from this choice and the fitness, health, awareness, care, and skill that I possess and use.

I further understand that the activities, programs, and services offered by _____ are sometimes conducted by personnel who may not be licensed, certified, or registered instructors or professionals. I accept the fact that the skills and competencies of some employees and/or volunteers will vary according to their training and experience and that no claim is made to offer assessment or treatment of any mental or physical disease or condition by those who are not duly licensed, certified, or registered and herein employed to provide such professional services.

I recognize that by participating in the activities, facilities, programs, and services offered by _____ _____, I may experience potential health risks such as transient light-headedness, fainting, abnormal blood pressure, chest discomfort, leg cramps, and nausea and that I assume willfully those risks. I acknowledge my obligation to immediately inform the nearest supervising employee of any pain, discomfort, fatigue, or any other symptoms that I may suffer during and immediately after my participation. I understand that I may stop or delay my participation in any activity or procedure if I so desire and that I may also be requested to stop and rest by a supervising employee who observes any symptoms of distress or abnormal response.

I understand that I may ask any questions or request further explanation or information about the activities, facilities, programs, and services offered by _____ at any time before, during, or after my participation.

I declare that I have read, understood, and agree to the contents of this informed consent agreement in its entirety.

Signature _____

Date of signing _____

Witness _____

*Note.* The law varies from state to state. No form should be adopted or used by any program without individualized legal advice.

■ **FIGURE 10.4** Informed consent agreement

| BOX 10.5 | *Assumption of the Risk* |
|---|---|

*Informed Consent:* An Assumption of the Risk or Informed Consent document essentially explains the risks of participating in physical activity to a prospective client. The client then agrees that he or she knowingly understands these risks, appreciates these risks, and voluntarily assumes responsibility for taking those risks.

*Release or Waiver of Liability:* A Waiver or Release of Liability document states that the client knowingly waives or releases the GEI from liability for any acts of negligence on the part of the GEI. In other words, the prospective client waives his or her right to sue the GEI, even if the GEI is negligent.

From Cotten DJ, Cotton MB. *Legal Aspects of Waivers in Sport, Recreation and Fitness Activities.* Canton (OH): PRC Publishing; 1997.

You need to consult an attorney in your location to determine which type of document is the standard practice for your state (14).

## PROFESSIONAL LIABILITY INSURANCE

In today's litigious environment, for the most protection, a GEI should carry professional liability insurance ($2 million per occurrence is the recommended amount), even when working in a business as an employee, where the GEI may be covered under the business owner's policy. The reason for this is that it is not unusual for a single claim to result in a million-dollar judgment. Purchasing the best protection enables you to perform your job responsibly and to feel confident your career will not be destroyed by one mishap. Most insurers of GEIs provide coverage for certified professionals. As a certified ACSM GEI, you are eligible to purchase liability insurance.

Professional liability insurance provides a broad spectrum of protection from claims such as those arising from negligence, breach of contract, or even sexual harassment, and it can provide coverage for both injuries to a person or to property. The risk is transferred to the insurer. Insurance professionals are experts at handling claims and will take care of all of the details, enabling the GEI to continue to operate his or her business (7).

## CERTIFICATION AND CONTINUING EDUCATION

An additional line of defense that many professionals don't consider risk management is the maintenance of your certifications and training. Since most certifications require continuing education and emergency preparedness such as regular CPR or AED trainings, simply remaining certified provides evidence that you are conducting yourself professionally and responsibly. Keep records of all training courses that you attend and certifications that you receive and provide copies to your employers.

## ADDITIONAL STRATEGIES

If, as a GEI, you own and operate your own business, incorporating the business is an important step to take to protect personal assets from any potential claims. Business owners should also consult local legal counsel to ensure that business practices meet the requirements of the specific location in which the business is located (7). Lastly, one of the most powerful strategies is to simply cultivate strong relationships with your clients and colleagues. While this may seem like a "soft" quality, it is actually extremely important according to experienced professionals. Fitness professionals and insurers alike agree that participants are much less likely to sue if they perceive a GEI as caring, responsible, and responsive to their needs.

## SUMMARY

*The exercise training industry is in a rapid state of growth and redefinition as more health care providers acknowledge the need for exercise training as part of a program of preventive health care. In addition, the wellness trend is encouraging more individuals to assume responsibility for their personal health and to use services such as those provided by GEIs to enhance the quality of their daily lives. The government, health and medical profession, and the growing wellness industry are supporting the use of exercise professional services to serve every segment of society—for youth and older adults, from athletes to the infirm, from low-income communities to Fortune 500 corporations. As a GEI, you have multiple opportunities to work in a variety of settings and to make a powerful difference in the lives of clients and of communities.*

*More professional opportunities, however, increase expectations of responsible professional conduct. More professional responsibility means more exposure to liability for failing to act responsibly. Today's GEI must understand these potential risk areas and the industry standards and guidelines that surround these issues to deliver services confidently and to proactively manage risk. This professionalism in all aspects of doing business not only increases the personal and professional rewards of life as a GEI, but also ensures lasting business success amid the growing complexity of our modern legal environment.*

*Ultimately, the purpose of liability is to protect individuals. The most successful GEIs understand that the essence of their role is to serve individuals and to provide leadership for the enjoyment of safe and effective exercises as part of a healthy lifestyle. If you fulfill these goals, you will optimize safety, effectively reduce liability, and improve lives.*

# References

1. ACSM Certified GEI SM Job Task Analysis. 2010.

2. American College of Sports Medicine. *ACSM's Certification Review.* 2nd ed. Baltimore (MD): Lippincott Williams & Wilkins; 2006.

3. American College of Sports Medicine. *ACSM's Health/Fitness Facility Standards and Guidelines.* 3rd ed. Champaign (IL): Human Kinetics; 2007.

4. American College of Sports Medicine. *ACSM's Guidelines for Exercise Testing and Prescription.* 8th ed. Baltimore (MD): Lippincott Williams & Wilkins; 2008.

5. American College of Sports Medicine. *ACSM's Resource Manual for Guidelines for Exercise Testing and Prescription.* 6th ed. Baltimore (MD): Lippincott Williams & Wilkins; 2010.

6. American College of Sports Medicine Code of Ethics for ACSM Certified and Registered Professionals; [cited 2010 June 19]. Available from: http://www.acsm.org/AM/Template.cfm?Section=Home_Page&TEMPLATE=/CM/HTMLDisplay.cfm&CONTENTID=2385

7. Archer S. Reward carries risk: a liability update. *IDEA Group Exercise Instructor.* 2004;15(4):30–4.

8. Archer S. Pilates equipment liability and safety. *IDEA Fitness Journal.* 2006;3(6):42–50.

9. Balady GJ, et al. Recommendations for cardiovascular screening, staffing and emergency policies at health/fitness facilities. *Circulation.* 1998;97(22):2283–93.

10. Balady GJ, et al. Automated external defibrillators in health/fitness facilities: supplement to the AHA/ACSM recommendations for cardiovascular screening, staffing and emergency policies at health/fitness facilities. *Circulation.* 2002;105(9):1147–50.

11. Cotten DJ, Cotton MB. *Legal Aspects of Waivers in Sport, Recreation and Fitness Activities.* Canton (OH): PRC Publishing; 1997.

12. Herbert DL, Herbert WG, Herbert TG. *Legal Aspects of Preventive, Rehabilitative and Recreational Exercise Programs.* 4th ed. Canton (OH): PRC Publishing; 2002.

13. Koeberle BE. *Legal Aspects of Personal Fitness Training.* 2nd ed. Canton (OH): PRC Publishing; 1994.

14. McInnis K, Herbert W, et al. Low compliance with national standards for cardiovascular emergency preparedness at health clubs. *Chest.* 2001;120(1):283–8.

# EXERCISE SCIENCE FOR THE GROUP EXERCISE INSTRUCTOR

PART

III

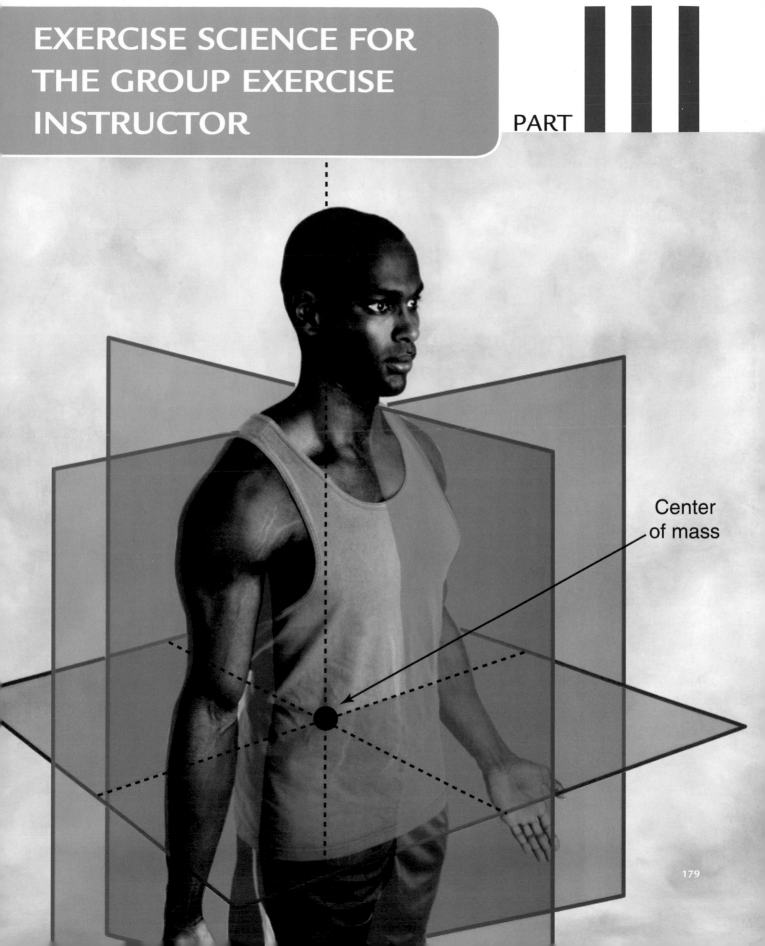

Center
of mass

# CHAPTER 11

# Exercise Physiology for Group Exercise Instructors

JERRY J. MAYO

## Objectives

**At the end of this chapter you will be able to:**
- Describe the functions and components of the cardiovascular and cardiorespiratory systems
- Describe the cardiovascular, respiratory, and metabolic responses to exercise
- Describe muscle structure and function
- Describe the function of the skeletal system
- Describe the basic structure and function of the joints in motion
- Describe the function of the neurological system
- Describe the relationship of cardiorespiratory fitness to health

A basic understanding of exercise physiology is vital to successful group exercise instruction. Exercise physiology principles not only are necessary for the development of safe and appropriate group exercise programs but also help instructors explain to clients the scientific processes that improve fitness. Often, there are occasions during a workout when group instructors need to precisely describe the physiology behind an exercise movement or activity.

In this chapter, we introduce some of the core concepts of exercise physiology. Specifically, key biological systems such as the cardiovascular (CV) system, respiratory system, energy system, musculoskeletal system, and neurological system and their function during exercise are presented.

## OVERVIEW OF EXERCISE PHYSIOLOGY

Among the exercise sciences, exercise physiology is the oldest, most widely studied discipline. Exercise physiology evolved from its parent discipline, physiology, and examines how the body systems work in concert to meet the increased demands of physical activity. Therefore, it is extremely important for all fitness professionals. Planning workouts, leading exercise routines, and progressing clients over time to achieve their goals all require a strong understanding of exercise physiology.

## DEFINITION OF EXERCISE PHYSIOLOGY

Exercise physiology is the study of how the body responds to acute (immediate) and chronic (long-term) bouts of exercise. Because physiological systems act in

unison during exercise stress, the discipline of exercise physiology includes the study of human physiology on both a system and a cellular level (5).

## CARDIOVASCULAR SYSTEM

The CV system is a major support system of the body. It is comprised of three important components: the heart (pump), the blood vessels (pipes), and the blood (fluid medium) (20). The CV system is a continuous closed circuit consisting of an estimated 60,000 miles of blood vessels with the origin and end point being the heart (13) (Fig. 11.1).

During rest and exercise, the primary goal of the CV system is to bring oxygen and nutrients to all body cells while removing carbon dioxide and other metabolic waste products (16). It also functions to support other systems by

- Transporting hormones and enzymes
- Maintaining fluid balance to avoid dehydration
- Regulating pH by controlling the blood's buffering capabilities
- Regulating body temperature by absorbing and redistributing heat
- Preventing infection from invading organisms

### THE HEART

The heart is a muscular pump that is responsible for circulating blood throughout the entire body. The adult heart is about the size of a closed fist and is positioned in the center of the thoracic cavity between the lungs in

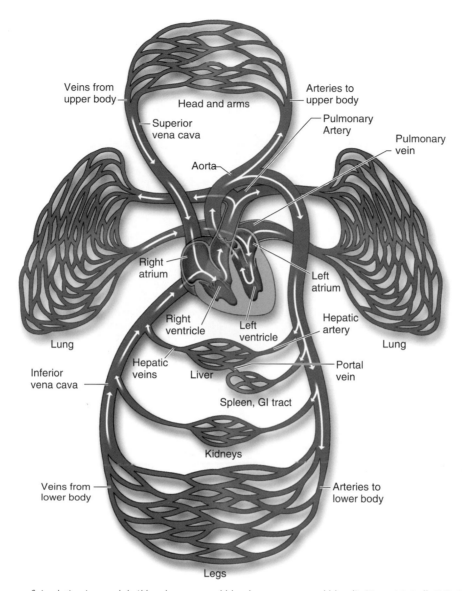

■ **FIGURE 11.1** Diagram of circulation in an adult (*blue*, deoxygenated blood; *gray*, oxygenated blood). (From McArdle WD, Katch FI, Katch VL. *Essentials of Exercise Physiology*. 2nd ed. Baltimore (MD): Lippincott Williams & Wilkins; 2000.)

an area called the mediastinum (16). A four-chambered organ, the heart has two upper (atria) and lower (ventricles) chambers (Fig. 11.2).

Because the heart is shaped like a blunt cone, it has an apex and a base. Interestingly, the apex or rounded point is found slightly below the base, which is broad and located at the superior aspect of the heart. When the heart contracts, blood is forced from the apex toward the base, like wringing out a wet towel.

## TISSUE COVERINGS AND LAYERS OF THE HEART

The heart is enclosed by a membranous sac known as the pericardium. The pericardium consists of two layers. The outer layer is tough (fibrous pericardium) while the inner layer is smooth (serous pericardium) (18). The serous

pericardium produces pericardial fluid that reduces friction while the heart moves within the pericardium. The heart wall consists of three distinct tissue layers: the epicardium, myocardium, and endocardium. The outermost layer of the heart is called the epicardium. It is a thin serous membrane that creates the smooth outer surface of the heart. The myocardium is the thick middle layer, which contains the cardiac muscle cells and is responsible for the heart's contraction. The smooth interior surface of the heart chambers is considered the endocardium.

## CHAMBERS, VALVES, AND BLOOD FLOW

Figure 11.2 illustrates the anatomy of the heart. The heart has four chambers (right and left atria and right and left ventricles) that are separated by a wall-like structure called a septum. Because of the separation,

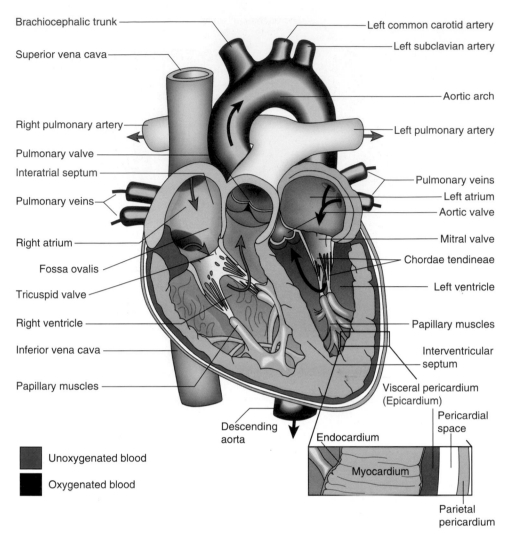

**■ FIGURE 11.2** The internal structures of the heart (anterior view). (From Smeltzer SCO, Bare BG. *Brunner and Suddarth's Textbook of Medical-Surgical Nursing*. 9th ed. Philadelphia (PA): Lippincott Williams & Wilkins; 2002.)

these chambers work as a two-cycle pump, with the right side of the heart (RA, RV) collecting deoxygenated blood from the body and pumping it to the lungs (pulmonary circuit) and the left side of the heart receiving oxygenated blood from the lungs and pumping it to all of the body tissues (systemic circuit) (13). The left ventricle is the largest, most muscular chamber because it is responsible for pumping blood to all regions of the body.

To maintain blood flow in one direction, the heart uses four valves. Two atrioventricular (AV) valves prevent the backflow of blood from the ventricles into the atria. The right AV valve has three cusps and is termed the tricuspid valve; the left AV valve only has two cusps and is referred to as the bicuspid or mitral valve. Chordae tendineae and the papillary muscles help ensure closure of the AV valves as the ventricles contract. The pulmonary and aortic (semilunar) valves block the reentry of blood flow into the ventricles from the pulmonary trunk and aorta, respectively.

From the RA, deoxygenated blood passes through the tricuspid valve into the RV. The RV pumps this oxygen-poor blood through the pulmonary valve into the pulmonary artery, which directs the blood to the lungs. In the lungs, oxygen is absorbed into the blood while carbon dioxide is removed. Once the lungs reoxygenate the blood, the pulmonary veins bring the oxygen-rich blood back to the left atrium. From the left atrium, oxygenated blood then passes through the bicuspid valve into the left ventricle. As the left ventricle contracts, blood passes through the aortic valve and out to all body tissues (16).

## THE BLOOD VESSELS

As blood flow leaves the heart, it enters the vascular system, which is a complex network of blood vessels (18). These vessels include arteries, arterioles, capillaries, venules, and veins. Arteries are strong elastic vessels that carry blood away from the heart, usually under large amounts of pressure. These vessels subdivide into

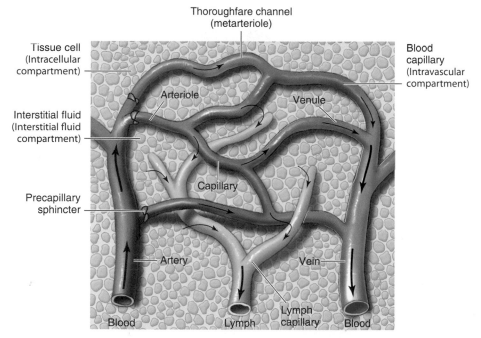

■ **FIGURE 11.3** Capillary blood flow. (Modified from Premkumar K. *The Massage Connection Anatomy and Physiology*. Baltimore (MD): Lippincott Williams & Wilkins; 2004.)

smaller muscular arteries then branch into even smaller arterioles. Characteristics of arterioles include lower pressure due to reduced vessel diameter and great amounts of smooth muscle tissue (less elastic tissue). The smooth muscle found in arterioles allows these vessels to become smaller (vasoconstrict) or larger (vasodilate) to control blood flow. Next, blood flows from arterioles to capillaries, where exchange of gases and nutrients occurs (Fig. 11.3). Capillaries form extensive "networks," sometime called capillary beds, in all body tissues. Capillaries are extremely small in diameter ($0.75\,\mu m$), forcing red blood cells to pass through them one at a time. From capillaries, blood flows into small venules, which converge into larger veins. The largest veins return blood to the heart.

## CARDIAC FUNCTION

The following cardiac terms describe how the heart functions at rest and during exercise. The terms heart rate (HR), blood pressure (BP), stroke volume (SV), and cardiac output (Q) will be described.

### Heart Rate

Heart rate (HR) is the number of times the heart beats per minute (bpm). A typical HR at rest is between 60 and 80 bpm (20). Due to their smaller heart size, the resting HR of women is approximately 10 bpm higher than that of men of the same fitness level. Children have higher HRs compared to adults, while older adults generally have lower HRs. A lower resting HR is observed in fit individuals. This is due to the trained heart's ability to increase SV,

therefore, requiring less bpm to achieve a given Q (10). HR can be measured in a number of ways including counting pulses or wearing an HR monitor.

### Blood Pressure

To meet the body's demand for oxygen, nutrients, and removal of waste, the CV system must maintain adequate blood flow. Flow is achieved by the heart's ability to work as a pump generating pressure. BP is the force exerted by the blood on vessel walls and is generally termed arterial BP (16). As the LV contracts, blood is propelled into the aorta with tremendous force. This pressure is the highest generated in the vessels and is termed systolic blood pressure (SBP). Diastolic blood pressure (DBP) is the lowest BP and occurs during ventricular relaxation. Normal resting BP is below 120 mm Hg for SBP and 80 mm Hg for DBP. Hypertension is a medical condition that occurs when SBP or DBP consistently exceeds 140 or 90 mm Hg, respectively (2).

### Stroke Volume

The volume of blood ejected by the LV in a single contraction is referred to as SV. At rest, approximately 60% of the blood filling the LV is ejected (20). SV is the difference between the amount of blood in the ventricle before and after contraction (5).

### Cardiac Output

Cardiac output (Q) is the volume of blood ejected by the ventricles per minute (16). It is calculated as a product of HR and SV. Resting Q for adults is around $4–5 \text{ L·min}^{-1}$,

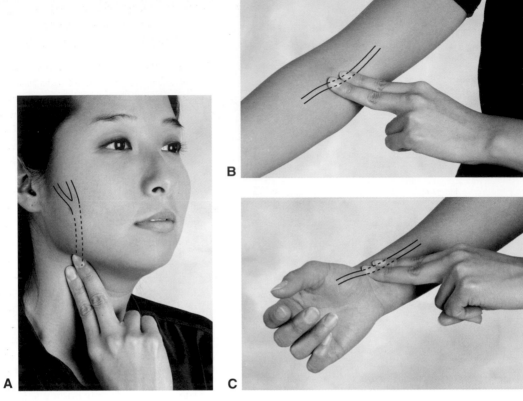

■ **FIGURE 11.4** The most common sites to palpate HR.

regardless of fitness level. However, a greater maximal Q is observed in fit individuals compared to unfit individuals.

## MEASURING PULSES

Contraction of the LV sends pressure waves or pulses throughout the body. These pulses can easily be palpated (felt) and provide important information about the heart, including HR. Radial, brachial, and carotid pulses are most often used to determine HR by palpation (9) (Fig. 11.4).

### Radial Pulse

The radial pulse is found in a groove on the lateral side of the wrist just below the base of the thumb.

### Brachial Pulse

The brachial artery is located on the medial side of the upper arm, slightly above the elbow and behind the biceps brachii.

### Carotid Pulse

The carotid pulse may be more visible and easily located than the radial or brachial pulse. This pulse can be found on the anterior side of the neck just lateral to the voice box.

### Taking Pulses

When measuring the pulse, lightly press the site using the index and middle fingers to prevent obstructing blood flow. The thumb should not be used to measure HR because it has a pulse of its own and could lead to an inaccurate reading. When palpating at the carotid site, do not apply too much pressure to the area. Baroreceptors in the carotid arteries detect this pressure and cause a reflex that slows HR (9). Using a stopwatch or the second hand on a wristwatch, count the number of pulses at rest for an entire minute. The pulse during exercise is usually measured over a 15-second period, with the count being multiplied by 4 to determine HR in bpm.

## ACUTE RESPONSE TO CARDIOVASCULAR EXERCISE

There are many CV changes that occur during a single bout of aerobic exercise. The goal of the CV system is to match the body's increased demand for oxygen, nutrients, and removal of carbon dioxide. This task is effectively managed by augmenting HR, SV, Q, blood flow, and BP.

### Heart Rate

During aerobic exercise, increases in HR are directly proportional to exercise intensity (13). HR response is related to numerous factors such as age, fitness level, mode of activity, medications, presence of disease, and environment (humidity and temperature). During submaximal exercise, a steady-state HR will be achieved after 3–5 minutes as the CV system meets the metabolic demands of the tissues. HR will eventually plateau with increasing work rates, indicating that HR has reached maximum. Maximum HR ($HR_{max}$) remains relatively stable from day to day but declines with age. The equation frequently used to estimate $HR_{max}$ in healthy men and women is "$HR_{max}$ = 220 − age." Because there is substantial variance with this equation (10–15 bpm), an alternate formula has been developed ($HR_{max}$ = 208 − (0.7 × age) (17).

## Stroke Volume

SV rises with increasing work rates until it plateaus at approximately 40%–60% of maximal aerobic capacity (5). During light to near-maximal CV exercise, SV and HR are responsible for the increase in Q. It is not uncommon for trained athletes to double or triple their SV during maximal exercise (from a resting SV of 80 mL to a maximal SV of 200 mL per beat). However, once SV reaches maximum, the increased need for oxygen is met by augmenting HR (5).

## Cardiac Output

Q increases in a linear fashion with work rate during CV exercise. Maximum Q varies based on age, body size, fitness level, and presence of disease. Maximal Q can increase from 5 L·min⁻¹ at rest to 40 L·min⁻¹ in elite endurance athletes. HR and SV both play a role in raising submaximal Q to about 60% of maximum, while higher levels of Q are achieved solely through elevated HRs.

## Blood Flow

During rest, only 15%–20% of Q is distributed to the muscles with the majority going to vital organs like the brain and heart (5). CV exercise requires that Q be redistributed to active skeletal muscle and shunted from areas such as the skin, liver, and stomach. For instance, cardiac blood flow increases fourfold with exercise, while the brain remains at resting levels. During maximal efforts, an estimated 80%–85% of Q is redirected to skeletal muscle.

## Blood Pressure

A linear relationship exists between SBP and exercise intensity (2). At maximal aerobic efforts, SBP may reach 200 mm Hg; however, maximal SBP becomes dangerously high at approximately 250 mm Hg. In contrast, an SBP that does not go up or even falls with increased work indicates a potential for a serious condition called exertional hypotension. DBP should remain unchanged or slightly decreases during exercise. This response is due to vasodilation of arterioles in active skeletal muscles creating a lower resistance to blood flow.

### ! *Take Caution*

## DESIGNING A SAFE WORKOUT EXPERIENCE

- Warm-up and cool-down are critical components of any group workout and should not be taken lightly. A proper dynamic warm-up serves to increases blood flow and muscle temperature. This prepares the body for exercise and may help reduce the chance of becoming dizzy (orthostatic hypotension) early in your exercise routine.
- Cool-down serves to prevent postexercise complications by returning blood back to the heart via muscular contractions. Abruptly stopping high-intensity exercise may bring about dizziness or in extreme cases cause a client to lose consciousness (pass out) due to inadequate blood flow to the brain. Also, a cool-down that contains general calisthenics and static stretching may reduce muscle soreness.
- Avoid dynamic changes in body position during workouts, especially with beginners or deconditioned individuals. Having clients move rapidly from a lying to standing position can lead to inadequate blood flow returning to the heart, rapidly lowering BP.
- During workouts, remind exercise participants to keep their heads up and not below their heart. This is a very frequent cause of dizziness and may occur during simple activities like bending over
  ▶ CLIP 11.1   to retie a shoe or to pick up weights from the floor.
- Adequate hydration is key, especially when exercising in a hot, humid environment. Dehydration will adversely affect exercise performance and increase the risk of heat-related illnesses.

## Maximal Oxygen Consumption

The gold standard for measuring CV fitness is maximal oxygen consumption or $VO_{2max}$ (20). $VO_{2max}$ is defined physiologically as the highest amount of oxygen the body can consume and utilize during an all-out aerobic effort. In terms of fitness, higher $VO_{2max}$ values are better. $VO_{2max}$ can be directly determined using indirect calorimetry (metabolic cart) or predicted from a submaximal exercise test. Assessing $VO_{2max}$ is important because it can be used to track fitness over time, helping to evaluate CV program effectiveness. Also, there is a distinct relationship between aerobic fitness (i.e., $VO_{2max}$) and disease. A higher $VO_{2max}$ indicates a reduced risk of CV disease. $VO_{2max}$ may decline with age but it may have more to do with physical inactivity than the aging process itself.

## RESPIRATORY SYSTEM

The structures of the respiratory system are presented in Figure 11.5. The main function of the respiratory system is to deliver oxygen and remove carbon dioxide using small air sacs in the lungs called alveoli (13). Also, the respiratory system serves as a filter, removing foreign particles from the air before reaching the lungs. The lungs are found within the thoracic cavity, just above the diaphragm. They are uniquely protected by the rib cage and chest muscles and are covered by a set of membranes called pleura.

## CONTROL OF BREATHING

Breathing or ventilation is the process of moving air into and out of the lungs (18). Normal rhythmic breathing is controlled by neurons in the brain that stimulate the respiratory muscles to contract. Increased muscle fiber recruitment and frequency of stimulation causes stronger respiratory muscle contraction, leading to increases in the depth and rate of respiration.

## DISTRIBUTION OF VENTILATION

Organs of the respiratory system can be divided into two groups, the upper and lower respiratory tracts, shown in Figure 11.5.

### Upper Respiratory Tract

The upper respiratory tract includes the nose and nasal cavity, pharynx, and larynx (18). Inhaled air is warmed, humidified, and cleaned by these structures before being conducted into the lower respiratory tract. During restful breathing, air moving through the nose is heated to body temperature and almost totally humidified.

The pharynx (throat) is a shared passageway for the respiratory and digestive systems. Air entering the nose combines with the air, food, and fluid from the mouth and moves past the pharynx. The epiglottis is a flap of elastic cartilage that covers the laryngeal opening and prevents food and fluid from entering the lower respiratory tract. The larynx contains the vocal cords, which create sound (speech) as air moves past them.

### Lower Respiratory Tract

The lower respiratory tract includes the trachea, the bronchi, and the lungs. The trachea or windpipe originates at the base of the neck and is located anterior to the esophagus. It is about 4–4.5 in (10–12 cm) in length, supported by 16–20 C-shaped cartilaginous rings. These cartilages are found on the anterior and lateral sides (horseshoe-shaped) of the trachea and help maintain an open passageway to the lungs. The trachea separates into

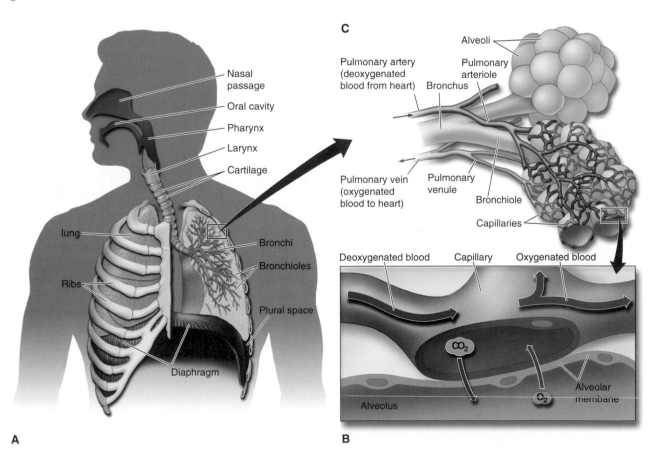

■ **FIGURE 11.5** The organs of the respiratory tract. **A:** Overview. **B:** Alveoli (air sacs) of the lungs and the blood capillaries. **C:** Transverse section through the lungs.

two primary bronchi, which allows airflow to the right and left lungs. The bronchi in each lung continue to branch until they eventually form terminal bronchioles. Terminal bronchioles repetitively divide to form respiratory bronchioles, alveolar ducts, and alveolar sacs. Alveolar sacs are composed of a large numbers of alveoli. The pulmonary capillaries surround an estimated 300 million alveoli, where gas exchange occurs through simple diffusion. The large numbers of alveoli serve to dramatically enhance the surface area for exchange of oxygen and carbon dioxide.

## VENTILATORY PUMP

The ventilatory pump consists of the chest wall, the respiratory muscles, and the pleural space.

### Chest Wall

The chest wall is comprised of the muscles of respiration (external intercostals, scalenes, pectoralis minor, and the diaphragm) and bones (ribs and sternum). The action of the chest wall facilitates inspiration and expiration by increasing or decreasing thoracic volume. Respiratory centers in the brain cause involuntary movement of the diaphragm and respiratory muscles, which begin inspiration. Inspiration is considered an active process, because it requires contraction of skeletal muscle. As the diaphragm contracts, it moves down (flattens), and respiratory muscles elevate the ribs and sternum to increase thoracic volume. This results in an expansion of the chest wall allowing the lungs to expand. As lung expansion occurs, it lowers the alveolar pressure, allowing air to move from the atmosphere through the respiratory passages to the alveoli. During expiration, which is a passive process, the diaphragm and respiratory muscles relax reducing thoracic volume causing air to move from the alveoli through the respiratory passage to the atmosphere.

### Respiratory Muscles

Interestingly enough, the muscles of respiration are the only skeletal muscles that are necessary for life. The dome-shaped diaphragm is the major muscle of inspiration. Two-thirds of the increase in thoracic volume during inspiration is due to the contraction of the diaphragm. Like a piston, the muscle fibers of the diaphragm continuously contract and relax. Other muscles that contribute to inspiration by elevating the ribs are the external intercostals, pectoralis minor, and scalenes. During exercise, inspiratory muscles become quite active, contracting forcefully to cause a greater increase in thoracic volume. Although expiration is a passive process, during labored breathing the internal intercostals and abdominal muscles contract powerfully to create a larger, more rapid decrease in thoracic volume.

### Pleura

The parietal (outer layer) and visceral (inner layer) pleura are thin membranes found between the chest wall and each lung. Between the parietal and visceral pleura lies the pleural cavity that contains pleural fluid produced by the two membranes. This fluid acts as a lubricant, allowing the membranes to slide past one another as the lung expands and relaxes. Another important role of pleural fluid is to hold the parietal and visceral membranes together. An analogy would be a thin layer of water between two sheets of glass; the glass slides easily back and forth but is difficult to separate (18).

### Pulmonary Ventilation

Pulmonary ventilation (VE) is the volume of air moved in and out of the lungs per minute. It is about $6\,L \cdot min^{-1}$ at rest in sedentary adult males but can increase 15- to 25-fold during maximal exercise (13). Pulmonary ventilation is regulated by the need for carbon dioxide removal more than oxygen consumption. Ventilation does not limit exercise capacity in healthy adults.

### Respiratory Changes

In healthy adults, the respiratory system does not appear to limit exercise performance. Ventilation increases linearly with $VO_2$ up to the ventilatory threshold where it becomes disproportionate to oxygen consumption (14). The increase in ventilation reflects a need to remove excess carbon dioxide. Unfit adults can improve maximal ventilation capacity by increasing fitness levels. When compared to sedentary adults, physically fit individuals demonstrate greater lung volumes and diffusion capacities at rest and during exercise. CV training has minimal if any affect on ventilation at rest or during submaximal exercise.

### Take Caution

#### STUDENTS WITH ASTHMATIC CONDITIONS

Exercise-induced asthma is a condition commonly seen during group exercise instruction. Although there are many different triggers and levels of severity, clients should always carry their inhalers to class and group exercise instructors should be ready to adapt exercises for these clients.

## ENERGY SYSTEMS

Energy is required to support all of the biological and chemical activities of the body. It is also crucial in producing the mechanical work needed to create movement of skeletal muscle. To release energy, carbohydrates, fats, and proteins are ingested, degraded to their simplest form through digestion, and absorbed into the bloodstream. These nutrients are distributed to skeletal muscle (among other tissues) where they are metabolized to yield a high-energy compound called adenosine triphosphate (ATP). The human body requires a continuous supply of ATP at rest and especially during intense physical activity. ATP is conveniently stored and utilized in the skeletal muscle cell. Unfortunately, ATP stores are very limited. There is only enough ATP stored in the muscle for about 5 seconds of movement. For movement to continue, there are three energy systems that supply the needed ATP: creatine phosphate (CP), anaerobic glycolysis, and aerobic oxidation.

## AEROBIC AND ANAEROBIC METABOLISM

As exercise commences, the three energy systems do not work in isolation. Each system contributes to help meet the total energy need; however, one of the three systems will predominate depending on the exercise intensity (Fig. 11.6). Two of these systems, CP and anaerobic glycolysis, are considered "anaerobic" because they occur without the presence of oxygen. CP is the most immediately available energy system. Anaerobic glycolysis uses carbohydrate stored in the muscle (as glycogen or glucose) to quickly manufacture ATP. Aerobic oxidation uses carbohydrates, fats, and minor amounts of protein to generate ATP via "aerobic metabolism." This energy system produces the most ATP along with the end products of carbon dioxide and water (5).

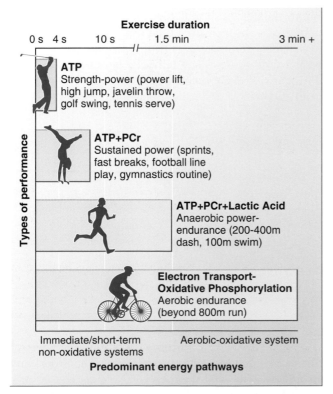

■ **FIGURE 11.6** Comparison of activity with the energy system used. (From Premkumar K. *The Massage Connection: Anatomy and Physiology*. 2nd ed. Baltimore (MD): Lippincott Williams & Wilkins; 2004.)

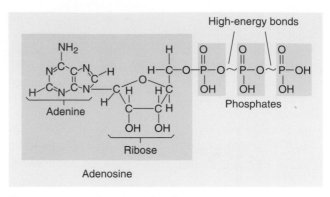

■ **FIGURE 11.7** Adenosine triphosphate.

## ADENOSINE TRIPHOSPHATE

ATP is considered the energy currency of the cell (Fig. 11.7). As ATP is hydrolyzed to adenosine diphosphate (ADP) and inorganic phosphate (Pi), energy is released to power contraction of skeletal muscle (14). The enzyme ATPase is used to facilitate this reaction. The body has a limited ability to store ATP, so it must continuously be resynthesized. There are three metabolic pathways (energy systems) that produce ATP during rest and exercise: CP, anaerobic glycolysis, and the aerobic oxidation of nutrients to water and carbon dioxide.

## CREATINE PHOSPHATE

The CP system donates a high-energy phosphate from CP to regenerate ATP from adenosine diphosphate. It is the simplest of the three energy systems because it only requires a one-step chemical reaction using the enzyme creatine kinase. The body stores about three to five times more CP than ATP, so the amount of ATP produced by this energy system is limited to all-out efforts from 10 to 30 seconds. Because this metabolic pathway occurs in the cytoplasm of the cell, oxygen is not involved, so it is considered anaerobic (without oxygen).

## ANAEROBIC GLYCOLYSIS

Glycolysis is the breakdown of carbohydrate using a series of complex chemical reactions. The metabolic process of glycolysis occurs in the cytoplasm of the muscle cell. Stored carbohydrates in the form of muscle glycogen or glucose from the blood are capable of rapidly producing small amounts of energy (2 or 3 ATP) without the use of oxygen (14) (Fig. 11.8). The end product of glycolysis is pyruvate. The fate of pyruvate is determined by the demand for ATP. If the exercise intensity is high, pyruvate is converted to lactate. This allows for more rapid generation of ATP but has the consequence of increasing H⁺ concentration eventually leading to cessation of exercise. When muscle glycogen or glucose is degraded to lactate, it is called "anaerobic glycolysis" or the "lactic acid system." This energy system can supply ATP for

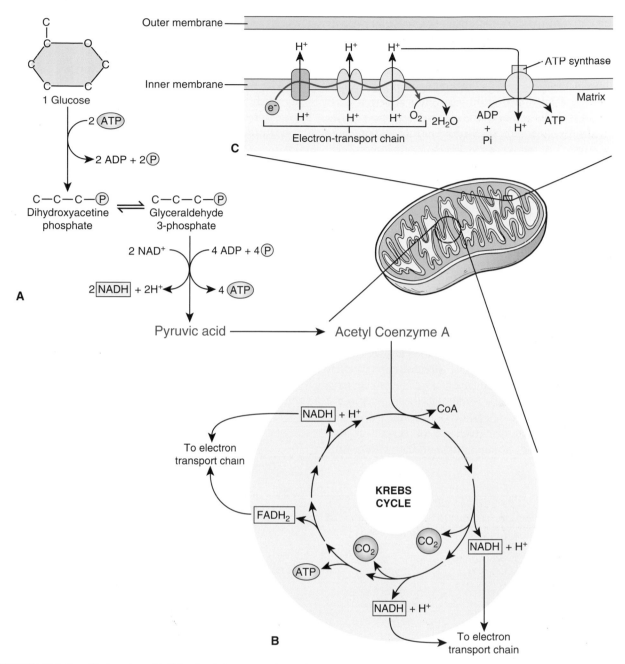

**■ FIGURE 11.8** Simplified version of (**A**) the glycolytic or anaerobic pathway where small amounts of energy are produced, (**B**) the aerobic pathway, where acetyl-CoA is produced from pyruvic acid and enters Krebs cycle and (**C**) the electron transport chain, in which the hydrogen (H⁺) ions and electrons (e⁻) from NADH + H⁺ complexes generated in the glycolytic and Krebs cycle are converted to ATP and water in the presence of oxygen ($O_2$).

high-intensity exercise lasting anywhere from 30 seconds to 2 minutes (13).

## AEROBIC OXIDATION

Aerobic metabolism generates ATP through the breakdown of carbohydrates, fats, and minor amounts of protein. This complex process is "aerobic," meaning oxygen is available to be used in the muscle cell. The presence of oxygen permits the carbon bonds in our food to be completely degraded to carbon dioxide. First, each nutrient is

broken down to their building block molecule; for carbohydrate it is glycogen or glucose and fats are degraded to fatty acids and proteins to amino acids. Each structure is then funneled to one common two-carbon molecule, acetyl coenzyme A (CoA), using a variety of metabolic pathways. Glycogen and glucose use glycolysis, fatty acids use beta-oxidation, and nitrogen is removed from amino acids allowing participation in ATP production. In the glycolytic pathway, with oxygen present, pyruvate moves into the mitochondria of the cell and is further degraded to acetyl-CoA. Fatty acids, which contain long chains of carbons, undergo beta-oxidation in the mitochondria as well. The two metabolic pathways for aerobic ATP production are the Krebs cycle and electron transport chain. These processes reside in the mitochondria as illustrated in Figure 11.8. As acetyl-CoA enters the Krebs cycle, carbon dioxide is produced and hydrogen is removed from four sites along the cycle. At the electron transport chain, these hydrogen atoms are split into electrons and protons. The electrons are passed down a chain of cytochromes, which ultimately allow for the generation of ATP. At the end of the chain, the hydrogen combines with oxygen to form water. Because the use of oxygen is coupled with the generation of ATP, the aerobic process is called oxidative phosphorylation (20). The complete aerobic oxidation of one glucose molecule produces 36–39 ATP, while one 16-carbon fatty acid may produce as much as 129 ATP. Finally, any activity maintained for >2 or 3 minutes requires the use of the aerobic system.

## RECOVERY FROM EXERCISE

Oxygen consumption ($VO_2$) remains elevated above resting levels for some time after the cessation of exercise (12). This is referred to as excess postexercise oxygen consumption (EPOC). Generally, the more intense and prolonged the exercise bout, the greater the energy expenditure after exercise because of several factors including higher body temperatures and larger amounts of circulating hormones.

## Take Caution

### HIGH-INTENSITY TRAINING

High-intensity training seen on popular TV shows and DVDs is not necessary for clients to successfully reach their goals. These workouts are inappropriate for novice exercisers or those with physical limitations (*i.e.*, extremely overweight, orthopedic problems), creating an increased chance of injury. A fitness regimen using moderate-intensity exercise will be more beneficial, especially in the initial weeks and months of training.

## MUSCULAR SYSTEM

Muscle is one of the four major types of tissue found in the human body. Three types of muscle exist in the human body: smooth, cardiac, and skeletal. It is skeletal muscle that attaches to bone and produces physical movements. Skeletal muscle has a "striated" appearance because its fibers have an alternating light and dark striped pattern. For the most part, skeletal muscle is under voluntary control, meaning it is controlled by conscious thought. Smooth muscle is found in blood vessels and other internal organs. Cardiac muscle is only

located in the heart. Unlike skeletal and smooth muscle, cardiac tissue is involuntary, under the control of the autonomic nervous system (ANS). Cardiac muscle does have a striped appearance; however, this banding pattern is absent in smooth muscle. All three types of muscle have the characteristics of contractility, excitability, extensibility, and elasticity (18). In this section, we concentrate on skeletal muscle because of its importance during exercise.

## SKELETAL MUSCLES (MACRO TO MICRO)

Skeletal muscle is made up of multiple connective tissue coverings. This is related to the function of skeletal muscle, which is to generate force by pulling on the bony levers of the body. Figure 11.9 presents the structure of skeletal muscle. The outermost connective tissue is referred to as the epimysium and covers the entire muscle. Skeletal muscle is composed of muscle fiber bundles called fasciculi. These bundles are covered and separated from other bundles by a connective tissue wrapping called the perimysium. One final connective tissue covering, the endomysium, separates individual muscle fibers. Directly beneath the endomysium, the sarcolemma (cell membrane) encloses the contents of the muscle fiber (20) (Fig. 11.10).

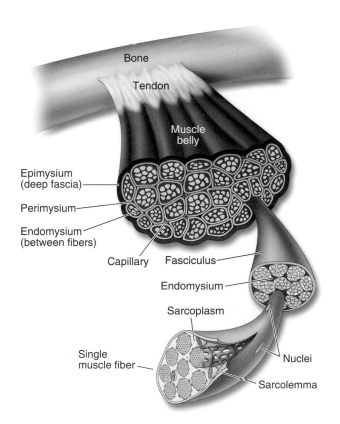

■ **FIGURE 11.9** Macroscopic structure of skeletal muscle. (From McArdle WD, Katch FI, Katch VL. *Essentials of Exercise Physiology*. 2nd ed. Baltimore (MD): Lippincott Williams & Wilkins; 2000.)

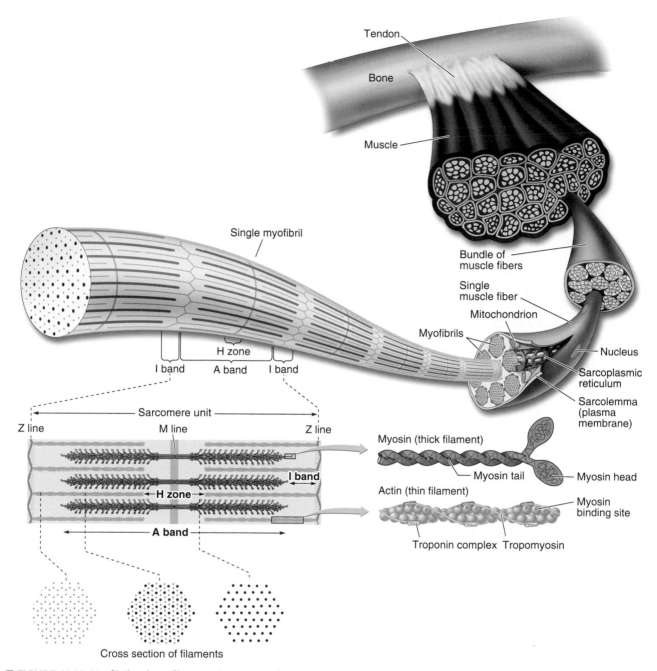

**■ FIGURE 11.10** Myofibril and myofilaments. (From McArdle WD, Katch FI, Katch VL. *Essentials of Exercise Physiology.* 2nd ed. Baltimore (MD): Lippincott Williams & Wilkins; 2000.)

Two important microstructures of skeletal muscles are the transverse tubules (T tubules) and the sarcoplasmic reticulum. T tubules pass laterally through the muscle fiber and have openings on the sarcolemma. The main function of the T tubules is to allow nerve impulses traveling down the sarcolemma to be spread quickly to the muscle's contractile proteins. The sarcoplasmic reticulum is a network of membranous channels that run parallel to the muscle fiber and store calcium, which is exceedingly important for muscle action (5).

## MUSCLE CONTRACTION (CROSS-BRIDGES)

The sarcomere is the smallest functional unit of skeletal muscle. A sarcomere consists of two primary muscle proteins, actin (thin filament) and myosin (thick filament). Two associated proteins, troponin and tropomyosin, are found on the actin molecule. Each myosin myofilament contains many cross-bridges that are used to bind with actin.

Three concepts that are vital to an understanding of how skeletal muscles contract include the sliding filament theory, the all-or-none principle, and muscle fiber recruitment. The sliding filament theory chronicles the events occurring at the sarcomere, in particular, the interaction between the protein filaments, actin and myosin. After receiving a nerve impulse, myosin cross-bridges attach to the actin filament, sliding it toward the center of the sarcomere. While tension is developed as the sarcomere shortens, no length change occurs in the actin or myosin filaments. This process takes place in sarcomeres all along the muscle fiber, allowing muscle to generate forceful contractions.

Skeletal muscle, when stimulated to contract by nerve impulses, exhibits an all-or-none response, meaning the sarcomere will contract maximally or not at all (16). Ultimately, the amount of force generated by a muscle is based on the number of muscle fibers recruited to contract. This can be accomplished by activating more motor units. A motor unit is a nerve and all the muscle fibers that it stimulates (15). In most cases, more than one motor unit is needed to stimulate an entire muscle to contract.

## MUSCLE CONTRACTION AND TRAINING

Muscular movement is usually classified into three different contraction types: static (isometric), concentric, and eccentric. During static contractions, a muscle or muscle group is held at constant length against resistance without changes in joint angle. Static training has been shown to provide significant increases in muscular strength; however, the gains are specific to the joint angles trained (6,11). As a result, the use of static training may provide little practical value, especially in improving functional strength. Functional strength is defined as gains in strength that translate to the real world, making common tasks easier (i.e., lifting boxes, sports activities). Static training has been found to cause dramatic, short-term elevations in BP, due to the substantial intrathoracic pressure developed during static contractions. Static training can be used effectively to maintain strength and prevent atrophy for those with immobilized limbs or those who are participating in physical rehabilitation (7,11).

Concentric contraction occurs as the muscle shortens, such as during the lifting phase of a biceps curl. Conversely, eccentric contraction happens through lengthening of the muscle (i.e., lowering phase of biceps curl). Collectively, concentric and eccentric muscle action is termed dynamic muscle contraction because joint movement occurs. Most dynamic resistance training exercises include concentric and eccentric action. Interestingly, greater loads can be moved eccentrically. This probably results from a slow movement velocity and increases in motor unit recruitment during eccentric exercise. Also, heavy eccentric loading exercise, like performing "negatives," seems to create more muscle soreness compared with concentric exercise.

## MUSCLE FIBER TYPES

The muscular system allows the body to perform a wide array of physical tasks that incorporate varying amounts of endurance, power, and speed. A single skeletal muscle is composed of different fiber types that are recruited to match the demands of the physical challenge. Although there is debate about the exact classification of muscle fibers, there is agreement that two general types of fibers exist: slow twitch (type I) and fast twitch (type 2) (20).

### Type I Muscle Fibers

Type I muscle fibers have the ability to use oxygen very well and are fatigue resistant. Because of this chief characteristic, type I fibers are often called "aerobic" fibers. These fibers are utilized for lower intensity (submaximal) activities such as walking and jogging. It is estimated that muscles of sedentary individuals are approximately 50% type I fibers (5). The percentage of type I fibers is higher in endurance athletes, but this is probably due to genetic predisposition. There is some evidence to support the notion that endurance training can alter fiber type. The most successful endurance athletes combine their genetic potential (high proportion of type I fibers) with a rigorous exercise training program.

### Type II Muscle Fibers

In contrast to type I fibers, type II fibers are recruited to perform anaerobic, higher-intensity exercise such as sprinting and weight training. These fibers fatigue easily but have the ability to develop tension considerably faster than type I fibers (19). These fibers are considered the "classic" fast-twitch, type IIb fibers. Type II fibers are associated with larger motor nerves; this results in higher conduction velocities and more muscle fibers stimulated per motor unit. Type II fibers also have a more developed sarcoplasmic reticulum, and myosin ATPase activity is higher, which contributes to a faster contraction speed when compared with type I fibers. In events lasting several minutes, a second kind of fast-twitch fiber, type IIa is recruited. This fiber is an intermediate fiber, meaning it does have some aerobic capacity while still being able to generate moderate amounts of force. Again, the distribution of fiber type is primarily due to genetics. This, however, does not ensure athletic success in strength and power sports. Factors such as training, motivation, body composition, CV function, and overall muscle size must be considered.

## NEUROMUSCULAR ACTIVATION

Physical activity involves purposeful movement; therefore, the stimulus for muscle activation originates in the brain (20). A signal is relayed through the brainstem to the spinal cord and is developed into a specific movement pattern.

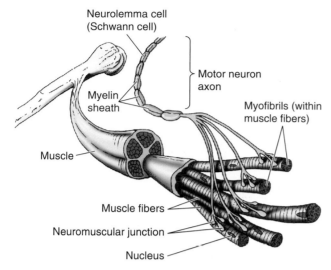

**■ FIGURE 11.11** The motor unit. (From Moore KL, Dalley AF II. *Clinical Oriented Anatomy*. 4th ed. Baltimore (MD): Lippincott Williams & Wilkins; 1999.)

The number of motor units recruited for a given task depends on the force necessary to complete the activity.

## MOTOR UNIT ACTIVATION

The functional unit of the neuromuscular system is the motor unit, which is illustrated in Figure 11.11 (15). It consists of the motor neuron (nerve) and the muscle fibers it stimulates. Motor units vary in size from a few to several hundred muscle fibers. Larger muscles are stimulated by multiple motor units, so it is possible for some muscle fibers within a given muscle to rest passively while adjacent fibers contract. Motor units follow an orderly recruitment pattern to stimulate contraction of skeletal muscle. Motor units are recruited based on the amount of force needed to complete the activity (18). Smaller motor units that stimulate type I fibers are recruited first. If more force is necessary, larger motor units that control type II fibers are called into action. For example, walking would require only type I fibers, whereas running 800 m would require not only type I fibers but also type IIa and possibly type IIb fibers at the finish (Fig. 11.11).

## SKELETAL SYSTEM

The skeletal system protects internal organs, produces blood cells, and stores nutrients. The skeletal system is comprised of 206 bones (Fig. 11.12). Bones are the rigid levers that work with skeletal muscle to create locomotion. The skull, vertebral column, sternum, and ribs are considered the axial skeleton; bones of the upper and lower limb make up the appendicular skeleton. A fibrous layer called the periosteum covers the bone and is continuous with tendons that anchor muscle to bone. Tendons are

likewise continuous with the epimysium, the outer layer of connective tissue covering muscle (13).

## STRUCTURE AND FUNCTION OF JOINTS IN MOVEMENT

Bones of the skeletal system articulate, meaning they join together to form joints (18). Joints are held together by tough connective tissue called ligaments. Joints are classified as fibrous, cartilaginous, or synovial. The most important for movement are the synovial joints, which are freely moving joints that unite bones of the appendicular skeleton. Synovial joints have cavities filled with synovial fluid that reduces friction, allowing movement to occur easier. The degree of movement at a joint is called range of movement. Joints are anatomically limited in range of movement, meaning articulation between the bones themselves prevents further movement. Also, movement of one joint may affect the extent of movement at adjacent joints because a large number of muscles and soft tissues cross two joints. For instance, wrist flexion decreases finger flexion, as muscles crossing the fingers and wrist cross multiple joints.

To facilitate appropriate movement patterns, joints have kinesthetic receptors that sense changes in joint angle and position in space. Through a process called proprioception, receptors at the joint send sensory information to the brain so that appropriate movement patterns can be accomplished and injury prevented.

## NEUROLOGICAL SYSTEM

The nervous system is without question one of the most complex systems in the human body. An overview of the nervous system is presented in Figure 11.13. It functions to provide communication and coordination of body tissues by receiving sensory input, integrating information, controlling glands, and maintaining mental activity (16). Also, the nervous system is essential to an understanding of human movement because, as mentioned previously, nerve impulses signal skeletal muscle to contract. The basic structural unit of the nervous system is the neuron; it contains three parts: the cell body (integration center), the dendrites (receives input), and the axon (sends nerve impulses). The nervous system consists of the brain, spinal cord, and peripheral nerves, and is divided into the central nervous system (CNS) and the peripheral nervous system (PNS). The CNS includes the brain and spinal cord, whereas the PNS consists of peripheral nerves of voluntary system (Fig. 11.13).

### CENTRAL NERVOUS SYSTEM

The CNS is the body's central command center where sensory input is received, integrated, analyzed, and interpreted, and finally relayed as nerve impulses are

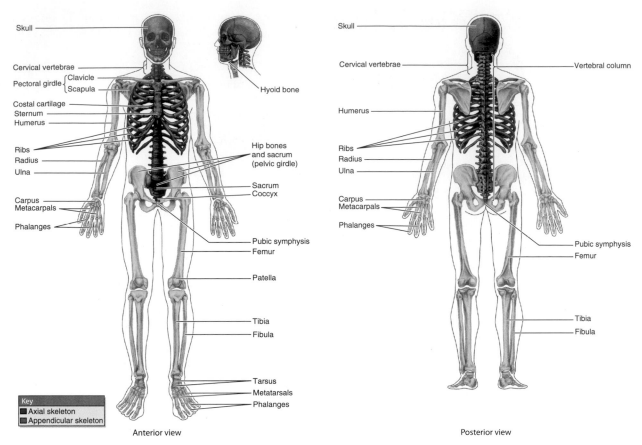

Anterior view

Key
Axial skeleton
Appendicular skeleton

Posterior view

■ **FIGURE 11.12** The skeletal system. (From Moore KL, Dalley AF II. *Clinically Oriented Anatomy*. 4th ed. Baltimore (MD): Lippincott Williams & Wilkins; 1999.)

sent to end organs (*i.e.*, muscles, glands, and heart). The brain is the most important component of the CNS and is encased and protected by the bony skull. The spinal cord is the extension of the brain, which runs down and is enclosed and protected by the vertebral column.

## PERIPHERAL NERVOUS SYSTEM

The PNS is made up of nerve cells and associated fibers that are located outside the brain and spinal cord. The PNS is the primary communication link between CNS and the rest of the body. There are two types of nerve fibers in the PNS, the sensory (afferent) fiber and the motor (efferent) fiber. The sensory nerve fiber is responsible for carrying nerve impulses from sensory receptors in the body to the CNS. Once sensory input is received by the CNS, the information is processed and analyzed. After the appropriate action is determined, a motor nerve fiber sends a response (nerve signal) from the CNS to the end organ. The PNS can be subdivided into two branches, the somatic nervous system (SNS) and the autonomic nervous system (ANS). Both systems are composed of a sensory division and a motor division. The somatic nervous system regulates the voluntary contraction of the skeletal muscles, whereas the autonomic system involves the motor activities that control internal organs such as the smooth (involuntary) muscles, cardiac muscle, and glands.

## AUTONOMIC NERVOUS SYSTEM

The ANS regulates involuntary internal activities such as HR, digestion, breathing, and the secretion of hormones. These activities operate subconsciously and continue to function throughout life. The ANS includes two major divisions, the sympathetic division and the parasympathetic division, which complement each other. The sympathetic division stimulates internal activities under stressful (or alarming) conditions, which results in acceleration of metabolism, HR, and breathing, and the release of adrenal hormones. Exercise can be treated as a stressful stimulus to the body that triggers the sympathetic nervous system for generating more energy and muscular force. When the stressful situation subsides, the parasympathetic nervous system brings the internal activities back to normal, *e.g.*, decreasing HR and respiratory rate, relaxing the muscles, and increasing gastrointestinal activities. The parasympathetic nervous system helps conserve and resume normal body function (5).

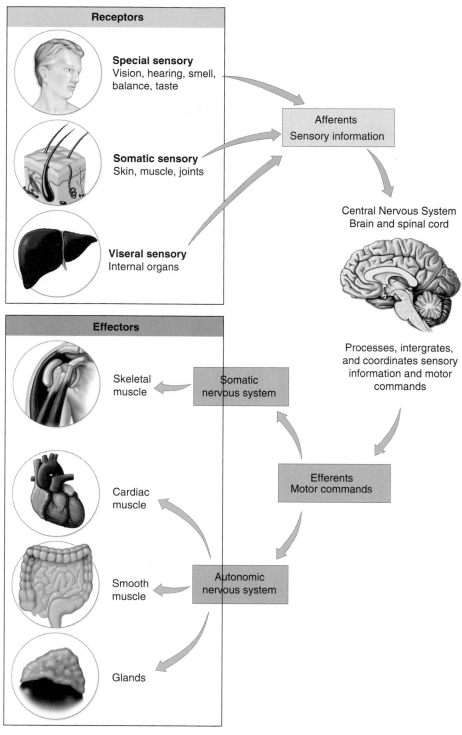

■ **FIGURE 11.13** Overview of nervous system. (From Premkumar K. *The Massage Connection Anatomy and Physiology*. Baltimore (MD): Lippincott Williams & Wilkins; 2004.)

## EXERCISE SYSTEM ADAPTATIONS: STRENGTH, CARDIOVASCULAR FUNCTION, FLEXIBILITY

Chronic exercise training is important to overall health, physical fitness, and general well-being. A properly designed exercise training program leads to long-term physiological changes, particularly improvement in muscular strength and endurance, CV function, and musculoskeletal flexibility. These improvements allow one to enhance athletic performance, enjoy active leisure-time pursuits, perform daily activities more easily, and maintain functional independence later in life.

## RESISTANCE TRAINING

Resistance training is an effective exercise mode to improve muscular strength and endurance. Strength improves when sufficient tension is applied to the muscle fiber and its contractile proteins. The tension required for strength gain is about 60%–80% of the muscle's maximum force. Fleck and Kraemer (6) recommended a range of 75%–90% of one repetition maximum contraction (1 RM) for optimizing strength gain. To enhance muscular fitness, the muscular system must be progressively overloaded (*e.g.*, increased resistance, repetitions, or sets). The most prominent adaptations to strength training include increases in muscle strength and muscular size, a condition called "hypertrophy."

The early strength gains from resistance training are due to neural factors such as increased neural drive to muscle, increased synchronization of motor units, and increased activation of the contractile proteins (20). After 6–8 weeks of progressive resistance training, fiber hypertrophy occurs primarily due to increases in the number of actin and myosin filaments. Another adaptation leading to improvements in strength include increases in CP and glycolytic enzyme activity.

## CHRONIC ADAPTATIONS TO CARDIOVASCULAR EXERCISE

Physical inactivity is now classified as a major contributing risk factor for heart disease, similar to that of elevated blood cholesterol level, cigarette smoking, and hypertension (2,1). Moreover, longitudinal studies have shown that higher levels of aerobic fitness are associated with lower mortality from heart disease even after statistical adjustments for age, coronary risk factors, and family history of heart disease (3,4).

Most exercise studies on healthy subjects demonstrate 20% (±10%) increases in $VO_{2max}$, with the greatest relative improvements among the most unfit (8). Because a fixed submaximal work rate has a relatively constant aerobic requirement, after regular CV training, the individual exercises at a lower percentage of maximum while at the same workload. Enhanced oxygen transport, particularly increased maximal SV and Q, has traditionally been regarded as the primary mechanism underlying the increase in $VO_{2max}$ with training (13).

After chronic CV training, the resting HR decreases by approximately 10–15 bpm as SV increases both at rest and during exercise. Q will increase during maximal exercise but will not change significantly at rest. Both resting SBP and DBP may decrease (if hypertensive prior to training) with long-term CV training.

## FLEXIBILITY

Flexibility is another important, yet often neglected, component of health-related physical fitness (2,1). The level of flexibility is greatly reduced with age and physical inactivity. Lower back problems have been associated with poor flexibility of the lower back and hamstring muscles and weak abdominal muscles.

After a flexibility enhancement program, both long- and short-term adaptations exist. For long-term adaptation, the range of movement of the joint is increased, resulting in a decrease in muscle soreness. Furthermore, an inverse relationship has been demonstrated between neuromuscular tension and musculotendon extendibility. Improving flexibility reduces the likelihood of strains, tears, and tightness that may result in muscular pain, spasm, and cramping. Flexibility training also lengthens the fascia, which supports and stabilizes the muscles, organs, and most body tissues.

## SUMMARY

*This chapter was designed to introduce the GEI to the discipline of exercise physiology. Emphasis is placed on CV physiology, pulmonary physiology, and muscle function because that is what the GEI works with every day. However, endocrine function and other body functions are also important, so it is suggested that as you come across new issues with your clients, you seek out additional references that can assist you in understanding the function of the human being under conditions of physical stress.*

## References

1. American College of Sports Medicine. *ACSM's Resources Manual for Guidelines for Exercise Testing and Prescription.* 6th ed. Baltimore (MD): Williams & Wilkins; 2009.
2. American College of Sports Medicine. *ACSM's Guidelines for Exercise Testing and Prescription.* 8th ed. Baltimore (MD): Lippincott Williams & Wilkins; 2009.
3. Blair SN, Kampert JB, Kohl HW III, et al. Influences of cardiorespiratory fitness and other precursors on cardiovascular disease and all-cause mortality in men and women. *JAMA.* 1996;276: 205–10.
4. Blair SN, Kohl HW III, Paffenbarger RS, et al. Physical fitness and all-cause mortality: a prospective study of healthy men and women. *JAMA.* 1989;262:2395–401.
5. Brown SP, Miller WC, Eason JM. *Exercise Physiology: Basis of Human Movement in Health and Disease.* Baltimore (MD): Lippincott Williams & Wilkins; 2006.
6. Fleck SJ, Kraemer WJ. *Designing Resistance Training Programs.* 3rd ed. Champaign (IL): Human Kinetics; 2004.
7. Gardner G. Specificity of strength changes of the exercised and nonexercised limb following isometric training. *Res Q.* 1963;34:98.

8. Haskell WL, Lee IM, Pate RR, et al. Physical activity and public health: updated recommendation for adults from the American College of Sports Medicine and the American Heart Association. *Med Sci Sports Exerc.* 2007;39:1423–34.

9. Heyward VH. *Advanced Fitness Assessment and Exercise Prescription.* Champaign (IL): Human Kinetics; 2010.

10. Karvonen MJ, Kentala E, Mustala O. The effects of training on heart rate: a longitudinal study. *Ann Med Exp Biol Fenn.* 1957;35:307.

11. Knapik JJ, Mawdsley RH, Ramos NU. Angular specificity and test mode specificity of isometric and isokinetic strength training. *J Orthop Sports Phys Ther.* 1983;5:58.

12. LaForgia J, Withers RT, Gore CJ. Effects of exercise intensity and duration on the excess post-exercise oxygen consumption. *J Sports Sci.* 2006;24:1247–64.

13. McArdle WD, Katch FI, Katch VL. *Essentials of Exercise Physiology.* 3rd ed. Baltimore (MD): Lippincott Williams & Wilkins; 2005.

14. McArdle WD, Katch FI, Katch VL. *Exercise Physiology, Energy, Nutrition, and Human Performance.* 7th ed. Baltimore (MD): Lippincott Williams & Wilkins; 2009.

15. Noth J. Motor units. In: Komi PV, editor. *Strength and Power in Sport.* Oxford (UK): Blackwell Scientific; 1992. 21–8 p.

16. Shier D, Butler JL, Lewis R. *Hole's Essentials of Human Anatomy and Physiology.* 12th ed. Boston (MA): McGraw-Hill; 2009.

17. Tanaka H, Monahan DK, Seals DR. Age-predicted maximal heart rate revisited. *J Am Coll Cardiol.* 2001;37:153–6.

18. VanPutte C, Regan J, Russo A. *Seeley's Essentials of Anatomy and Physiology.* 7th ed. Boston (MA): McGraw-Hill; 2010.

19. Vrbova G. Influence of activity on some characteristic properties of slow and fast mammalian muscles. *Exerc Sport Sci Rev.* 1979;7:181–213.

20. Wilmore JH, Costill DL, Kenney WL. *Physiology of Sport and Exercise.* Champaign (IL): Human Kinetics; 2008.

# 12

# Kinesiology, Anatomy, and Biomechanics

## GAVIN MOIR • TERI L. BLADEN

*Objectives*

At the end of this chapter you will be able to:
- Use basic anatomical terminology to describe movements
- Describe basic biomechanical concepts
- Describe the muscular, skeletal, and articular systems
- Describe how muscles produce movement
- Describe the factors affecting muscular tension
- Identify the major muscles of the upper and lower extremities
- Describe common injuries incurred by the group exercise instructor

With a better understanding of the physiological aspects of exercise from Chapter 11, let's now look at how we can analyze movements. A solid knowledge of kinesiology, anatomy, and biomechanics is fundamental to the success and safety of teaching group exercise. Though these areas can be intimidating to the new group exercise instructor, think of them more as building blocks to success. By understanding the structures of the body and their role in human motion, you have key components in the formula for creating safe and effective workouts. If a participant were to ask you why you chose a move or pattern of moves, could you explain your reasoning? Being able to explain to a participant the "why" in addition to the "how" of your exercise routines not only aids in his or her success in movement, it demonstrates your competency as a fitness professional. Put in the time to acquire a solid understanding of these principles; it will take some stress out of creating safe and effective group exercise workouts.

Though you may not always use anatomical or biomechanical terminology with your participants (can you imagine saying, "contract the pectoralis major to perform horizontal shoulder adduction in the transverse plane" instead of "chest fly"?), this terminology is the common language of exercise professionals used to describe and understand human motion. So, even though you may not use it every day with your participants, it helps us all speak with a common language. Let's begin with some basic definitions. Kinesiology can be defined as the study of human movement. Anatomy is the study of the structure of biological organisms, whereas biomechanics is concerned with the action of forces in the study of anatomical and functional aspects of biological organisms. The objective of this chapter is to highlight the importance of kinesiology for the group exercise instructor through the exploration of basic anatomical and biomechanical principles applied to exercise.

## BASIC ANATOMY AND ANATOMICAL PRINCIPLES

### ANATOMICAL POSITION

The anatomical position is a universally accepted reference position that is used in kinesiology to describe spatial relations between body segments and to identify orientations of the body segments during specific movements. In the anatomical position, the body is upright with the feet together and the arms hanging at the sides, the palms facing forward with the fingers extended and the thumbs facing away from the body (Fig. 12.1). Table 12.1 contains some common anatomical terms used to describe spatial relations and position of anatomical structures in relation to the anatomical position. When instructing your class, you are most likely to use terms such as *posterior*, *anterior*, *supine*, *prone*, *unilateral*, and *bilateral*.

### PLANES OF MOTION AND AXES OF ROTATION

All movements of individual body segments occur in a plane of motion and around an axis of rotation. There are three imaginary planes that pass through the body (Fig. 12.2). The sagittal plane divides the body into left and right halves; the frontal plane (also called the coronal plane) divides the body into anterior and posterior halves (front and back); the transverse plane (also called

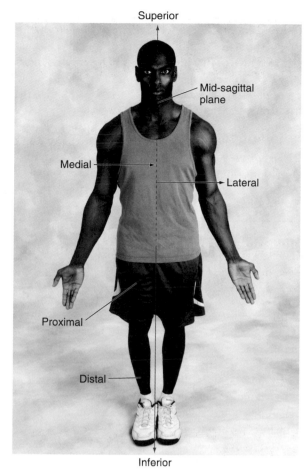

Superior

Mid-sagittal plane

Medial

Lateral

Proximal

Distal

Inferior

■ **FIGURE 12.1** The body in the anatomical position. (From Thompson WR, edition. ACSM's Resources for the Personal Trainer. 3rd ed. Baltimore (MD): Lippincott Williams & Wilkins; 2010.)

| Table 12.1 | TERMINOLOGY USED TO DESCRIBE SPATIAL RELATIONS AND POSITION OF ANATOMICAL STRUCTURES |
|---|---|
| **TERM** | **DEFINITION** |
| Anterior | The front of the body; ventral |
| Posterior | The back of the body; dorsal |
| Proximal | Closer to any reference point |
| Distal | Farther from any reference point |
| Superior | Toward the head; higher (cephalic) |
| Inferior | Away from the head; lower (caudal) |
| Medial | Toward the midline of the body |
| Lateral | Away from the midline of the body |
| Superficial | Located close to or on the body surface |
| Deep | Below the surface |
| Ipsilateral | On the same side |
| Contralateral | On the opposite side |
| Unilateral | One side |
| Bilateral | Both sides |
| Prone | Lying face down |
| Supine | Lying face up |

*From Mayer JM. Anatomy, kinesiology, and biomechanics. In: Thompson WR, Baldwin KE, Pire NI, Niederpruem M, eds. ACSM's Resources for the Personal Trainer. 2nd ed. Baltimore (MD): Lippincott Williams & Wilkins; 2007:109–76.*

Table 12.2 lists specific joint motion terminology that will be used throughout this chapter.

the cross-sectional, axial, or horizontal plane) divides the body into superior and inferior halves.

**CLIP 12.1** As mentioned earlier, each anatomical plane has an associated axis of rotation, which acts perpendicular to the plane. Each of these axes has a specific name: the mediolateral axis (also called the frontal axis) is perpendicular to the sagittal plane; the anteroposterior axis (also called the sagittal axis) is perpendicular to the frontal plane; the longitudinal axis (also called the vertical axis) is perpendicular to the transverse plane. Some practical examples will help. When a dumbbell is raised and lowered during a biceps curl, the forearm rotates relative to the arm about the elbow joint. The segments move in the sagittal plane with the rotation of the segments occurring about a mediolateral axis. During a lateral raise, the arm segment rotates relative to the trunk, constituting rotation about an anteroposterior axis with the motion of the arm occurring in the frontal plane.

## JOINT MOTION TERMINOLOGY

The motion at a joint is described by the spatial orientation of body segments relative to one another and typically uses the anatomical position as the starting point.

## BASIC BIOMECHANICAL PRINCIPLES

In the biomechanical study of movement, we are interested in the motion of a body and also the factors that affect the motion of the body. The motion of the body is described using kinematic variables that reference spatial (the position that a body occupies in space) and temporal (the change in position of a body with respect to time) characteristics. Kinematic variables include the velocity and acceleration of the body. Kinetic variables, such as forces and torques, provide information about the causes of any changes in motion that are observed. An understanding of both kinematic and kinetic variables is required to accurately describe movements.

## TYPES OF MOTION

When a body is in the process of changing its position in space, it is described as being in motion. A change in position of a body divided by the time taken to change position is known as the velocity of the body. The rate at which velocity changes is known as an acceleration. In biomechanics, we use the velocity of a body to determine the motion possessed by the body with the motion of a body being described in either linear or angular terms. Linear motion, also called translation, refers to movement of a body along a virtual path that is either straight or curved. Angular motion, also called rotation, refers to the

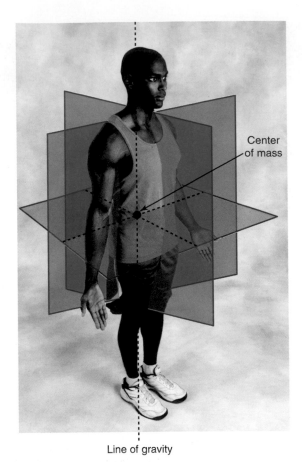

**■ FIGURE 12.2** Anatomic position showing CM and anatomic planes of motion. (Adapted from Thompson WR, edition. *ACSM's Resources for the Personal Trainer.* 3rd ed. Baltimore (MD): Lippincott Williams & Wilkins; 2010.)

movement of a body that is restricted to move around a fixed axis, resulting in the body following a circular path.

The body represents a linked segmental system whereby the body segments are constrained to rotate about axes of rotation defined by anatomical joints. Therefore, even if the motion of a barbell during a bench press exercise follows a linear path (linear motion), this is only achieved by the rotation of the arm and forearm segments during the movement (angular motion). In this manner, all of our voluntary movements during exercise are the result of angular motion, the rotation of body segments. The observed angular motion is usually the consequence of skeletal muscles acting across the joints.

## CENTER OF MASS

When describing the motion of a body, biomechanists analyze a virtual point known as the center of mass (CM).[1]

Mass is a measure of the quantity of matter contained within a body, and the CM is the point about which the mass of a body is equally distributed. The CM is located around the area of the navel for a human stood in the anatomical position. However, by changing the position of the body segments, the location of the CM can be changed, and during some movements the CM actually lies outside of the body. As well as using the CM to describe the motion of a body, the position of the CM relative to the external forces acting on a body can provide important information about the outcome of a given movement.

## THE EFFECT OF FORCES ON MOTION

A force is simply an agent that changes or tends to change the motion of a body (some forces may not be sufficiently large to actually change the motion of a body, but they *tend* to change the motion of the body). A change in motion of a body is known as acceleration. Examples of agents that we encounter that change our motion include gravity,[2] air resistance, and, of course, muscular forces. In general, forces produce either pushing actions, where we refer to compressive forces, or pulling actions, where we refer to tensile forces. For example, during upright posture, the femur experiences compressive forces due to the gravitational force acting down while muscles produce tensile forces when they contract.

Newton's three laws of motion tell us about the interaction of forces acting on a body:

1. Law of inertia. A body will remain in its present state of rest or motion unless acted upon by unbalanced external forces.
2. Law of acceleration. The change in motion of a body is proportional to and in the same direction as the applied force, but inversely proportional to the mass of the body. A rearrangement of this law informs us that a force is the product of mass and acceleration.
3. Law of reaction. When we apply a force to another body, that body applies an equal force back onto us.

A practical example can demonstrate the application of Newton's three laws of motion. When we stand stationary on a set of bathroom scales, we are in a state of rest; *i.e.,* our CM does not change its motion. Given that we are within a gravitational field, we know that gravity is trying to accelerate our CM toward that of the earth. From Newton's second law of motion, gravity produces a force acting down that is proportional to our mass being accelerated, resulting in a force that we call bodyweight that acts at the CM.

---

[1]The terms center of mass and center of gravity are often used interchangeably in biomechanics. Mechanically, the CM of an object is defined as the virtual point about which all of the mass is equally distributed, while the center of gravity is the virtual point where the gravitational force acts on an object. We can assume that humans operate within a constant gravitational field, and therefore the locations of the CM and the center of gravity of the human coincide. The term CM will be used throughout this chapter for clarity.

[2]Gravity is an attractive force whereby objects that possess mass are attracted to one another. From Newton's law of universal gravitation, the force of attraction depends on the masses involved and inversely as the square of the distance between the objects. As the earth is the most massive object in our locale, every object that possesses mass is attracted to the earth's center and therefore experiences an acceleration, a change in linear motion, in a downward direction.

| Table 12.2 | JOINT MOTION TERMINOLOGY | |
|---|---|---|
| **TERM** | **DESCRIPTION** | **EXAMPLE EXERCISES** |
| Flexion | Movement resulting in a decrease in joint angle<br>The segment typically rotates in the sagittal plane | Shoulder joint: upward movement a during a front raise<br>Elbow joint: upward movement of the dumbbell during a biceps curl<br>Hip joint: the descent during a squat<br>Knee joint: the descent during a squat<br>Spine: bending from the anatomical position to touch toes |
| Extension | Movement resulting in an increase in joint angle<br>The segment typically rotates in the sagittal plane | Shoulder joint: downward movement during a front raise<br>Elbow joint: downward movement of the dumbbell during a biceps curl<br>Hip joint: the ascent during a squat<br>Knee joint: the ascent during a squat<br>Spine: rising from touching toes to the anatomical position |
| Abduction | Movement away from the midline of the body<br>The segment rotates in the frontal or transverse planes | Shoulder joint: upward movement of the bar during a lat pull<br>Hip joint: movement of the thigh away from the body during hip abduction |
| Adduction | Movement toward the midline of the body<br>The segment rotates in the frontal or transverse planes | Shoulder joint: downward movement of the bar during a lat pull<br>Hip joint: movement of the thigh toward the body during hip adduction |
| Medial rotation | Rotation toward the midline of the body<br>The segment rotates in the transverse plane | Shoulder joint: movement of the hand toward the body during a cable internal row<br>Hip joint: rotation of the hip of the back foot during back-swing of golf swing |
| Lateral rotation | Rotation away from the midline of the body<br>The segment rotates in the transverse plane | Shoulder joint: movement of the hand away from the body during a cable internal row<br>Hip joint: rotation of the hip of the back foot during downswing of golf swing |
| Pronation[a] | Rotation of the radius on the ulna resulting in the hand moving from the palm-up to the palm-down position<br>The forearm rotates in the transverse plane | Radioulnar joint: rotation of the dumbbell from the anatomical position to begin a hammer curl |
| Supination[b] | Rotation of the radius on the ulna resulting in the hand moving from the palm-down to the palm-up position<br>The forearm rotates in the transverse plane | Radioulnar joint: opposite to above |
| Dorsiflexion | Movement of the ankle joint resulting in a decrease in joint angle<br>The foot rotates in the sagittal plane[c] | Ankle joint: the descent during a squat |
| Plantarflexion | Movement of the ankle joint resulting in an increase in joint angle<br>The foot rotates in the sagittal plane[c] | Ankle joint: the ascent during a squat |
| Horizontal abduction | Movement of the arm in the transverse plane away from the midline of the body | Shoulder joint: downward movement of the barbell during a bench press |
| Horizontal adduction | Movement of the arm in the transverse plane toward the midline of the body | Shoulder joint: upward movement of the barbell during a bench press |
| Elevation | Upward or superior movement of the scapula | Shoulder girdle: upward movement during shoulder-shrug exercises |
| Depression | Downward or inferior movement of the scapula | Shoulder girdle: downward movement during shoulder-shrug exercises |
| Upward rotation | Rotating the scapula so that the glenoid fossa moves upward<br>The shoulder girdle rotates in the frontal plane | Shoulder girdle: grasping the bar to begin a lat pull-down exercise |
| Downward rotation | Rotating the scapula so that the glenoid fossa moves downward<br>The shoulder girdle rotates in the frontal plane | Shoulder girdle: pulling the bar down during a lat pull-down exercise |

[a]Pronation also occurs at the ankle as a combination of ankle dorsiflexion, subtalar eversion, and forefoot abduction.
[b]Supination also occurs at the ankle as a combination of ankle plantarflexion, subtalar inversion, and forefoot adduction.
[c]Because the foot is fixed against the floor during movements such as the squat, it appears that the leg rotates in the sagittal plane.

Despite the downward force of bodyweight, we remain stationary. From Newton's first law of motion, this situation means that there must be another force that opposes bodyweight acting in the opposite direction; i.e., the forces acting on us must be balanced because we are not changing motion. The force that acts in the opposite direction to bodyweight is called a reaction force, from Newton's third law of motion. As this reaction force is produced by the ground, we call this the ground reaction force (GRF).

The GRF is an important force during many human movements. It is because of the GRF that we are able to move around our environment. In order to do this, we need the GRF to exceed any forces that may oppose a change in our motion. When we stand stationary on the bathroom scales, the GRF is equal to bodyweight. However, by repeatedly flexing and extending the knee joints, we should notice that the reading of the scales changes; our bodyweight remains the same, yet the GRF is changing. The consequence of changing the GRF is that the two forces acting on us are unbalanced, producing a change in motion of the CM. Our up and down movements are the changes in motion of the CM. In this example, we are able to change the magnitude of the GRF by changing the motion of our body segments through contracting the muscles that cross the joints associated with the segments. Under certain circumstances, we can flex and extend our knee joints and contract our muscles so forcefully that we produce a GRF large enough to change the motion of the CM to such an extent that we leave the ground. This situation occurs when we jump.

As the GRF acts to change the motion of the CM when we are in contact with the ground, the size of the force can determine the outcome of many sporting movements. For example, the best sprinters produce the greatest GRFs (64). It is no coincidence that the fastest sprinters also demonstrate high levels of muscular strength (44). While it appears that producing very large GRFs is important in sport, there are situations where reducing the magnitude of the GRF is beneficial, particularly during impacts associated with landings, as you might use in a step or boot camp class format. This impact force will be transmitted throughout the body and could cause injury if sufficiently large. This situation is likely to occur during high-impact forms of group exercise where both feet leave the ground during the execution of the movements (55).

These forces can be lessened by flexing the hip, knee and ankle joints upon landing, minimizing the size of the GRF and therefore the potential for injury. This is important when performing a plyometric move off the step or during a sports conditioning or boot camp class format. "Absorb the shock" is a verbal cue you might use in those cases. Appropriately selected footwear can also reduce the forces associated with impacts during exercise movements (1). Conversely, fatigue can result in greater impact forces being experienced by the performer (8). The magnitude of impact forces have been shown to increase with both step height and stepping frequency during step routines (39,55). Therefore, the group exercise instructor needs to consider the selection of exercises and equipment as well as the state of fatigue of the participants to account for possible injuries from impact forces.

Recently there has been an interest in the performance of exercise regimes in an aquatic environment both for clients with disabilities and healthy individuals (50,61). Biomechanical analyses of jumping movements performed in an aquatic environment have shown that the impact forces are actually reduced due to the buoyant force produced by the water (63). Interestingly, the GRFs are also greater during the propulsive phase of jumps performed in water with the increased resistance caused by water the likely cause (63). Therefore, performing exercises in a water fitness class may benefit those participants for whom impact forces pose a problem such as elderly or injured clients, while still providing sufficient stimulus to allow adaptation.

The GRF can be broken down into three components: a vertical component that acts perpendicular to the supporting surface and two horizontal components that act parallel to the supporting surface. The vertical component acts to oppose gravity, while the horizontal components are due to friction. Friction is a force that is induced when two surfaces act to slide across one another. When we change direction in sport, we do so usually by planting our foot away from the CM. The foot wants to slide across the ground, and the reaction to this potential motion, from Newton's third law of motion, is a frictional force that acts in the opposite direction. It is the frictional force therefore that acts to accelerate the CM horizontally and cause us to change direction.

In most sports we select footwear and surfaces that optimize frictional forces: track and field athletes wear spiked shoes on rubberized tracks, and soccer players wear cleats on grass to maximize the frictional force; skiers use waxed skis on snow to minimize frictional force. Therefore, the selection of footwear and the condition of the surface can have significant implications for exercise. For example, wet surfaces have been shown to slow rapid changes of motion (43). As such, the group exercise instructor needs to consider the surface condition (e.g., remove sweat, dust, etc.) in order to aid the performance of his or her participants.

## STABILITY AND BALANCE

When standing in an upright posture, the line of action of gravity (the line of action associated with the bodyweight force) should fall within the **base of support**, defined as the area around those body parts that are in contact with the ground (Fig. 12.2). With the gravity line within the base of support, the body is described as being in a stable position. **Stability** is the ability to resist a change in motion, while **balance** is defined as the ability to maintain a stable position. The closer the gravity line moves toward the edge of the base of support, the more unstable the body becomes. In practical terms, the closer the gravity line falls to the edge of the base of support, the less distance that the body has to be moved through in order to have the gravity line fall outside of the base of support. Once the gravity line falls outside of the base of support, the force of bodyweight acts to rotate the body about an axis defined by the edge of the base of support (Fig. 12.2).

In situations where a force acts at a distance from an axis of rotation, a **torque** is induced that acts to rotate the body. A torque is simply the product of a force and the distance that the force acts from an axis of rotation (see Fig. 12.11). If the torque associated with bodyweight remains unopposed, then the body will change its motion until the forces acting on the body are balanced once again; *i.e.*, the person will fall. Persons who find themselves in this situation can prevent a possible fall by reestablishing the gravity line within the base of support. However, such an action requires rapid movements of the limbs, and some individuals, such as elderly participants, may lack sufficient muscular strength and reaction time to reestablish the base of support within the limited time constraints (24). The ability to maintain balance can also be compromised by muscular fatigue (48).

As you might expect, the stability of the body is related to the size of the base of support; the larger the area of the base of support, the more stable the body. This is important because we can easily increase the size of our base of support simply by increasing the distance between our feet when we are standing. However, the vertical position of the CM also affects the stability of the body by influencing the distance that the body must be moved through in order to move the gravity line outside of the base of support. The greater the vertical position of the CM from the base of support, the less distance the body has to be moved through before the gravity line falls outside of the base of support and therefore the less stable the body. As such, the stability of the body can be increased if the person crouches down. However, performing exercises on one leg such as during a one-legged squat, or with a load placed overhead such as during an overhead squat, or performing exercises on an unstable surface such as a physioball or a balance board can provide significant challenges to balance (Fig. 12.3).

## PRACTICAL IMPLICATIONS FOR THE GROUP EXERCISE INSTRUCTOR

- Changes in motion occur when unbalanced forces act on the human body.
- The GRF represents an important external force that humans use to change motion and therefore influences exercise performance.
- The GRF can be altered by
  - Producing more forceful contractions of the muscles
  - Changing the posture adopted during the movement
  - Changing the frequency at which the exercises are performed

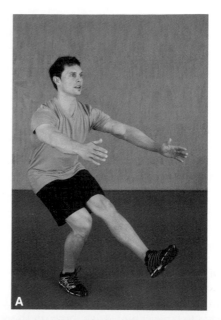

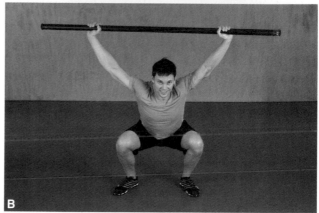

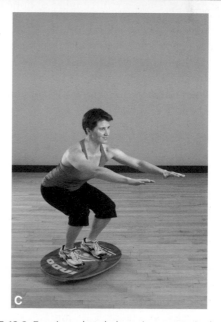

■ **FIGURE 12.3** Exercises where balance is compromised. **A:** During a single-leg squat, the base of support is reduced. **B:** During an overhead squat, the extra mass held above the head causes CM to be located high above the base of support. **C:** During squats on an unstable surface, it is difficult to maintain balance.

○ Changing the environment in which the exercises are performed (dry land versus aquatic)
○ Changing footwear
○ Changing the condition of the floor surface
• Balance can be enhanced by increasing the size of the base of support or crouching down during movements.
• Performing exercises with a load held overhead provides a significant challenge to balance during the movement.

## SKELETAL SYSTEM

The human skeleton comprises more than 200 bones (Figs. 12.4 and 12.5). The bones with the human skeleton serve many important functions. Some important functions for the group exercise instructor to understand are

• **Support** — The long bones of the body such as the femur and tibia act to support the mass of the body segments during upright posture. These bones are subjected to large compressive forces in this endeavor.
• **Attachment for muscle** — The scapulae are broad and flat bones that are ideal for the attachment of the muscles responsible for movements about the shoulder joints.
• **Levers** — Bones act as levers in the production of movements.
• **Calcium reservoir** — Bone tissue contains minerals including calcium. All cells require calcium for normal functioning and in particular muscular contractions would not occur without calcium.

### HISTOLOGY OF BONE

Bone is a type of connective tissue being composed of bone cells and a matrix. There are three types of bone cells.

1. **Osteoblasts** — These cells build up bone tissue by laying down bone matrix.
2. **Osteocytes** — These cells are osteoblasts that have been surrounded by bone matrix.
3. **Osteoclasts** — These cells break down bone matrix in a process known as resorption.

Bone matrix has an organic and an inorganic component. The organic component comprises proteins (collagen fibers, proteoglycans) and contributes to the strength of bone (10). The inorganic component of bone matrix comprises minerals salts (calcium, phosphate, sodium, magnesium) and provides stiffness to the bone (10). Bone tissue also contains a significant amount of fluid.

### STRUCTURE OF BONE

Figure 12.6 shows a typical long bone. The **diaphysis** is the main shaft of the bone, while the **medullary cavity** is the space inside the diaphysis and contains the marrow. A membrane known as the **endosteum** lines the inner surface of the medullary cavity and contains the bone cells that are responsible for growth and repair of the bone (osteoblasts and osteoclasts). The **periosteum** is a fibrous membrane that covers the exterior of the bone and contains bone cells as well as blood vessels that serve the bone. The periosteum also provides an attachment for tendons and ligaments (Fig 12.6). The ends of the long bone, the **epiphyses**, are covered with **articular cartilage** that reduces friction during joint motion and also contributes to absorbing contact forces. The **epiphyseal disk** is a region where growth of the bone takes place and is often assumed to be the weak biomechanical link in the skeletal system of the growing child (35). Exercises that produce undue forces at these sites are to be avoided because disruption of the epiphyseal disk during childhood and adolescence can adversely affect growth. However, participation in weight-bearing exercises that will stimulate bone growth for the young is recommended and so the group exercise instructor is encouraged to follow published guidelines on workout design (25).

There are two types of bone tissue, **compact bone** (also known as cortical bone) and **spongy bone** (also known as cancellous or trabecular bone). Compact bone comprises tightly packed tissue and forms the external layer of all bones as well as the diaphyses of long bones (Fig. 12.7). The architecture of compact bone provides resilience to bending forces (10). Spongy bone is much less dense and comprises a latticework of bars and plates of bone tissue known as **trabeculae** (Fig. 12.7). These trabeculae provide the strength to resist the forces typically experienced by the bone while reducing the weight of the bone. The trabeculae are able to align themselves with the direction that the forces are applied to the bone (10).

### ADAPTABILITY OF BONE

Bone is a relatively strong material, although because it is a metabolically active tissue its strength continually changes. Bone strength is dependent upon the direction that the forces are applied with the greatest strength demonstrated in the direction that the greatest forces are typically experienced by the bone (10). The process of **bone remodeling** allows the bone to adapt its strength and is due to the activity of the coupled activity of the bone cells (osteoclasts and osteoblasts), which can be stimulated by forces applied to the bone (52). GRFs and forces associated with muscular contractions are applied to the bones during exercise and represent potent stimuli for bone remodeling (58).

It has been shown that dynamic loading of bone is required to induce positive adaptations, with static loading shown to be ineffectual (52). Moreover, the magnitude and the rate at which the loads are applied during the exercise regime appear to be more important than the number of repetitions performed (52,58). However, through repeated force application, the strength of the bone may be reduced such that relatively small forces can

**Anterior view**

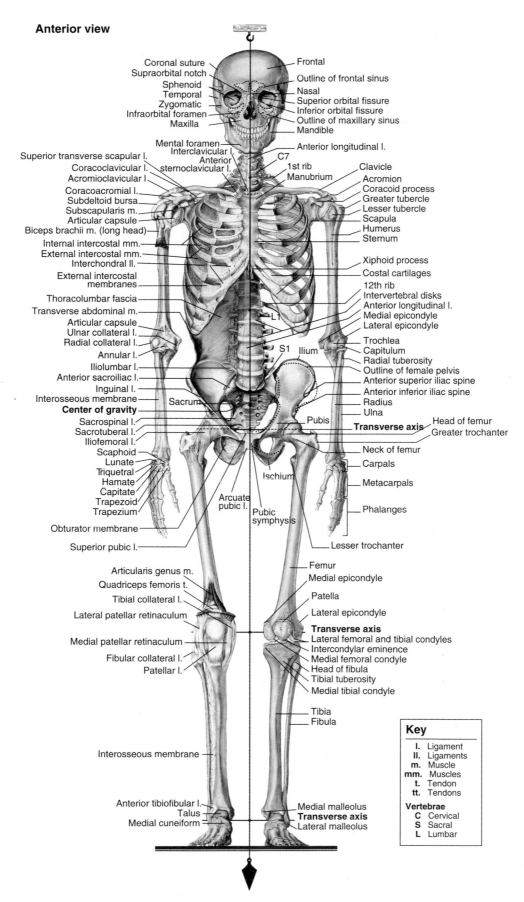

■ **FIGURE 12.4** An anterior view of the skeletal system. (Asset provided by Anatomical Chart Co.)

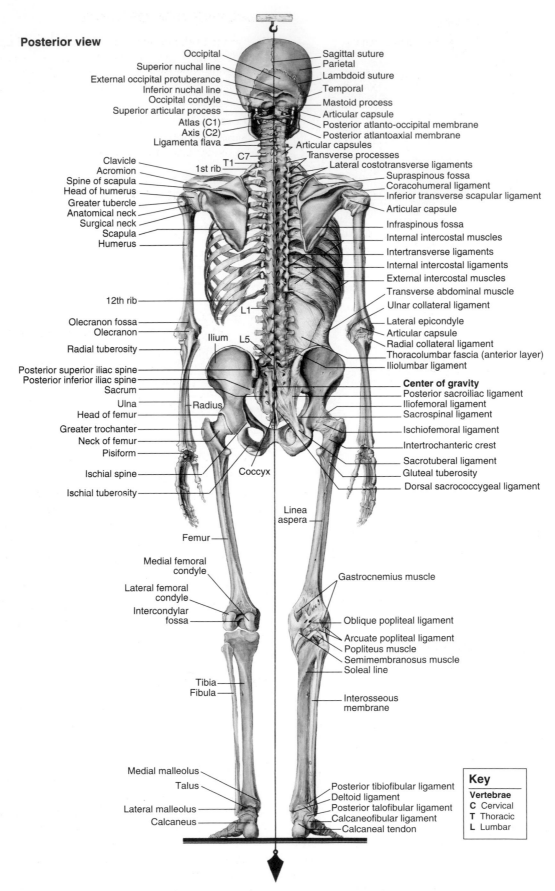

**Posterior view**

Occipital
Superior nuchal line
External occipital protuberance
Inferior nuchal line
Occipital condyle
Superior articular process
Atlas (C1)
Axis (C2)
Ligamenta flava

Sagittal suture
Parietal
Lambdoid suture
Temporal
Mastoid process
Articular capsule
Posterior atlanto-occipital membrane
Posterior atlantoaxial membrane
Articular capsules
Transverse processes
Lateral costotransverse ligaments

Clavicle
Acromion
Spine of scapula
Head of humerus
Greater tubercle
Anatomical neck
Surgical neck
Scapula
Humerus

C7
T1
1st rib

Supraspinous fossa
Coracohumeral ligament
Inferior transverse scapular ligament
Articular capsule

Infraspinous fossa
Internal intercostal muscles
Intertransverse ligaments
Internal intercostal ligaments
External intercostal muscles
Transverse abdominal muscle
Ulnar collateral ligament

12th rib

L1

Olecranon fossa
Olecranon
Radial tuberosity

Ilium
L5

Lateral epicondyle
Articular capsule
Radial collateral ligament
Thoracolumbar fascia (anterior layer)
Iliolumbar ligament

Posterior superior iliac spine
Posterior inferior iliac spine
Sacrum
Ulna
Head of femur
Greater trochanter
Neck of femur
Pisiform
Ischial spine
Ischial tuberosity

Radius

Coccyx

**Center of gravity**
Posterior sacroiliac ligament
Iliofemoral ligament
Sacrospinal ligament
Ischiofemoral ligament
Intertrochanteric crest
Sacrotuberal ligament
Gluteal tuberosity
Dorsal sacrococcygeal ligament

Linea
aspera

Femur

Medial femoral
condyle

Lateral femoral
condyle

Intercondylar
fossa

Gastrocnemius muscle

Oblique popliteal ligament
Arcuate popliteal ligament
Popliteus muscle
Semimembranosus muscle
Soleal line

Tibia
Fibula

Interosseous
membrane

Medial malleolus
Talus

Lateral malleolus
Calcaneus

Posterior tibiofibular ligament
Deltoid ligament
Posterior talofibular ligament
Calcaneofibular ligament
Calcaneal tendon

**Key**
_Vertebrae_
**C** Cervical
**T** Thoracic
**L** Lumbar

■ **FIGURE 12.5** A posterior view of the skeletal system. (Asset provided by Anatomical Chart Co.)

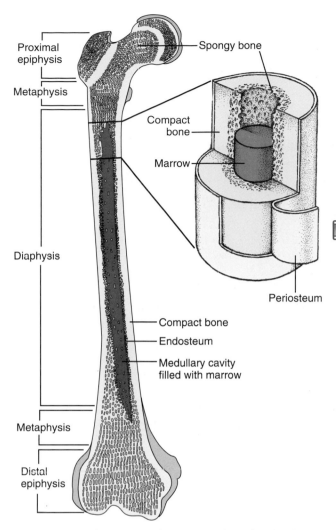

■ **FIGURE 12.6** The structure of a typical long bone found in the skeleton. (From Thompson WR, editor. *ACSM's Resources for the Personal Trainer*. 3rd ed. Baltimore (MD): Lippincott Williams & Wilkins; 2010.)

produce significant damage. This is the case with **stress fractures** (29).

## PRACTICAL IMPLICATIONS FOR THE GROUP EXERCISE INSTRUCTOR

- Bones adapt to the forces applied to them and alter their strength accordingly.
- A potent stimulus for the adaptation is the dynamic force associated with exercise.
- The magnitude and the rate at which the forces are applied during the exercise regime appear to be more important than the number of repetitions performed.

## ARTICULAR SYSTEM

The articulation of two or more bones constitutes an anatomical joint that allows movement. The articular system includes bones, joints, and their associated structures (Fig. 12.8).

## CLASSIFICATION OF JOINTS

The joints of the body can be classified based upon their structure, with the consideration of the presence of a joint cavity, the shape of the bones, and the nature of the tissue connecting the bones included. Although there are many types of joints in the body, we are interested in the freely moveable synovial joints, and Table 12.3 summarizes the common classification system for synovial joints and provides examples in the body.

## JOINT MOVEMENTS

CLIP 12.2    Joint movement is a combination of rolling, sliding, and spinning of the articulating surfaces. The degree of movement at a given joint about a specific axis of rotation is called the **range of motion** (ROM) of the joint. The movements available at the major joints of the body are shown in Table 12.4. It should be noted that the ROM at a specific joint can be assessed actively (the range produced by voluntary contraction of muscles crossing the joint) or passively (the range produced by external means), both of which will be limited by the structures surrounding the joint (muscles, tendons, ligaments, bones, etc.). These structures can explain some of the individual differences observed in joint ROM.

The muscles crossing a joint can provide a significant limitation to ROM, and **flexibility exercises** target this tissue. In response to a single flexibility session, there is likely to be a reduction in passive muscle stiffness, allowing the joint to move through a greater ROM, while depression of reflex activity, resulting in a greater relaxation of the muscles crossing the joints, also contributes to the observed increase in ROM (13). The increases in ROM following a single flexibility session are likely to be augmented by repeated sessions. However, an increase in the ability of the participant to tolerate the discomfort associated with the stretch is an important adaptation that contributes to increase ROM following long-term flexibility training (13).

## JOINT STABILITY

The stability of a joint refers to its ability to resist the action of forces that displace the bones. Five factors account for joint stability (19).

- **Bony structures** — The bones that constitute the joint affect its stability. For example, the shoulder and hip joints are both ball-and-socket joints, yet the greater depth of the acetabulum of the pelvic bone compared to the shallow glenoid fossa of the scapula confers greater stability to the hip joint.
- **Ligamentous arrangements** — Ligaments are connective tissue composed primarily of collagen fibers that connect adjacent bones. They act to prevent joint

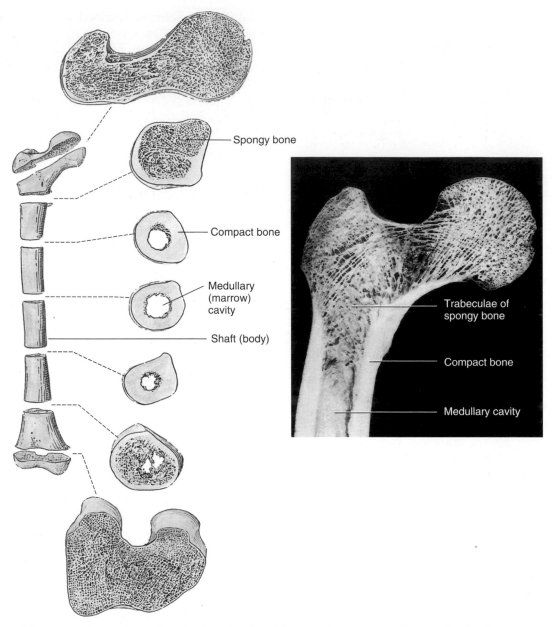

Spongy bone

Compact bone

Medullary (marrow) cavity

Shaft (body)

Trabeculae of spongy bone

Compact bone

Medullary cavity

■ **FIGURE 12.7**  Compact and spongy bone. Note that the trabeculae of the spongy bone are aligned in particular directions, corresponding to the direction of the typical forces experienced by the bone. (From Moore KL, Agur A. *Essential Clinical Anatomy*. 2nd ed. Philadelphia (PA): Lippincott Williams & Wilkins; 2002.)

motion beyond normal ranges and so contribute significantly to the stability of a joint.

• **Musculotendinous arrangements** — The muscles and tendons that span a joint provide substantial support for a joint, particularly one lacking appropriate bony structures. For example, the rotator cuff muscles are important stabilizers of the shoulder joint, acting to maintain the humeral head within the glenoid fossa during normal motion.

• **Fascia and skin** — Fasciae are composed of fibrous connective tissue that surrounds muscle. The iliotibial tract of the tensor fasciae latae combined with thick skin provides stabilization for the knee joint.

• **Atmospheric pressure** — The difference in pressure across a joint capsule can create a vacuum that acts to hold the heads of long bones in their sockets. This occurs at the shoulder and hip joints.

The factors affecting the stability of a joint may be more or less important depending upon the joint. For example, the knee joint lacks significant bony structures that enhance stability and experiences forces during sporting movements that might exceed the capacity of the ligamentous structures, and so relies on the muscles spanning the joint to provide stability (66). However, should the appropriate activation of the muscles be altered,

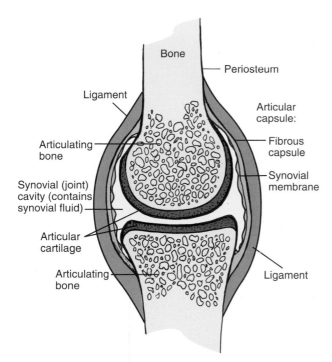

**■ FIGURE 12.8** An example of a synovial joint. (From Oatis CA. *Kinesiology: The Mechanics and Pathomechanics of Human Movement.* Baltimore (MD): Lippincott Williams & Wilkins; 2003.)

through fatigue, *e.g.*, the stability of the joint can become compromised, predisposing the stabilizing structures, particularly the ligaments, to injury (6). Following an injury, any damage to the stabilizing structures such as ligaments or muscles could compromise the stability of a joint (66). Therefore, joint instability can be regarded as both a cause and a result of injury.

## PRACTICAL IMPLICATIONS FOR THE GROUP EXERCISE INSTRUCTOR

- The movements available at joints are limited by the stabilizing structures surrounding the joint such as bony congruency, ligaments, muscles, and the joint capsule.
- Differences in the characteristics of the stabilizing structures means that the ranges of motion available at a specific joint are likely to differ between individuals.
- The stability of a joint can be regarded as a risk factor for injury and can be compromised as a result of an injury.

## MUSCULAR SYSTEM

While the skeleton is important in providing support and leverage, controlled motion about the joints of the skeleton would be impossible without muscles. The human body contains more than 600 skeletal muscles, and many of the superficial muscles are shown in Figures 12.9 and 12.10.

Skeletal muscles are attached to the periosteum of bone via **tendons**. Tendons are similar to ligaments in that they contain a large amount of collagen fibers arranged in parallel, although they are slightly less elastic. When a skeletal muscle contracts, it produces a tensile or pulling force. The **tension** developed by the muscle is transmitted to the bone via the tendon, which can then produce motion about the joint if the tension is sufficiently large. The proximal attachment of a skeletal muscle is called the **origin**, while the distal attachment is called the **insertion**.

## HOW MUSCLES PRODUCE MOVEMENT

### Torque and Lever Systems

The human body represents a linked segmental system whereby the body segments rotate about axes defined by the joints. Therefore, even linear motion is achieved by the rotation of body segments. Typically, the cause of the angular motion of the body segments is the action of skeletal muscles acting across anatomical joints. Because muscles cause the body segments to rotate about joints, we need to consider the rotational effect of the force, something called the **torque**. A torque is calculated as the product of a force and the perpendicular distance between the line of action of the force and the axis of rotation. The perpendicular distance between the line of action of the force and the axis of rotation is known as the **moment arm** of the force.

Figure 12.11 shows the schematic representation of a muscle torque ($F_M \times M_M$) and an opposing torque associated with the dumbbell being held in the hand ($F_R \times M_R$). Notice that these two torques are attempting to rotate the forearm in opposite directions. If the muscular torque exceeds that associated with the dumbbell, then the elbow joint will flex. Should the torque associated

| Table 12.3 | CLASSIFICATION OF SYNOVIAL JOINTS IN THE HUMAN BODY |
|---|---|
| **JOINT CLASSIFICATION** | **FEATURES AND EXAMPLES** |
| Plane | Gliding and sliding movements (*e.g.*, acromioclavicular joint) |
| Hinge | Uniaxial movements (*e.g.*, elbow joint) |
| Ellipsoidal | Biaxial joint (*e.g.*, radiocarpal joint) |
| Saddle | Unique joint that permits movements in all planes (*e.g.*, carpometacarpal joint of the thumb) |
| Ball-and-socket | Multiaxial joint that permits movements in all planes (*e.g.*, shoulder and hip joints) |
| Pivot | Uniaxial joint that permits rotation (*e.g.*, humeroradial joint) |

*From Mayer JM. Anatomy, kinesiology, and biomechanics. In: Thompson WR, Baldwin KE, Pire NI, Niederpruem M, eds. ACSM's Resources for the Personal Trainer. 2nd ed. Baltimore (MD): Lippincott Williams & Wilkins; 2007:109–76.*

| Table 12.4 | MOVEMENTS AT THE MAJOR JOINTS, PLANES OF MOTION, AND RANGES OF MOTION | | | |
|---|---|---|---|---|
| **JOINT** | **JOINT TYPE** | **JOINT MOVEMENT** | **PLANE OF MOTION** | **RANGE OF MOTION** |
| Shoulder girdle (Scapulothoracic) | Not a true joint | Elevation-depression Upward-downward rotation Protraction-retraction | Frontal Frontal Frontal | 55 degrees 60 degrees 25 degrees |
| Shoulder (Glenohumeral) | Synovial: ball-and-socket | Flexion-extension Abduction-adduction Horizontal abduction-adduction Internal-external rotation | Sagittal Frontal Transverse Transverse | 170–180-degree flexion; 40–60-degree extension[a] 170–180-degree abduction; 75-degree adduction[a] 45-degree horizontal abduction; 140–150-degree horizontal adduction[a] 70–90 degrees |
| Elbow (Humeroulnar) | Synovial: hinge | Flexion-extension | Sagittal | 145–150-degree flexion; 5–10-degree hyperextension |
| Proximal radioulnar | Synovial: pivot | Pronation-supination | Transverse | 80–90 degrees |
| Wrist | Synovial: ellipsoidal | Flexion-extension Abduction-adduction | Sagittal Frontal | 70–90-degree flexion; 65–85-degree extension 15–25-degree abduction; 25–40-degree adduction |
| Metacarpophalangeal | Synovial: ellipsoidal | Flexion-extension Abduction-adduction | Sagittal Frontal | 85–100-degree flexion; 0–40-degree extension |
| Proximal and distal interphalangeal | Synovial: hinge | Flexion-extension | Sagittal | 80–120 degrees |
| Intervertebral | Cartilaginous | Flexion-extension Lateral flexion Rotation | Sagittal Frontal Transverse | T1-T12: 12 degrees; L vertebrae: ~13–15 degrees T1-T12: 8 degrees; L vertebrae: ~3–6 degrees T vertebrae: ~3–8 degrees; L vertebrae: ~2–5 degrees |
| Hip | Synovial: ball-and-socket | Flexion-extension Abduction-adduction Medial-lateral rotation | Sagittal Frontal Transverse | 0–130-degree flexion; 0–30-degree extension 0–35-degree abduction; 0–30-degree adduction 0–45-degree medial rotation; 0–50-degree lateral rotation |
| Knee | Synovial: modified hinge | Flexion-extension Medial-lateral rotation | Sagittal Transverse | 0–140-degree flexion; 10-degree extension 0–15-degree medial rotation; 0–30-degree lateral rotation |
| Ankle: talocrural | Synovial: hinge | Flexion-extension[b] | Sagittal | 15–20-degree dorsiflexion; 50-degree plantarflexion |

[a]Values include shoulder girdle motion. T, thoracic; L, lumbar.
[b]These actions are referred to as dorsiflexion and plantarflexion, respectively, at the ankle joint.
Data from Floyd RT. Manual of Structural Kinesiology. New York: McGraw-Hill; 2009; Mayer JM. Anatomy, kinesiology, and biomechanics. In: Thompson WR, Baldwin KE, Pire NI, Niederpruem M, edition. ACSM's Resources for the Personal Trainer. 2nd ed. Baltimore (MD): Lippincott Williams & Wilkins; 2007:109–76; McGill SM. Low Back Disorders. 2nd ed. Champaign (IL): Human Kinetics; 2007.

with the dumbbell exceed that of the muscle, the elbow will extend. Finally, if the two opposing torques equal one another, there will be no change in motion of the dumbbell.

To better understand how skeletal muscles produce rotations of body segments requires knowledge of lever systems. A **lever system** comprises an **axis of rotation**, a lever that rotates about the axis (usually defined as a rigid body), and a pair of forces named the **effort force** and the **resistance force** and their associated moment arms, which result in opposing torques acting on the lever (Fig. 12.11).

An understanding of the mechanical characteristics of lever systems can aid the group exercise instructor in many exercises. For example, during lateral dumbbell raises, the muscular torque developed by the deltoid that abducts the shoulder must exceed the torque associated with the dumbbell. Each of the torques has a moment arm, and if the elbow joint is held in extension during the exercise, the moment arm associated

with the dumbbell will be maximized when the joint reaches 90 degrees of abduction. The torque associated with the dumbbell will be at its greatest at this point, and the participant is likely to find the exercise difficult. By flexing the elbow during the movement, the dumbbell (resistance force) will be moved closer to the shoulder joint (axis of rotation), reducing the associated moment arm and therefore the torque that the shoulder abductors must overcome. Obviously, another option to reduce the torque associated with a weight is to select a lighter dumbbell, in which case the resistance force is reduced.

## Muscle Roles

It is important to consider that several muscles are likely to be responsible for the motion at any given joint. Remember that muscles produce tensile, or pulling forces; they cannot push. Therefore, muscles tend to be arranged in opposing pairs such as flexor-extensor,

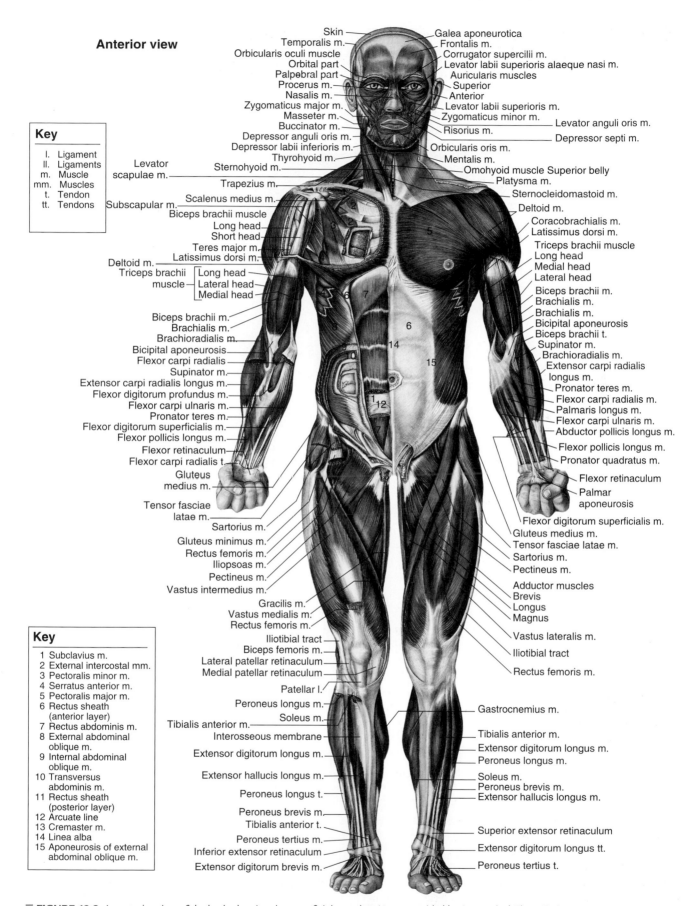

**Anterior view**

**Key**
- I.   Ligament
- II.  Ligaments
- m.   Muscle
- mm.  Muscles
- t.   Tendon
- tt.  Tendons

**Key**
1. Subclavius m.
2. External intercostal mm.
3. Pectoralis minor m.
4. Serratus anterior m.
5. Pectoralis major m.
6. Rectus sheath (anterior layer)
7. Rectus abdominis m.
8. External abdominal oblique m.
9. Internal abdominal oblique m.
10. Transversus abdominis m.
11. Rectus sheath (posterior layer)
12. Arcuate line
13. Cremaster m.
14. Linea alba
15. Aponeurosis of external abdominal oblique m.

**■ FIGURE 12.9** An anterior view of the body showing the superficial muscles. (Asset provided by Anatomical Chart Co.)

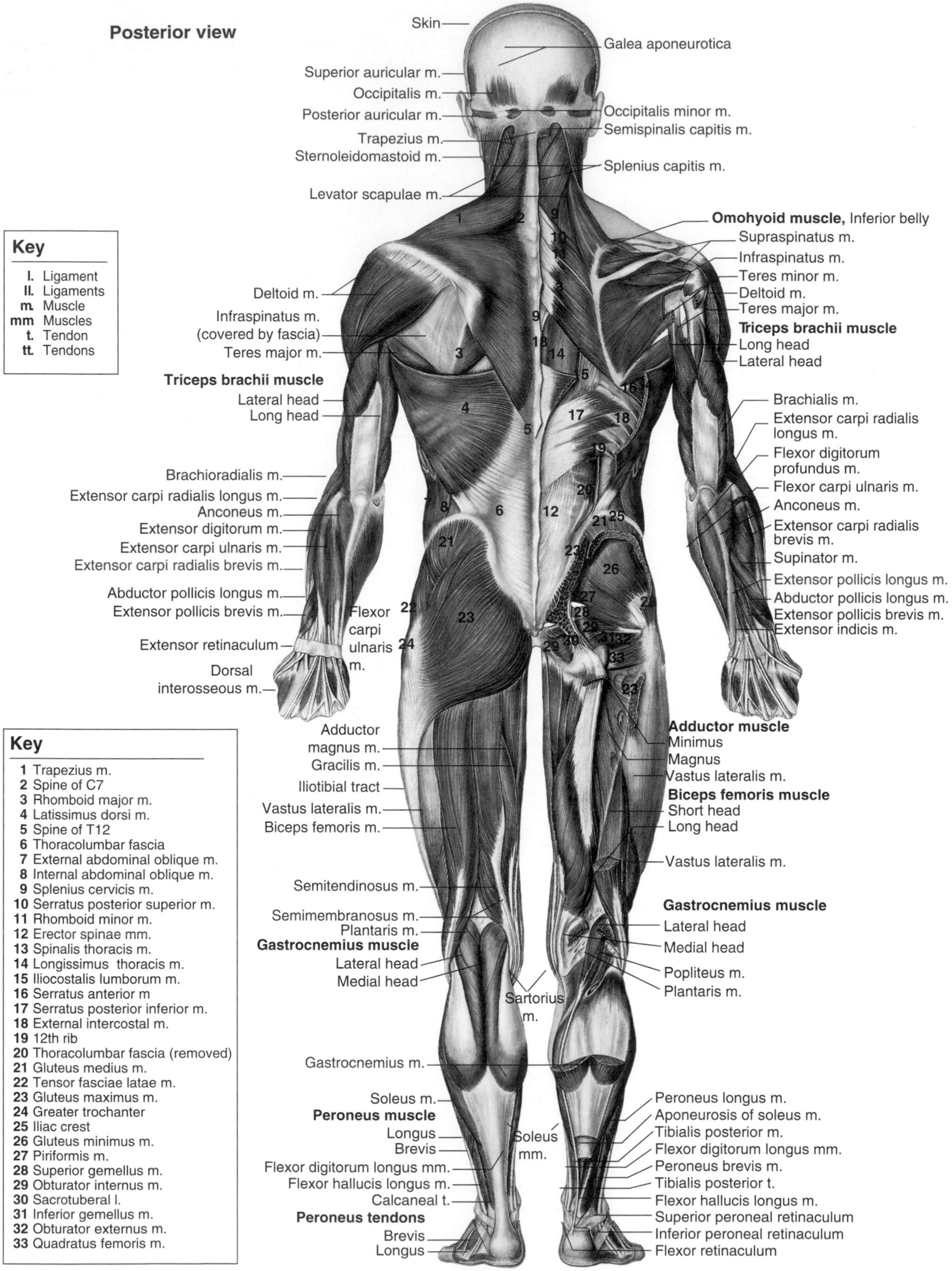
Posterior view
Skin
Galea aponeurotica
Superior auricular m.
Occipitalis m.
Posterior auricular m.
Occipitalis minor m.
Semispinalis capitis m.
Trapezius m.
Sternoleidomastoid m.
Splenius capitis m.
Levator scapulae m.
Omohyoid muscle, Inferior belly
Supraspinatus m.
Infraspinatus m.
Teres minor m.
Deltoid m.
Teres major m.
Triceps brachii muscle
Long head
Lateral head
Key
l. Ligament
ll. Ligaments
m. Muscle
mm Muscles
t. Tendon
tt. Tendons
Deltoid m.
Infraspinatus m. (covered by fascia)
Teres major m.
Triceps brachii muscle
Lateral head
Long head
Brachialis m.
Extensor carpi radialis longus m.
Flexor digitorum profundus m.
Flexor carpi ulnaris m.
Anconeus m.
Extensor carpi radialis brevis m.
Supinator m.
Extensor pollicis longus m.
Abductor pollicis longus m.
Extensor pollicis brevis m.
Extensor indicis m.
Brachioradialis m.
Extensor carpi radialis longus m.
Anconeus m.
Extensor digitorum m.
Extensor carpi ulnaris m.
Extensor carpi radialis brevis m.
Abductor pollicis longus m.
Extensor pollicis brevis m.
Extensor retinaculum
Dorsal interosseous m.
Flexor carpi ulnaris m.
Key
1 Trapezius m.
2 Spine of C7
3 Rhomboid major m.
4 Latissimus dorsi m.
5 Spine of T12
6 Thoracolumbar fascia
7 External abdominal oblique m.
8 Internal abdominal oblique m.
9 Splenius cervicis m.
10 Serratus posterior superior m.
11 Rhomboid minor m.
12 Erector spinae mm.
13 Spinalis thoracis m.
14 Longissimus thoracis m.
15 Iliocostalis lumborum m.
16 Serratus anterior m
17 Serratus posterior inferior m.
18 External intercostal m.
19 12th rib
20 Thoracolumbar fascia (removed)
21 Gluteus medius m.
22 Tensor fasciae latae m.
23 Gluteus maximus m.
24 Greater trochanter
25 Iliac crest
26 Gluteus minimus m.
27 Piriformis m.
28 Superior gemellus m.
29 Obturator internus m.
30 Sacrotuberal l.
31 Inferior gemellus m.
32 Obturator externus m.
33 Quadratus femoris m.
Adductor magnus m.
Gracilis m.
Iliotibial tract
Vastus lateralis m.
Biceps femoris m.
Adductor muscle
Minimus
Magnus
Vastus lateralis m.
Biceps femoris muscle
Short head
Long head
Vastus lateralis m.
Semitendinosus m.
Semimembranosus m.
Plantaris m.
Gastrocnemius muscle
Lateral head
Medial head
Gastrocnemius muscle
Lateral head
Medial head
Popliteus m.
Plantaris m.
Sartorius m.
Gastrocnemius m.
Soleus m.
Peroneus muscle
Longus
Brevis
Soleus mm.
Flexor digitorum longus mm.
Flexor hallucis longus m.
Calcaneal t.
Peroneus tendons
Brevis
Longus
Peroneus longus m.
Aponeurosis of soleus m.
Tibialis posterior m.
Flexor digitorum longus mm.
Peroneus brevis m.
Tibialis posterior t.
Flexor hallucis longus m.
Superior peroneal retinaculum
Inferior peroneal retinaculum
Flexor retinaculum

■ **FIGURE 12.10** A posterior view of the body showing the superficial muscles. (Asset provided by Anatomical Chart Co.)

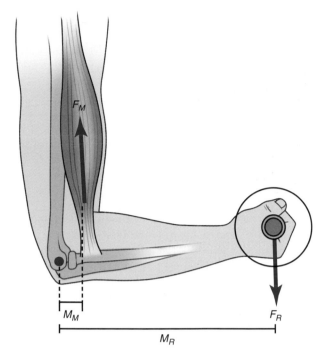

**■ FIGURE 12.11** Schematic representation of a muscular torque acting at a joint. ($F_M$, muscular force; $F_R$, resistance force; MM, moment arm associated with $F_M$; $M_R$, moment arm associated with $F_R$.) (From Harman E. Biomechanics of resistance training. In: Baechle TR, Earle RW, eds. *Essentials of Strength Training and Conditioning.* Champaign (IL): Human Kinetics; 2008:66–91pp.)

internal-external rotator or abduction-adduction combinations. Muscles can be classified according to their roles during movements.

### Prime Movers or Agonists

A muscle that is directly responsible for the motion at a given joint is known as a prime mover or an agonist. There may actually be a number of muscles that are agonists during a movement. For example, during a biceps curl (elbow flexion), the agonists are biceps brachii, brachialis, and brachioradialis, which all produce flexion of the elbow joint.

### Antagonists

Muscles that have an effect opposite to that of the agonists are classified as antagonists. The antagonist muscles during a given movement are located on the opposite side of a joint from the agonists. For example, the antagonists during elbow flexion associated with a biceps curl are triceps brachii and anconeus. Antagonists relax in order to allow the agonists to produce the desired joint motion and then may contract to arrest the motion. However, there may be times when both the agonists and antagonists are activated concurrently. During such **coactivation**, the stability of the joint will be enhanced, although mobility will be compromised.

### Synergists

A muscle may perform a synergetic role to aid the agonists by stabilizing a body part to allow the agonist to produce the appropriate joint motion. For example, the rhomboid muscles stabilize the scapulae to permit the teres major to effectively adduct the arm. Without the activation of the rhomboid muscles, teres major would produce upward rotation of the scapulae as it adducted the arm, producing inefficient motion. Synergetic muscles also neutralize undesired joint motion as a result of muscle contraction. For example, if a muscle both extends and externally rotates a given joint when contracted, but only extension is desired, an internal rotator must also be activated concurrently to neutralize the unwanted motion. For example, the trapezius muscles act to adduct and upwardly rotate the scapulae, while the rhomboid muscles act to produce adduction and downward rotation of the scapulae. The combined activity of these muscles produces adduction of the scapulae while neutralizing any upward or downward rotation.

### Biarticular Muscles

Many of the muscles in the body actually span more than one joint. For example, gastrocnemius crosses both the ankle and knee joints, and so its activation can produce motion at both of these joints. This type of muscle is referred to as a biarticular muscle, while muscles, such as soleus, that cross only one joint, are referred to as monoarticular. Other biarticular muscles of note are the hamstrings group (biceps femoris, semitendinosus, semimembranosus) that cross the hip and knee joints, rectus femoris that crosses the hip and knee joints, and biceps brachii and triceps brachii, both of which cross the shoulder and elbow joints.

## FACTORS AFFECTING MUSCULAR TENSION

### Muscle Action

A muscle can develop tension either under static conditions (muscle length remains constant) or under dynamic conditions (the muscle changes length). When the tension is developed and muscle length remains constant, the muscle is said to be performing an **isometric** contraction. Under dynamic conditions the muscle can contract **eccentrically**, where tension is developed as the muscle lengthens, or **concentrically**, where tension is developed as the muscle shortens.

The force developed by a muscle while operating isometrically is dependent upon the muscle length (51). This length dependence of isometric force production, known as the **length-tension relationship**, is essentially due to changes in the overlap of the **actin** and **myosin** myofilaments within the muscle fiber with force being reduced at long and short muscle lengths. The practical significance of this relationship is that muscular force will vary with muscle length, which in turn will vary with the joint angle selected in a given movement.

While the length-tension relationship can be used to describe the force developed under isometric conditions, this relationship cannot be used to describe the behavior of muscle contracting dynamically. Rather, the **force-velocity relationship** describes the force developed by a muscle when contracting eccentrically or concentrically. This relationship shows that muscle force decreases as the speed at which concentric contractions are performed increases, yet muscle force increases as the speed of eccentric contractions increase. While the decrease in force development associated with concentric contractions can be explained in terms of chemical reaction rates associated with actin-myosin cycling (30), the rise in force associated with eccentric muscle contractions cannot be easily explained. However, the force-velocity relationship demonstrates that eccentric contractions are associated with greater forces than isometric contractions, while isometric contractions are associated with greater forces than concentric contractions (30).

Previous researchers have demonstrated that the force developed during a concentric contraction can be enhanced when it is preceded by an eccentric contraction (14). This sequencing of concentric and eccentric muscle contractions is termed the **stretch-shortening cycle** and has been shown to enhance concentric force development through mechanisms including elastic energy contributions, reflex activation, and architectural changes within the active muscles (26). An example of this cycle is seen when performing a vertical jump for maximal height and participants "dip down" before jumping. By doing so, they incorporate the stretch-shortening cycle into the movement and enhance their jump height.

### Muscle Cross-sectional Area and Pennation Angle

The cross-sectional area of a muscle is related to the number of actin and myosin filaments arranged in parallel, and therefore, greater force is developed during a contraction (40). Despite the importance of cross-sectional area to the force capabilities of a muscle, the relationship is affected by the **pennation angle**, defined as the angle between the orientation of the muscle fibers and the line of action of the force associated with the muscle. In such situations, the **physiological cross-sectional area** should be considered (30) (see Fig. 12.12). Larger pennation angles are associated with greater force capabilities of the muscle (22) because more muscle fibers can be packed into a given volume of muscle. However, the range over which the entire muscle shortens is limited in pennate muscles.

### Line of Action and Angle of Attachment

In Figures 12.9 and 12.10, we can see the lines of action of many of the superficial muscles. When the body is in the anatomical position, we can infer the joint motions that a given muscle would produce at the joint it crosses. However, the resultant joint motion produced by a muscle may change as the posture and segment orientation alters during exercise movements. For example, the pectoralis major acts as an adductor and flexor of the shoulder joint. However, when the arm is abducted beyond 90 degrees, the line of action of the pectoralis major changes and the upper fibers now contribute to abduction at the shoulder joint. The line of action of a muscle may be altered by bony structures. For example, the peroneus longus muscle passes posteroinferiorly to the maleollus of the fibula that alters its line of action.

### Neural Influences

The central nervous system has a profound effect on muscular tension. Increasing the number of muscle fibers activated during a voluntary contraction can increase the magnitude of muscular force (11). The activation of muscle fibers during a given movement has been shown to be affected by the orientation of the body segments (5). This implies that the magnitude of muscular force will be influenced by the posture adopted during a given movement.

The muscular torque developed at a specific joint is the result of the interaction of the force developed by groups of muscles. From a simplified representation of a joint served by an antagonistic pair of muscles, it is clear that the force associated with the contraction of the agonist is influenced by the activity of the antagonist. Therefore, the overall torque developed by the muscles crossing a joint will be dependent upon the degree of **coactivation** between the antagonistic pair of muscles. It is known that athletes exhibit less coactivation during muscular strength tests compared to untrained individuals (3), which may partly explain the greater strength values recorded for well-trained subjects. As already mentioned, coactivation of muscles can increase the stability of a joint, albeit at the expense of its mobility.

Muscular strength can be defined as the ability of a muscle or group of muscles to voluntarily produce a force or torque against an external resistance under specific conditions defined by muscle action, movement velocity, and posture. **Maximal muscular strength** is then the ability to voluntarily produce a maximal force or torque under specific conditions defined by muscle action, movement velocity, and posture, while the ability to voluntarily produce force or torque repeatedly against submaximal external resistances and resist fatigue is the defining characteristic of **muscular endurance**.

## PRACTICAL IMPLICATIONS FOR THE GROUP EXERCISE INSTRUCTOR

The force produced by a muscle is affected by the following:

- The type of muscle contraction with more force being developed during an eccentric as opposed to a concentric contraction

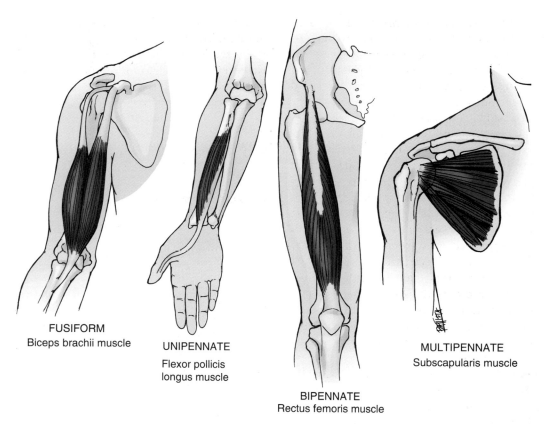

FUSIFORM
Biceps brachii muscle

UNIPENNATE
Flexor pollicis
longus muscle

BIPENNATE
Rectus femoris muscle

MULTIPENNATE
Subscapularis muscle

■ **FIGURE 12.12** Muscles with different fiber alignments. (From Thompson WR, edition. *ACSM's Resources for the Personal Trainer*. 3rd ed. Baltimore (MD): Lippincott Williams & Wilkins; 2010.)

- The velocity of movement with an increase in velocity during a concentric contraction, resulting in a reduction in force development
- The posture adopted such that a client who is strong on a leg press machine may not be strong during a back squat

What we observe in tests of strength are actually the torques produced by the lever systems of the human body, and so the distances that both the muscle forces and resistance forces act relative to the axis of rotation need to be considered. The group exercise instructor should recognize that a participant who demonstrates great strength in one movement (*e.g.*, leg press) may not be strong in another movement (*e.g.*, back squat) even though the active muscles are similar.

## MUSCLES OF THE UPPER AND LOWER EXTREMITIES

We need to address the action of specific muscles that the group exercise instructor should be familiar with. Because the muscles that we are interested in operate across joints, we will discuss the muscle in relation to the main joints of the human body including the shoulder, elbow, hip, knee and ankle joints, as well as those of the spine.

## MUSCLES OF THE UPPER EXTREMITY

### The Shoulder Girdle

The bones that comprise the shoulder girdle are the sternum, clavicles, and scapulae (Figs. 12.4 and 12.5). The shoulder girdle acts to facilitate motion at the shoulder joint. Indeed, the movement of the shoulder girdle allows approximately 80 degrees of greater flexion and abduction, and 15 degrees of greater horizontal abduction at the shoulder joint than if the shoulder girdle did not move (15). Similarly, many of the muscles that produce motion at the shoulder joint have their origin on the scapula. Therefore, the shoulder girdle provides a foundation from which shoulder joint motion occurs. Table 12.5 lists the motion produced by each muscle and the exercises that can strengthen them.

### SHOULDER JOINT

The shoulder joint is the articulation between the head of the humerus and the glenoid fossa of the scapula (Figs. 12.4 and 12.5). It is a ball-and-socket joint that permits a wide ROM in the three anatomical planes (Table 12.4), although this comes at the expense of stability that is compromised at the shoulder joint. There are a large number of muscles responsible for the motion at the shoulder joint, and Table 12.6 lists the motion produced

| **Table 12.5** | **THE MAJOR MUSCLES OF THE SHOULDER GIRDLE** | |
|---|---|---|
| **MUSCLE** | **ACTION** | **STRENGTHENING EXERCISES** |
| Trapezius | Upper fibers: elevation of scapula | Shoulder-shrug exercises |
| | Middle fibers: elevation, upward rotation and adduction of scapula | Bent-over rows |
| | Lower fibers: depression, adduction, and upward rotation of scapula | Parallel dips |
| Rhomboid | Elevation, adduction, and downward rotation of scapula | Chin-ups |
| | | Parallel dips |
| | | Bent-over rows |
| Levator scapulae | Elevation of scapula | Shoulder-shrug exercises |
| Serratus anterior | Abduction and upward rotation of scapula | Push-ups |
| | | Bench-press |
| Pectoralis minor | Abduction, downward rotation, and depression of scapula | Push-ups |
| | | Bench-press |

by each of the muscles crossing the shoulder joint and the exercises that can strengthen them.

## ELBOW JOINT

The elbow joint is formed by the articulation between the distal portion of the humerus and the trochlear notch on the ulna (Figs. 12.4 and 12.5). This is a hinge-type joint allowing only flexion and extension (Table 12.4). However, in close proximity to the elbow joint, the radius bone articulates with the ulna to form the proximal **radioulnar joint**. It is at this joint that we get pronation and supination of the forearm. Table 12.7 lists the motion produced by the major muscles of the elbow joint and the exercises that can be used to strengthen them.

## MUSCLES OF THE LOWER EXTREMITY

### Hip Joint

The head of the femur articulates with the acetabulum of the pelvic bone at the hip joint (Figs. 12.4 and 12.5). This ball-and-socket joint permits a wide ROM in the three anatomical planes (Table 12.4), with the stability of the joint enhanced by the joint capsule and a number of ligaments, as well as many muscles as listed in Table 12.8.

### Knee Joint

The knee joint is a modified hinge joint (combining the function of hinge and pivot joints) formed by the articulation of the femur with the tibia (Figs. 12.4 and 12.5). Flexion and extension as well as internal and external rotation are possible at the knee joint (Table 12.4). The major muscles responsible for the motion at the knee joint are listed in Table 12.9.

### Ankle Joint

The articulation between the distal tibia and talus of the foot forms the ankle joint (Figs. 12.4 and 12.5). The joint is a hinge joint that allows plantarflexion (extension) and dorsiflexion (flexion) in the sagittal plane (Table 12.4). The major muscles responsible for the motion at the joint are shown in Table 12.10.

### Spine and Pelvis

The spine is composed of 33 vertebrae arranged in a column arranged into the four following regions, beginning superior and moving inferior: **cervical**, **thoracic**, **lumbar**, and **sacrococcygeal** (Figs. 12.4 and 12.5). Each of the four regions of the spine has an associated curve when viewed in the sagittal plane. These curves facilitate the strength of the vertebral column and the "spring-like" behavior of the spine in response to loading.

Of the 33 vertebrae of the spine, only 24 are moveable (cervical, thoracic, and lumbar vertebrae) and contribute to the considerable ROM of the spine (Table 12.4). The nine remaining vertebrae are fused to form the **sacrum** and **coccyx**, with the sacrum articulating with the iliac bones of the pelvis allowing a certain amount of motion, although this varies considerably between individuals. During trunk motion, such as that observed when an individual bends forward from the anatomical position to touch his or her toes, there is synchronization between the spine and the pelvis whereby flexion of the spine is accompanied by anterior tilt of the pelvis. There are many muscles that are responsible for the motion of the spine and pelvis. A few of these are listed in Table 12.11.

## TRAINING FOR THE "CORE"

The core is a concept that has received much attention in exercise and fitness literature, yet it is often ill defined and poorly understood. The focus of the exercise and fitness literature has been on the musculature of the core because the stabilization of the core region is provided mainly by active muscles (41). The core has been variously defined as the musculature of the lumbar spine and

**Table 12.6  THE MAJOR MUSCLES OF THE SHOULDER JOINT**

| MUSCLE | ACTION | STRENGTHENING EXERCISES |
|---|---|---|
| Deltoid | Anterior fibers: abduction, flexion, horizontal adduction and medial rotation | Dumbbell press; |
|  | Middle fibers: abduction | Lateral dumbbell raises |
|  | Posterior fibers: abduction, extension, horizontal abduction, and lateral rotation | Anterior: bench-press |
|  |  | Posterior: bent-over rows |
| Pectoralis major | Medial rotation, adduction (abduction once arm adducted beyond 90 degrees), horizontal adduction and flexion | Push-ups |
|  |  | Dumbbell flies |
|  |  | Bench-press |
| Latissimus dorsi | Adduction, extension, medial rotation and horizontal abduction | Lat pull-downs |
|  |  | Seated rows |
| Teres major | Extension, medial rotation, and adduction | Lat pull-downs |
|  |  | Seated rows |
| Biceps brachii[a] | Weak flexion | Bent rows |
|  | Abduction of the laterally rotated shoulder |  |
| Triceps brachii[a] | Long head: extension, adduction, and horizontal abduction | Dumbbell press |
| Subscapularis[b] | Medial rotation, adduction, and extension | Lat pull-downs |
|  | Stabilization of the humeral head in the glenoid fossa | Medial or internal rotation |
| Supraspinatus[b] | Abduction | Lateral dumbbell raises |
|  | Stabilization of the humeral head in the glenoid fossa |  |
| Infraspinatus[b] | Lateral rotation, horizontal abduction, and extension | Lat pull-downs |
|  | Stabilization of the humeral head in the glenoid fossa | Lateral or external rotation |
| Teres minor[b] | Lateral rotation, horizontal abduction, and extension | Lat pull-downs |
|  | Stabilization of the humeral head in the glenoid fossa | Lateral or external rotation |

[a]These are biarticular muscles that also cross the elbow joint.
[b]These are the rotator cuff muscles.

the pelvis, the definition expanded to include the muscles of the hip and even the upper-body musculature (59).

The stability of the core has received significant attention in recent years. We have already introduced the concept of stability as it relates to the whole body and individual joints and defined it as the ability to resist a change in motion, or a resistance to a displacement caused by forces. Hodges and Richardson (20) noted that the spine was inherently unstable and required support from a number of mechanisms (ligaments, facet articulations, muscle tension, neural feedback), the main source of which was muscular tension. The muscles involved in providing stability of the core are shown in Table 12.12.

The interest in the stability of the core has developed from the assertion that it is an important prerequisite in providing a foundation for movement of the upper and lower extremities during exercise (2). Moreover, the role of the core musculature has been implicated in low back pain (12) and groin injuries (34). This has led to an interest in exercises that can strengthen the musculature of the core to enhance stability, thus improving

performance and minimizing injury. However, sufficient stability can be achieved through modest levels of muscle activity (41). Therefore, performing exercises against heavy external loads may not be necessary. Similarly, the stability of the core is dependent upon the coordinated activation of a number of muscles, dispelling the myth of a single muscle as the most important "core stabilizer"; rather the relative importance of the muscles in stabilizing the core is posture dependent. The practical implications for the group exercise instructor are that a variety of exercises designed to improve the coordination of core muscles as well as increase their strength should be included within the exercise sessions of an individual. It also appears that muscular endurance rather than maximal muscular strength is important for the core musculature, particularly in injury prevention (41). For specific exercises, the reader is referred to McGill (41) (also see clip 12.3).

Performing exercises on an unstable surface, such as that provided by a physioball, has been proposed to produce greater stimulus for core musculature (4). The efficacy of such exercises is based upon the assumption

| Table 12.7 | THE MAJOR MUSCLES OF THE ELBOW JOINT | |
| --- | --- | --- |
| **MUSCLE** | **ACTION** | **STRENGTHENING EXERCISES** |
| Biceps brachii[a] | Flexion of the humeroulnar joint | Biceps curl with forearm supinated |
| | Supination of the radioulnar joint | |
| Brachialis | Flexion of the humeroulnar joint | Biceps curl |
| Brachioradialis | Flexion of the humeroulnar joint | Hammer curl |
| | Pronation of the radioulnar joint from supinated to neutral | Biceps curl |
| | Supination of the radioulnar joint from pronated to neutral | |
| Triceps brachii[a] | Extension of the humeroulnar joint | Triceps kickbacks |
| | | Cable push-downs |
| Anconeus | Extension of the humeroulnar joint | Triceps kickbacks |
| | | Cable push-downs |

[a]Long head of triceps brachii is biarticlar muscles that also cross the shoulder joint.

that when whole body stability is compromised, postural adjustments, which likely require stabilization of the core, are required (Fig. 12.13). Despite these proposals, research has failed to support the efficacy of unstable surfaces compared to exercises performed on a stable surface in terms of the activation of the core musculature (67). It should be noted that exercises performed on unstable surfaces reduce the ability of the participant to produce large forces through the extremities (arms and legs) and therefore may limit the adaptive stimulus to the exercise. However, this should not prohibit the group exercise instructor from utilizing exercises performed on an unstable surface. Indeed, the inclusion of such exercises has been shown to improve the ability of the performer to control fast changes of direction, which may limit the potential for injury (9).

## PRACTICAL IMPLICATIONS FOR THE GROUP EXERCISE INSTRUCTOR

- The stability of the core is highly dependent upon the tension developed by a large number of muscles as well as their coordinated activity.
- Because the activity of the core musculature is dependent upon posture, a variety of exercises should be employed to elicit improvements.
- The focus of the exercises for the core musculature should be on developing muscular endurance.
- An unstable surface is not always required to activate the core musculature.

## VERBAL CUES FOR TEACHING EXERCISES

In this section we highlight some execution and form cues that the group exercise instructor can use to aid the performers in their class. We will use the example of the squat as it is an excellent exercise in group exercise as it challenges balance, uses joints and large muscle groups of the lower body frequently used in daily activities, doesn't take much space to perform, and uses the resistance of bodyweight, therefore requiring no extra equipment (Table 12.13).

## COMMON INJURIES

While a number of authors have reported the injuries incurred by group exercise instructors and their participants, the research is confounded by methodological issues. For example, the style of exercise undertaken is not always sufficiently detailed, while little attention is given to previous injuries sustained by the participants,

| Table 12.8 | THE MAJOR MUSCLES OF THE HIP JOINT | |
| --- | --- | --- |
| **MUSCLE** | **ACTION** | **STRENGTHENING EXERCISES** |
| Iliopsoas | Iliacus: flexion and lateral rotation | |
| | Psoas major: flexion and lateral rotation | Leg raises; flexion (tubing or cables) |
| Rectus femoris[a] | Flexion | |
| Sartorius[a] | Flexion, abduction, and lateral rotation | |
| Gracilis[a] | Adduction | Adduction (cable or machine); ball squeezes |
| Adductor magnus | Adduction | |
| Gluteus maximus | Extension and lateral rotation | |
| | Lower fibers: adduction | |
| Tensor fasciae latae[a] | Abduction and flexion | Squats; step-ups; dead lift; good morning |
| Gluteus medius | Abduction | Abduction (tubing or cables) |
| | Anterior fibers: medial rotation | |
| | Posterior fibers: lateral rotation | |
| Biceps femoris[a] | Long head: extension and adduction | Abduction (tubing or cables); one-legged stance will activate muscle |
| Semitendinosus[a] | Extension and medial rotation | Dead lift; good morning |
| Semimembranosus[a] | Extension and medial rotation | |

[a]These are biarticular muscles that also cross the knee joint.

| Table 12.9 | THE MAJOR MUSCLES OF THE KNEE JOINT | |
|---|---|---|
| **MUSCLE** | **ACTION** | **STRENGTHENING EXERCISES** |
| Vastus lateralis | Extension | Squats; step-ups |
| Vastus intermedius | Extension | |
| Vastus medialis | Extension | |
| Rectus femoris[a] | Extension | |
| Sartorius[a] | Flexion and internal rotation | Dead lift; good morning; leg curls |
| Biceps femoris[a] | Flexion and external rotation | |
| Semitendinosus[a] | Flexion and internal rotation | |
| Semimembranosus[a] | Flexion and internal rotation | |

*[a]These are biarticular muscles that also cross the hip joint.*

environmental factors (e.g., footwear, floor surface) and any other activities that they may be engaged in concurrently (17). Similarly, the retrospective design of the research should also be considered when interpreting the relevant findings. Despite these limitations, some important information can be gleaned that will be useful for the group exercise instructor.

There are many exercises that the group exercise instructor and his or her participants may encounter, from step aerobics to indoor cycling. Research has shown that each of these exercise modes have different patterns of injury associated with them. For example, low-impact dance exercise routines and step aerobics tend to produce pain and discomfort in the foot, lower-leg, back (thoracic and lumbar regions), and shoulder regions (17,56,62), while indoor cycling classes are associated with a higher prevalence of knee injuries (33). Scharff-Olson et al. (56) noted a high prevalence of voice disorders in group exercise instructors, but such injuries will not be discussed here. Despite the reported injuries associated with these types of activities, the injury rates are much lower than those associated with activities such as running (56). Similarly, the severity of injuries reported following dance exercise routines and step aerobics are relatively minor being limited to acute injuries such as low-grade muscle strains and delayed-onset muscle soreness (DOMS) (56). However, Malliou et al. (37) recently reported a high incidence of more chronic, overuse injuries in group exercise instructors, although the exact type of overuse injuries were not noted. Thompson et al. (62) noted that almost 40% of injuries reported by group exercise instructors were general inflammation and muscle strains, whereas almost 17% were stress fractures, and 9% were overuse injuries of the tendons (tendinopathy).

It might be expected that group fitness instructors would incur a greater number of injuries than their participants, given their greater frequency of exposure to potentially injurious exercise situations. Indeed, a higher frequency of exercise sessions has been reported by those individuals enrolled in indoor cycling classes who also reported suffering from knee injuries (33). Despite earlier research identifying a greater number of injuries reported by group exercise instructors compared to their students (56), more recent research has failed to reveal this relationship, with instructors actually reporting fewer injuries (17,62). The reasons for this relationship are perhaps due to the greater technical competence and fitness levels of the instructors, as well as the increased diversity of classes taught by group exercise instructors.

Malliou et al. (37) reported that the duration of the warm-up and cool-down performed by group exercise instructors was inversely related to injury rate. Specifically, 15 minutes of warm-up and cool-down resulted in fewer reported injuries compared to spending only 5 minutes in both warm-up and cool-down. It remains unclear whether this finding is due to the direct effects of performing a warm-up and a cool-down or simply due to spending less time performing the higher intensity exercises during the actual session. However, injury rates were shown to be further reduced when the instructors performed a private warm-up prior to their instructional session.

An important consideration for group exercise instructors is the proposed role of eating disorders as a causative factor in injuries. A history of eating disorders has been reported by more than one third of group exercise instructors (21,57). The reduced energy availability associated with disordered eating can affect menstrual status and significantly increase the risk of injury, particularly stress fractures (38). Indeed, Thompson et al. (62) reported that injury rates were related to past eating disorders in female group exercise instructors, although the associations were weak. While the research on eating disorders with group exercise instructors has focused on women, one should recognize that eating disorders also affect men (45).

| Table 12.10 | THE MAJOR MUSCLES OF THE ANKLE JOINT | |
|---|---|---|
| **MUSCLE** | **ACTION** | **STRENGTHENING EXERCISES** |
| Tibialis anterior | Dorsiflexion | Dorsiflexion (tubing or cables) |
| Extensor digitorum longus | Dorsiflexion | |
| Extensor hallucis longus | Dorsiflexion | |
| Peroneus longus | Plantarflexion | Seated calf raises |
| Gastrocnemius[a] | Plantarflexion | |
| Soleus | Plantarflexion | |

*[a]This is a biarticular muscle that also crosses the knee joint.*

**Table 12.11**    SOME OF THE MUSCLES OF THE SPINE AND PELVIS.

| MUSCLE | ACTION | STRENGTHENING EXERCISES |
|---|---|---|
| Spinalis[a] | Extension, rotation, and lateral flexion of spine | Back extension; seated row; dead lifts; good morning |
| Longissimus[a] | Extension, rotation, and lateral flexion of spine | |
| Iliocostalis[a] | Extension, rotation, and lateral flexion of spine | |
| Rectus abdominis | Flexion of lumbar spine; lateral flexion | Sit-ups; curl-ups |
| Psoas[b] | Flexion and lateral flexion of the spine; anterior tilt of the pelvis | |
| External oblique | Flexion of lumbar spine; lateral flexion; rotation | Twisting sit-ups |
| Iliacus[b] | Anterior tilt of the pelvis | Supine leg raises |
| Rectus femoris[b] | Anterior tilt of the pelvis | |
| Gluteus maximus[b] | Posterior tilt of the pelvis | Squats; dead lifts; good morning |
| Biceps femoris[b] | Posterior tilt of the pelvis | |
| Semitendinosus[b] | Posterior tilt of the pelvis | |
| Semimembranosus[b] | Posterior tilt of the pelvis | |
| Gluteus medius[b] | Lateral tilt of the pelvis | Hip abduction (tubing or cables); one-legged stance will activate muscle |

[a]These belong to the erector spinae group.
[b]These muscles also cross the hip joint.

## COMMON ACUTE INJURIES OF GROUP EXERCISE INSTRUCTORS

### Acute Muscle Strain

The tissue damage associated with an acute muscle strain is caused by overstretching a passive muscle or dynamically overloading an active one, with the severity of the damage dependent upon the rate and magnitude of the applied force as well as the strength of the musculotendinous structures (65). Clinically, muscle strains can be categorized into three grades depending on the severity of the damage (32).

- Grade I muscle strain — mild strain that is symptomatic (tenderness and mild pain) but results in no impairment (full ROM and no loss of strength)
- Grade II muscle strain — moderate impairment, marked tenderness, decreased ROM of the associated joint, and a noticeable loss of strength
- Grade III muscle strain — immediate pain, as well as a palpable defect in the muscle surrounded by swelling (edema), indicating rupture of fibers or the whole muscle

Low-grade muscle strains are common among group exercise instructors (56,62).

### Preventive Measures

Increasing the temperature of skeletal muscle can enhance its ability to withstand higher forces before failure (46), and so may protect the muscle against certain grades of acute strain. Therefore the completion of an appropriate warm-up, whereby the temperature of the tissue is increased, may reduce the chance of an acute muscle strain injury. In addition, McHugh and Cosgrave (42) recently reported that the occurrence of acute muscle strain injuries may be reduced as a result of performing static stretches within a warm-up routine. For information on developing an appropriate warm-up regime, the reader is directed to Jeffreys (23).

In contrast to the possible protective effect of increased tissue temperature and stretching, fatigue such as that experienced during an exercise session can increase the likelihood of incurring an acute muscle strain injury (36). Given this knowledge, the group exercise instructor should consider programming variables of intensity, duration, and volume of the exercise sessions, as well as the form of exercise in order to avoid this type of injury.

### Treatments

The treatment of an acute muscle strain is dependent upon the grade of injury sustained. For low-grade muscle strains, standard conservative treatment involves rest, ice, compression, and elevation of the affected muscle (32).

### Delayed-onset Muscle Soreness

DOMS is a symptom of exercise-induced muscle damage that is peculiar to acute bouts of eccentric exercise and is accompanied by muscle weakness, stiffness, and swelling (47). The pain associated with DOMS increases in intensity within the first 24 hours following the exercise bout, peaks in intensity between 24 and 72 hours, and subsides and disappears by 5–7 days after the exercise (7). DOMS has been reported as a common injury with group exercise instructors (56).

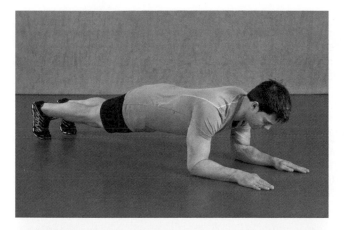

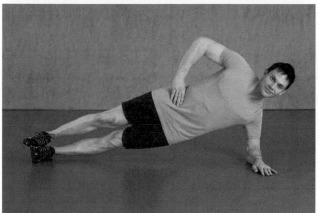

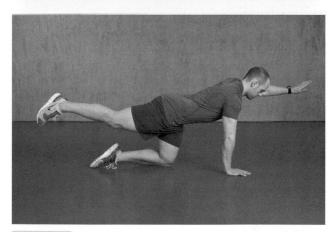

 CLIP 12.3

■ **FIGURE 12.13** Some core stabilization exercises. **A:** Plank, **B:** side bridge, **C:** bird dog.

The etiology of DOMS appears to be related to damage to the muscle fibers or the connective tissue associated with the muscle caused by the greater forces experienced during eccentric contractions (47). The inflammatory response resulting from the damage explains the delay in pain experienced by the participant. Although DOMS may not be considered a serious injury that results in a long-term cessation of exercise, one should consider that more serious injuries may be incurred due to alterations in muscular performance and changes in movement patterns that could accompany DOMS if the individual continues their exercise participation.

*Preventive Measures*

The efficacy of the proposed methods of preventing DOMS is limited. For example, stretching and an increase in muscle temperature prior to exercise have failed to alleviate the symptoms of DOMS (7). What has been shown is a reduction in the severity of the symptoms following repeated exposure to the same exercise bout, a phenomenon known as the **repeated-bout effect** (47). This protective mechanism can be effective even when the bouts are separated by several weeks, and it reflects adaptations that either attenuate further tissue damage or enhance the recovery process (47).

*Treatments*

Similar to the preventive methods for DOMS, the efficacy of the treatments proposed for DOMS are limited with ice application, stretching, and massage administered afterward having little effect (7).

## COMMON OVERUSE INJURIES OF GROUP EXERCISE INSTRUCTORS

### Stress Fractures

A stress fracture is a partial or incomplete fracture of a bone as a result of repeated cycles of applied forces (53). It is important to note that the magnitude of the forces required to produce a stress fracture can be below that required to produce complete failure of the bone. As already noted in this chapter, the forces applied to bone as a result of exercise provide an important stimulus to which the tissue adapts. However, if insufficient time is provided between loading cycles to allow the bone to adapt, then a stress fracture can result (29). Given this knowledge, consideration of the programming variables including intensity, duration, and volume of the exercise sessions could protect against incurring stress fractures. Stress fractures tend to be the most common type of overuse injury reported by group exercise instructors (62).

The forces applied to bone that are responsible for stress fractures can come from repeated muscular contractions or ground contacts experienced during exercise (53). Concerning ground contact forces, stress fractures of the tibia have been associated with greater GRFs in female runners (18). Such an association is important for the group exercise instructor because we have already shown that GRFs are increased by increasing step height and step frequency during step aerobic routines. As previously mentioned, impact forces can also be lessened through appropriate technique (increasing joint flexion upon landing) and footwear and by minimizing fatigue in the performer.

Sex differences in the risk of stress fractures have not been found in athletic populations (53). However, menstrual irregularities such as those resulting from disordered eating have been shown to increase the risk of stress fracture (38). The situation may be compounded by the fact that exercise instructors with an

| Table 12.12 | THE MUSCULATURE OF THE CORE | |
|---|---|---|
| **CORE REGION** | **MUSCLE** | **PROPOSED ROLE IN CORE STABILITY** |
| Superior wall | Diaphragm | Increases intra-abdominal pressure |
| Inferior wall | Psoas major | Stabilizes lumbar spine during hip flexion; provides compression of lumbar spine |
| | Pelvic floor | Modulates intra-abdominal pressure |
| Posterior wall | Multifidus | Lumbar extensor |
| | Longissimus | Thoracolumbar extensor |
| | Iliocostalis | Thoracolumbar extensor |
| | Intertransversarii | Neural feedback (proprioception) |
| | Quadratus lumborum | Stabilizes lumbar spine to protect against lateral buckling when spine is compressed |
| | Rotatores | Neural feedback (proprioception) |
| | Transverse abdominis | Increases intra-abdominal pressure, stabilizes sacroiliac joint; coactivation with internal oblique limits translation and rotation; attachment to linea semilunaris allows tension to be transmitted to rectus abdominis |
| | Gluteus maximus | Trunk extensor when lower extremities are stationary |
| Anterior wall | Rectus abdominis | Trunk flexor, controls extension |
| | External oblique | Trunk flexor, controls extension; contralateral rotator, controls ipsilateral rotation; ipsilateral lateral flexor, controls contralateral flexion; attachment to linea semilunaris allows tension to be transmitted to rectus abdominis |
| | Internal oblique | Trunk flexor, controls extension; ipsilateral rotator, controls controlateral rotation; contralateral lateral flexor, controls ipsilateral flexion; attachment to linea semilunaris allows tension to be transmitted to rectus abdominis |

*From Dale RB, Lawrence R. Principles of core stabilization for athletic populations. Athletic Therapy Today. 2005;10:12–8; McGill S. Low Back Disorders. Champaign (IL): Human Kinetics; 2007.*

active eating disorder have reported a greater weekly exercise load (21), further increasing the risk of incurring a stress fracture.

### Preventive Measures

There are currently no firm conclusions as to the most effective preventive measures to avoid stress fractures, although methods to lessen the forces experienced by the tissue (*e.g.*, footwear with appropriate "shock absorption, proper flooring, etc.") have been suggested (54). However, given that the proposed etiology of stress fractures involves excessive and repetitive cycling of forces, an effective countermeasure to avoid such injuries would appear to be an appropriately designed exercise regimen. The American College of Sports Medicine provides recommendations for the duration, intensity, and frequency of exercise required for cardiorespiratory and muscular fitness as well as bone health in adults (25,49), which should provide the bases for developing safe and effective exercise programs.

### Treatments

It is essential to eliminate the forces from the affected bone following the diagnosis of a stress fracture and therefore altering or ceasing exercise activities is essential. Conservative treatments that promote osteosynthesis, including extracorporeal shock-wave therapy and low-intensity ultrasound, have been suggested as effective treatments (29). Surgical techniques such as bone drilling, autograft

transplantation, and internal fixation are recommended in cases where conservative methods fail or there is an associated dislocation of the bone (29).

### Tendinopathy

Tendinopathy is the term used to describe both acute and chronic pain in the tendon, and unlike both tendinosis (tendon degeneration) and tendinitis (tendon inflammation) does not require histopathological examination (16). Tendinopathy is generally considered as an injury resulting from overuse although the exact etiology is unknown

| Table 12.13 | EXECUTION AND FORM CUES THAT CAN BE USED DURING THE SQUAT EXERCISE | |
|---|---|
| **CONSIDERATIONS** | **VERBAL CUE** |
| Set participant up with a solid base | "Stand with feet hip-width apart, knees soft" |
| Coach participants through downward movement | "With your weight on your heels, push your hips back; squat down like you're going to sit in a chair" |
| Coach stability | "You can lift your arms out to the front to balance out the hips, keep your abs contracted, breathe" |
| Coach upward movement | "Pushing from the heels, straighten the legs without locking the knees, contracting the gluteals; exhale" |

and a wide range of both intrinsic and extrinsic factors have been forwarded, including excessive force applied to the tendon, repetitive cycling of forces, and inappropriate footwear and exercise surfaces (16). The most common tendons afflicted in athletic populations are the patellar and Achilles tendons (28,31). Tendinopathy is relatively common in group exercise instructors (62).

### Preventive Methods

As with stress fractures, the appropriate development of exercise sessions that avoid excessive and repetitive cycling of forces is likely to provide an effective countermeasure to avoid tendinopathy. However, a further consideration with tendinopathy is that increases in tendon strength appear to lag behind that of muscle in response to an exercise regimen (27). The group exercise instructor should therefore be aware of effective and appropriate methods of progressing the exercise sessions to account for these differences in tissue adaptation rates.

### Treatments

Unloading of the affected tissue is the first treatment in tendinopathy. This can be achieved by altering the exercises performed, altering the biomechanics of the exercises through the use of orthoses, or simply by ceasing the activities. Conservative treatments such as extracorporeal shock-wave therapy, nitric oxide therapy, and eccentric exercises have been shown to be effective in the treatment of certain tendinopathies (60). Various surgical treatments, such as excision (removal of abnormal tissue), have also been shown to be effective (60), although these are used only after the injury fails to respond to conservative methods.

## PRACTICAL IMPLICATIONS FOR THE GROUP EXERCISE INSTRUCTOR

- The main acute injuries incurred by the group exercise instructor tend to be low-grade muscle strains.
- More serious are the overuse injuries such as stress fractures that are reported by group exercise instructors.
- The countermeasures available to group exercise instructors to prevent injuries both to themselves and to their participants include the following:
  ○ Appropriate supervision
  ○ Correct exercise technique
  ○ Appropriate exercise programming (intensity, duration, and volume of exercise sessions)
  ○ Appropriate warm-up and cool-down
  ○ Appropriate equipment and flooring
  ○ Appropriate clothing/footwear

## SUMMARY

*This chapter has provided an overview of basic biomechanics and functional anatomy of the musculoskeletal system. An understanding of biomechanics and functional anatomy provides the framework in which movements can be analyzed and can aid group exercise instructors in developing safe and effective exercise sessions for themselves and their participants. Although many of the concepts presented here are complex, the group exercise instructor is encouraged to master these skills by continuing to read the scientific literature.*

## References

1. Aguinaldo A, Mahar A. Impact loading in running shoes with cushioning column systems. *J Appl Biomech.* 2003;19:353–60.
2. Akuthota V, Nadler SF. Core strengthening. *Arch Phys Med Rehabil.* 2004;85:S86–92.
3. Amiridis I, Martin A, Morlon B, et al. Co-activation and tension-regulating phenomena during isokinetic knee extension in sedentary and highly skilled humans. *Eur J Appl Physiol Occup Physiol.* 1996;73:149–56.
4. Boyle M. *Functional Training for Sports.* Champaign (IL): Human Kinetics; 2004.
5. Brown DA, Kautz SA, Dairaghi CA. Muscle activity patterns altered during pedaling at different body orientations. *J Biomech.* 1996;29:1349–56.
6. Chappell JD, Herman DC, Knight BS, Kirkendall DT, Garrett WE, Yu B. Effect of fatigue on knee kinetics and kinematics in stop-jump tasks. *Am J Sports Med.* 2005;33:1022–9.
7. Cheung K, Hume PA, Maxwell L. Delayed onset muscle soreness. Treatment strategies and performance factors. *Sports Med.* 2003;33:145–64.
8. Christina KA, White SC, Gilchrist LA. Effect of localized muscle fatigue on vertical ground reaction forces and ankle joint motion during running. *Hum Mov Sci.* 2001;20:257–76.
9. Cochrane JL, Lloyd DG, Besier TF, Elliott BC, Doyle TLA, Ackland TR. Training affects knee kinematics and kinetics in cutting maneuvers in sport. *Med Sci Sports Exerc.* 2010;42:1535–44.
10. Downey PA, Siegel MI. Bone biology and the clinical implications for osteoporosis. *Phys Ther.* 2006;86:77–91.
11. Duchateau J, Semmler JG, Enoka RM. Training adaptations in the behavior of human motor units. *J Appl Physiol.* 2006;101:1766–75.
12. Duncan RA, McNair PJ. Factors contributing to lower back pain in rowers. *Br J Sports Med.* 2000;34:321–2.
13. Enoka RM. *Neuromechanics of Human Movement.* 4th ed. Champaign (IL): Human Kinetics; 2008.
14. Finni T, Ikegawa S, Komi PV. Concentric force enhancement during human movement. *Acta Physiol Scand.* 2001;173:369–77.
15. Floyd RT. *Manual of Structural Kinesiology.* 17th ed. New York: McGraw Hill; 2009.

16. Fredburg U, Stengaard-Pedersen K. Chronic tendinopathy tissue pathology, pain mechanisms, and etiology with a special focus on inflammation. *Scand J Med Sci Sports*. 2008;18:3–15.

17. Garnham A, Finch C, Salmon J. An overview of the epidemiology of aerobics injuries. *Int Sport Med J*. 2001;2:1–11.

18. Grimston SK, Engsberg JR, Kloiber R, Hanley DA. Bone mass, external loads and stress fractures in female runners. *Int J Sports Biomech*. 1991;7:292–302.

19. Hamilton N, Weimar W, Luttgens K. *Kinesiology. Scientific Basis of Human Motion*. 11th ed. New York: McGraw Hill; 2008.

20. Hodges PW, Richardson CA. Contraction of the abdominal muscles associated with movement of the lower limb. *Phys Ther*. 1997;77:132–42.

21. Höglund K, Normén L. A high exercise load is linked to pathological weight control behavior and eating disorders in female fitness instructors. *Scand J Med Sci Sports*. 2002;12:261–75.

22. Ichinose Y, Kanehisa H, Ito M, Kawakami Y, Fukunaga T. Relationship between muscle fiber pennation and force generation capability in Olympic athletes. *Int J Sports Med*. 1998;19:541–6.

23. Jeffreys I. Warm-up and stretching. In: Baechle TR, Earle RW, ed. *Essentials of Strength Training and Conditioning*. Champaign (IL): Human Kinetics; 2008:295–324pp.

24. Kemoun G, Thoumie P, Boisson D, Guieu JD. Ankle dorsiflexion delay can predict falls in the elderly. *J Rehabil Med*. 2002;34:278–83.

25. Kohrt WM, Bloomfield SA, Little KD, Nelson ME, Yingling VR. ACSM position stand. Physical activity and bone health. *Med Sci Sports Exerc*. 2004;36:1985–96.

26. Komi PV. Stretch-shortening cycle. In: Komi PV, ed. *Strength and Power in Sport*. 2nd ed. Oxford, (UK): Blackwell Science Ltd; 2003:184–202.

27. Kubo K, Ikebukuro T, Yata H, Tsunoda N, Kanehisa H. Time course of changes in muscle and tendon properties during strength training and detraining. *J Strength Cond Res*. 2010;24:322–31.

28. Kujala UM, Sarna S, Kaprio J. Cumulative incidence of Achilles tendon rupture and tendinopathy in male former elite athletes. *Clin J Sports Med*. 2005;15:133–35.

29. Lassus J, Tulikoura I, Konttinen YT, Salo J, Santavirta S. Bone stress injuries of the lower extremities. A review. *Acta Orthop Scand*. 2002;73:359–68.

30. Leiber L. *Skeletal Muscle Structure, Function, and Plasticity. The Physiological Basis of Rehabilitation*. Baltimore (MD): Lippincott, Williams and Wilkins; 2002.

31. Lian O, Dahl J, Ackermann PW, Frihagen F, Engebretsen L, Bahr R. Pronociceptive and antinociceptive neuromediators in patellar tendinopathy. *Am J Sports Med*. 2006;34:1801–8.

32. Lovering RM. Physical therapy and related interventions. In: Tiidus PM, ed. *Skeletal Muscle Damage and Repair*. Champaign (IL): Human Kinetics; 2008:219–30.

33. Lubetzky-Vilnai A, Carmeli E, Katz-Leurer M. Prevalence of injuries among young adults in sport centers: relation to the type and pattern of activity. *Scand J Med Sci Sports*. 2009;19:828–33.

34. Maffey L, Emery C. What are the risk factors for groin strain injury in sport? A systematic review of the literature. *Sports Med*. 2007;37:881–94.

35. Maffulli N, Baxter-Jones DG. Common skeletal injuries in young athletes. *Sports Med*. 1995;19:137–49.

36. Mair SD, Seaber AV, Glisson RR, Garrett WE. The role of fatigue in susceptibility to acute muscle strain injury. *Am J Sports Med*. 1996;24:137–43.

37. Malliou P, Rokka S, Beneka A, Mavridis G, Godolias G. Reducing risk of injury due to warm up and cool down in dance aerobic instructors. *J Back Musculoskelet Rehabil*. 2007;20:29–35.

38. Manore MM, Ciadella Kam L, Louks AB. The female athlete triad: components, nutrition issues, and health consequences. *J Sports Sci*. 2007;25:S61–71.

39. Maybury MC, Waterfield J. An investigation into the relation between step height and ground reaction forces in step exercise: a pilot study. *Br J Sports Med*. 1997;31:109–13.

40. McComas AJ. *Skeletal Muscle: Form and Function*. Champaign (IL): Human Kinetics; 1996.

41. McGill SM. *Low Back Disorders*. Champaign (IL): Human Kinetics; 2007.

42. McHugh MP, Cosgrave CH. To stretch or not to stretch: the role of stretching in injury prevention and performance. *Scand J Med Sci Sports*. 2010;20:169–81.

43. Menant JC, Steele JR, Menz HB, Munro BJ, Lord SR. Rapid gait termination: effects of age, walking surfaces and footwear characteristics. *Gait Posture*. 2009;30:65–70.

44. Mero A, Komi PV, Gregor RJ. Biomechanics of sprint running: a review. *Sports Med*. 1992;13:376–92.

45. Morgan JF. *The Invisible Man. A Self-help Guide for Men with Eating Disorders, Compulsive Exercising and Bigorexia*. London, (UK): Routledge; 2008.

46. Noonan TJ, Best TM, Seaber AV, Garrett WE. Thermal effects on skeletal muscle tensile behavior. *Am J Sports Med*. 1993;21:517–22.

47. Nosaka K. Muscle soreness and damage and the repeated-bout effect. In: Tiidus PM, edition. *Skeletal Muscle Damage and Repair*. Champaign (IL): Human Kinetics; 2008:59–76.

48. Parijat P, Lockhart TE. Effects of quadriceps fatigue on the biomechanics of gait and slip propensity. *Gait Posture*. 2008;28:568–73.

49. Pollock ML, Gaesser GA, Despres JP, Dishman RK, Franklin BA, Garber CE. ACSM position stand. The recommended quantity and quality of exercise for developing and maintaining cardiorespiratory and muscular fitness, and flexibility in healthy adults. *Med Sci Sports Exerc*. 1998;30:975–91.

50. Pöyhönen T, Keskinen KL, Kyröläinen H, Hautala A, Savolainen J, Mälkiä E. 2001. Neuromuscular function during therapeutic knee exercise under water and dry land. *Arch Phys Med Rehabil*. 2001;82:1446–52.

51. Rassier DE, MacIntosh BR, Herzog W. Length dependence of active force production in skeletal muscle. *J Appl Physiol*. 1999;86:1445–57.

52. Robling AG, Castillo AB, Turner CH. Biomechanical and molecular regulation of bone remodeling. *Annu Rev Biomed Eng*. 2006;8:455–98.

53. Romani WA, Gieck JH, Perrin DH, Saliba EN, Kahler DM. Mechanisms and management of stress fractures in physically active persons. *J Athl Train*. 2002;37:306–14.

54. Rome K, Handoll HG, Ashford RL. Interventions for preventing and treating stress fractures and stress reactions of bone of the lower limbs in young adults. *Cochrane Database Syst Rev*. 2005;2:1–49.

55. Scharff-Olson MR, Williford HN, Blessing DL, Moses R, Wang T. Vertical impact forces during bench-step aerobics: exercise rate and experience. *Percept Mot Skills*. 1997;84:267–74.

56. Scharff-Olson MR, Williford HN, Brown JA. Injuries associated with current dance-exercise practices. *J Dance Med Sci*. 1999;3:144–50.

57. Scharff-Olson MR, Williford HN, Richards LA, Brown JA, Pugh S. Self-reported eating disorder inventory by female aerobic instructors. *Percept Mot Skills*. 1996;82:1051–58.

58. Scott A, Khan KM, Duronio V, Hart DA. Mechanotransduction in human bone. *In vitro* cellular physiology that underpins bone changes with exercise. *Sports Med*. 2008;38:139–60.

59. Sherry M, Best T, Heiderscheit B. The core: where are we and where are we going? *Clin J Sports Med*. 2005;15:1–2.

60. Tan SC, Chan O. Achilles and patellar tendinopathy: Current understanding of pathophysiology and management. *Disabil Rehabil*. 2008;30:1608–15.

61. Thein JM, Brody LT. Aquatic-based rehabilitation and training for the elite athlete. *J Orthop Sports Phys Ther*. 1998;27:32–41.

62. Thompson SH, Case AJ, Sargent RG. Factors influencing performance-related injuries among group exercise instructors. *Women Sport Phys Activ J*. 2001;10:125–42.

63. Triplett NT, Colado JC, Benavent J, et al. Concentric and impact forces of single-leg jumps in an aquatic environment versus on land. *Med Sci Sports Exerc.* 2009;41:1790–96.

64. Weyand PG, Sternlight DB, Bellizzi MJ, Wright S. Faster top running speeds are achieved with greater ground forces not more rapid leg movements. *J Appl Physiol.* 2000;89:1991–9.

65. Whiting WC, Zernicke RF. *Biomechanics of Musculoskeletal Injury.* Champaign (IL): Human Kinetics; 2008.

66. Wikstrom EA, Tillman MD, Chmielewski TL, Borsa PA. Measurement and evaluation of dynamic joint stability of the knee and ankle after injury. *Sports Med.* 2006;36:393–410.

67. Willardson JM. Core stability training: applications to sports conditioning programs. *J Strength Cond Res.* 2007;21:979–85.

# 13 Introduction to Nutrition for Group Exercise Instructors

## FELICIA D. STOLER

**Objectives**

At the end of this chapter you will be able to:

- Understand the GEI's scope of practice limitations as they relate to nutrition education
- Be able to convey some basic nutrition information to their class participants
- Identify sports nutrition, hydration, and eating disorder issues
- Understand how to provide some basic advice about weight management and fad diets

## ROLE OF GROUP EXERCISE PROFESSIONALS

As a group exercise professional, it is important to keep advice within your scope of practice. Know that nutrition is going to be a multifaceted concern for most clients whom you work with. This chapter will provide you with some credible basic information that you may share with your class participants. However, it is recommended that you refer your clients to a registered dietitian (RD) whenever they are in need of more in-depth guidance or are dealing with a health-related condition that requires clinical nutrition intervention.

✔ **RECOMMENDED RESOURCES:**

**To find a nutritional professional in your community, go to the American Dietetic Association Web site at http://www.eatright.org**

The nutrition in this chapter is simplified to its most basic principles. There are many courses and degrees that can be attained if you are interested in expanding your knowledge base. The American Dietetic Association (ADA) and the American College of Sports Medicine (ACSM) have a number of joint position papers that are updated regularly. The recommendations are based upon the science, as demonstrated in peer-reviewed journals, the Dietary Guidelines, and generally accepted principles of medicine.

There is a plethora of misinformation in the media. Although your clients may ask you about a number of these new "findings," it is far better to refer them to credible resources and professionals than to say something you may be unsure of.

## UNDERSTANDING NUTRITION: BASIC CONCEPTS AND DEFINITIONS

Nutrition is the nourishment that is provided to an organism to allow it to function. Often it is referred to by many as "diet," which is the sum of one's usual intake and how it impacts one's body. Some people perceive the word diet to represent an eating pattern that someone will start and stop or that yields a particular outcome.

Humans do not intuitively eat the right combinations of nutrients (carbohydrates, protein, fat, vitamins, minerals, and water) (2). People often misinterpret a "craving" for a food as a deficiency of the nutrient(s) that may be contained in the food they have a burning urge to eat. This is just one chapter on nutrition. It does not make you an expert, but it will help you to provide basic information for your clientele. Here are some basic definitions.

- *Food* is any substance that your body can take in and assimilate that will enable it to function (Fig. 13.1).
- *Nutrition* is the study of the nutrients in foods and in the body and also the study of human behaviors that are related to food.
- *Diet* is all foods that are consumed, usually through the mouth.
- *Essential nutrients* are those nutrients that must be ingested (brought into the body) since they cannot be created in sufficient amounts by the body. Examples of essential nutrients are carbohydrates, essential fatty acids, essential amino acids, vitamins, minerals, and water.

Nutrition is a relatively new science. Understand, too, that science is always changing. Epidemiologists are scientists who study the relationship between disease and lifestyle behaviors to try to find a link. For instance, it's

| BOX 13.1 | *Registered Dietitians* |
|---|---|

If you would like more assistance with nutrition matters, contact a RD. Be aware that all dietitians are nutritionists, but not all nutritionists are dietitians. All but four states have licensure for dietitians/nutritionists. There are some who state they are "certified nutritionists," with self-education, claims of continuing education hours, and misrepresentation of credentials. This does not give credibility. Dietetics professionals are part of a nationally recognized professional association that is approved to be one aspect of the multidisciplinary health care team that is covered by insurance.

RDs have a minimum of a bachelor's degree, completed a minimum of 900 hours of a supervised dietetic internship and have successfully passed a national registration exam. Those in private practice carry malpractice insurance, just as physicians do. RDs use evidence-based practice that is supported by publication in scientific journals, not driven by supplement manufacturers' sales. RDs understand the anatomy and physiology of the body, its systems, disease states, drug-nutrient interactions, and behavior modification.

well established that smoking can cause lung cancer (6). This doesn't mean that every person who has lung cancer was a smoker or that every person who ever smoked will develop lung cancer. Similarly, dietary intake habits and physical activity can affect the following diseases/conditions (7):

- Cancer
- Cardiovascular disease
- Depression
- Diabetes
- Gallstones
- High cholesterol
- Hypertension
- Joint and orthopedic problems
- Obesity
- Osteoporosis
- Sleep apnea

According to the American Cancer Society, many cancer deaths could be prevented if people ate healthier foods,

exercised more, discontinued smoking, and received the recommended cancer screenings (4). What's known about nutrition and exercise is that it can be the least expensive, least invasive, and most effective way to prevent, treat, and delay the onset of many diseases. Food choice definitely can play an important role in one's health. After all, prevention is the best medicine. Being well nourished helps your immune system to function properly. When humans are malnourished, they're at risk for diseases and illnesses. Dietary intake that is rich in fruits, vegetables, and whole grains and low in fat is better for health promotion.

## ENERGY AND METABOLISM

All organisms require energy to function — from plants to people. Once again, we do not inherently know the amount of caloric energy that we each need in a day (5).

Energy Balance = Energy In (Food) – Energy Out
(Metabolic Rate + Physical Activity)

### WHAT IS A CALORIE?

A calorie is the amount of heat that is required to increase 1 g of water 1°C. It is commonly used as a unit measure of food energy (Fig. 13.2). All foods are made up of either one or more of three macronutrients: carbohydrates, proteins, and fats. The amount of calories that each of these nutrients supplies to the body is as follows:

- Carbohydrates = 4 cal/g
- Protein = 4 cal/g
- Fat = 9 cal/g

Note that alcohol provides 7 cal/g, but will not be included in our discussion on macronutrients.

Whether a person's goal is weight loss or weight gain, there are safe ways to do this. One should aim for no more

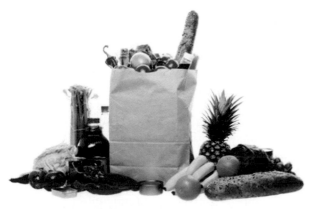

k4947543 www.fotosearch.com

■ **FIGURE 13.1** Food is any substance that your body can assimilate and that will enable it to function.

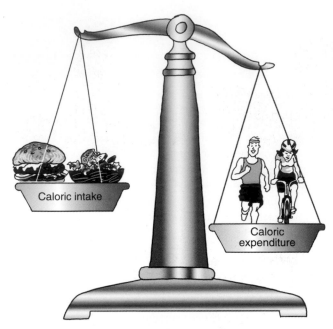

■ **FIGURE 13.2** Calories In = Calories Out (From Roitman JL, LaFontaine T. *The Exercise Professional's Guide to Optimizing health: Strategies for preventing and Reducing Chronic Disease.* Baltimore (MD): Lippincott Williams Wilkins; 2012 p.145.)

than 2 lb/week for weight loss. How can that happen? It should be a combination of reducing caloric intake with increases in physical activity. The "rule" for the mathematical component is shown in Table 13.1. There are several formulas for calculating caloric intake.

### Take Caution

#### MONITOR CALORIC INTAKE

Nobody should consume <1,200 kcals per day. It is important that calculations be made to determine caloric intake needs, so that adjustments can be made to meet health goals.

 **RECOMMENDED RESOURCES:**

*As a group fitness professional, you will be giving out general and not specific diet information. You can easily direct your students to www.mypyramid.gov for more detailed information.*

| Table 13.1 | 3500 KCAL = 1 LB | |
|---|---|
| **TO GAIN/LOSE (LB PER WEEK)** | **MODIFY DAILY CALORIES BY (KCALS PER DAY)** |
| ½ | 250 |
| 1 | 500 |
| 1½ | 750 |
| 2 | 1,000 |

## GETTING YOUR NUTRIENTS FROM THE FOOD SUPPLY

Are all calories created equal? The answer is no. People consume calories (energy), which are used to fuel body functions. Metabolism is a process that breaks down nutrients from carbohydrates, protein, and fat along with oxygen to yield energy (for activity), carbon dioxide, and water. Nutrients are the components of food that are indispensable for body functions. They provide energy, serve as building material, help maintain or repair body parts, and support growth. The six nutrients are carbohydrates, protein, fat, vitamins, minerals, and water (Fig. 13.3).

## CARBOHYDRATES

The preferred fuel for most body functions is carbohydrate. The brain relies exclusively on carbohydrates for its fuel. With the exception of dairy products, carbohydrates are foods that originate from plants. Carbohydrates are also referred to as "sugars." The simple building blocks of all carbohydrates are sugar molecules; the form used in the body is called "glucose." Generally, your body stores carbohydrate in the form of glycogen in the muscles and liver. Regardless of food origin, once a carbohydrate is absorbed through the lining of the small intestine, it goes directly to the liver. It cannot leave the liver to be used elsewhere in the body as anything except glucose. Which of the food groups have carbohydrates? They're found in breads, rice, cereal, pasta, whole grains, fruits, vegetables, and dairy products. Humans have a very limited capacity to store carbohydrates in their bodies (only enough fuel to last about 6–7 hours).

Carbohydrates should make up about 50%–60% of the diet (5). When carbohydrates are consumed by themselves, they can be digested and absorbed quickly by the body. However, during a mixed-nutrient meal (with protein and fat) or in the presence of fiber, digestion and absorption can be slowed down. Fiber is an important type of carbohydrate, found only in foods of plant origin, which may also contain phytochemicals and antioxidants.

### Fiber

Fiber is beneficial because it provides satiety (the feeling of fullness), helps with bowel function, and can decrease total cholesterol. There are two types of fiber: soluble and insoluble. Soluble fibers can be broken down completely and digested by human enzymes. Examples of soluble fibers are found in oat bran, barley, and kidney beans. Insoluble fibers are those parts of plants that cannot be broken down by human enzymes and absorbed by the body (such as the strings in celery). This type of fiber does not contribute a significant amount of calories to one's body because it utilizes even more calories to move it through the digestive system. Examples of insoluble fibers are wheat bran, vegetables, and whole grains.

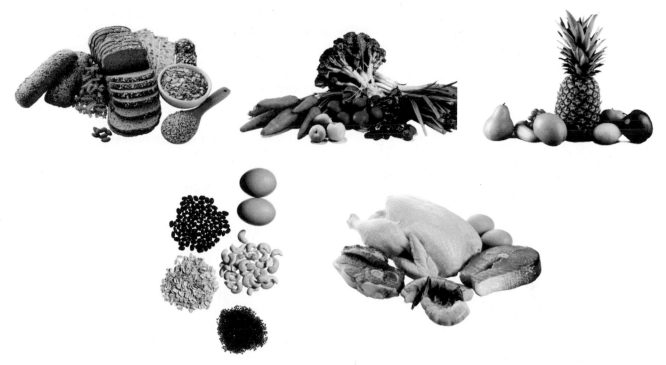

■ **FIGURE 13.3** Combining all food groups in their appropriate amounts ensures optimal nutrition.

## PROTEIN

Protein is used for tissue building and repair, which is why we need it but don't generally use it as a source of energy for activity. This nutrient is made up of molecules called "amino acids" (which are often referred to as "the building blocks of protein"). Amino acids are found in grains, vegetables, dairy products, meat, poultry, fish, eggs, nuts, seeds, beans, legumes, and soy products — pretty much all foods except for fruits. Protein is frequently found with fat in its food of origin (or in the cooking process). Many people have greater satiety after eating protein foods because they take longer to be digested and absorbed.

Like carbohydrates, protein also provides 4 cal/g. Protein is considered to be an "expensive" form of energy and, thus, is normally used only to provide energy as a last resort. Also, the human body has limited storage capacity for protein. Contrary to popular belief, eating more protein doesn't increase muscle mass (exercise does). About 15%–20% of the diet should be protein (5). We have a genetically predetermined amount of muscle mass that we can attain (naturally), so overconsuming protein just puts a strain on the liver and kidneys — it does not equate to muscle mass.

## FAT

Fat provides 9 cal/g — more than twice that of carbohydrates and protein. Fats can be classified based on the saturation of the molecule: monounsaturated, polyunsaturated, or saturated. Other terms with which you may be familiar are "trans" or "hydrogenated" oils. Hydrogenation comes from adding hydrogen, which makes the fat more solid. Trans comes from the type of chemical bond formed during the hydrogenation process. The trans fats act like a saturated fat in the body and are considered more dangerous to health than even the saturated fats. Saturated and trans fats can have a direct impact on one's blood cholesterol levels (both total cholesterol as well as triglycerides).

Science has shown that consuming saturated and trans fats on a regular basis is more dangerous to health than the consumption of cholesterol. While on the subject, cholesterol does have important roles in the body. For one thing, it is the building block for other substances in your body such as bile, steroid hormones and much more. But since the body can create cholesterol, it isn't considered to be an essential nutrient.

There are essential fatty acids that we need. You may have heard of omega-3 and omega-6 fatty acids. These "good" fats can be found in fish, nuts, seeds, soy, olive oil, and avocados. Fats are found in dairy products and meats as well as two fruits: avocados and coconuts. As the ADA likes to emphasize, "All foods can fit in moderation." Fat should be no more than about 30% of the diet (with <10% coming from saturated fat) (5).

## GLYCEMIC INDEX

This can be an overwhelming topic to discuss. In simple terms, glycemic index is the rate at which carbohydrate foods are broken down during digestion and absorbed into the blood stream. It was first noted in the 1980s by researchers studying diabetes. Foods are then ranked in comparison to a loaf of white bread. For a diabetic taking insulin, this is important information. For the rest of us, this can be too much information to help a person make sound food choices because most people eat a mixed macronutrient meal — so it will probably have some carbohydrates, protein, fat, and maybe even some fiber.

## VITAMINS AND MINERALS

Vitamins and minerals are essential to human body processes (Table 13.2). They are components of the foods supply and are found in nature. However, some people choose to take supplements to augment their dietary intake. Vitamin and mineral supplements are not a replacement for food. The Recommended Dietary Allowances and Dietary Reference Intake Values are established by scientific advisory committees under the auspices of the U.S. Department of Agriculture (USDA). You may commonly see these numbers on the Nutrition Facts panel. There are values established for intake levels to maintain health and prevent deficiency symptoms for healthy individuals. The specific values vary by sex and age.

Vitamin and mineral levels vary from person to person. There are no tests that have been proven to be accurate or precise to measure vitamin and mineral levels in each person (*i.e.*, scanners, blood or saliva test, or hair sampling). Vitamins are divided into two categories—fat soluble and water soluble. Excess intake of fat-soluble vitamins can be stored, and are therefore potentially toxic, while the water-soluble vitamins are NOT stored, but excreted in the urine. The fat-soluble vitamins are A, D, E, and K. They are found in foods which contain fat/oils, are transported in the body in fat molecules, and are stored in fat tissues. Water-soluble vitamins are transported in the body in water and are easily excreted from the body in water. Hence it is often noted that Americans have the most expensive urine in the world from all the extra supplements that are consumed here.

## WEIGHT LOSS PROGRAMS

Your clients may or may not speak with you directly about their weight or weight loss goals. It is best to refer them to a RD for specific, individualized advice. It is not within your scope of practice to be providing energy calculations or meal plans as a group fitness instructor. However, what you need to know is that safe weight loss is considered by ACSM and the ADA to be *no more than* 2 lb per week. For many clients, simply encouraging them to watch their portions may be helpful. The USDA's Mypyramid.gov web site provides great resources that are quite easy to use (www.mypyramid.gov). It can be unsafe for people to consume *very* low-calorie diets (<1,200 cal), and most people who are at least 5 ft tall need at least 1,600 cal per day. The best recommendations for eating that you could provide to your clients is to not skip meals or eliminate food groups. Start from the ground up and encourage them to eat whole grains, fruits and vegetables, low-fat or fat-free dairy products, lean protein, and fats in moderation (Fig. 13.4).

It is a common practice for busy people to skip meals. However, skipping meals will tend to make a person eat more at his or her next "feeding" opportunity. There is the concept of Thermic Effect of Eating or Feeding, which is related to the amount of calories that one burns through the act of digestion. By skipping a meal, an individual decreases the amount of calories that his or her body would expend. In addition, by skipping a meal, blood glucose levels decrease and drive up hunger urges, which may cause a person to binge. By keeping your brain and body "happy" by maintaining adequate caloric intake throughout the day, you can ensure that you will be feeding your brain and your body appropriately.

## COMMON EATING DISORDERS

Anorexia nervosa is the first thing that pops into most people's minds when you say the term eating disorder. Anorexia nervosa is a mental illness associated with a person's unrealistic body image and unwillingness to maintain an appropriate body weight. It may involve

| Table 13.2 | VITAMINS AND MINERALS |
|---|---|
| **NUTRIENT** | **FOOD SOURCES** |
| **Fat-Soluble Vitamins** | |
| Vitamin A | Dark green, yellow and orange fruits and vegetables, liver |
| Vitamin D | Fortified dairy products |
| Vitamin E | Vegetable oils, nuts, leafy vegetables |
| Vitamin K | Green vegetables, dairy products |
| **Water-Soluble Vitamins** | |
| Vitamin C | Citrus fruits, tomatoes |
| Thiamine | Enriched grains, pork |
| Riboflavin | Meats, liver, grains |
| Niacin | Meat, nuts, legumes |
| Vitamin $B_6$ | Poultry, fish, liver, eggs |
| Folate | Leafy vegetables, liver |
| Vitamin $B_{12}$ | Animal proteins |
| **Minerals** | |
| Calcium | Dairy products, dark greens |
| Phosphorus | Meats |
| Magnesium | Seafood, legumes, grains |
| Iron | Meats, eggs, grains |
| Zinc | Meats, seafood, eggs |
| Iodine | Iodized salt, seafood |
| Selenium | Seafood, liver, meats |

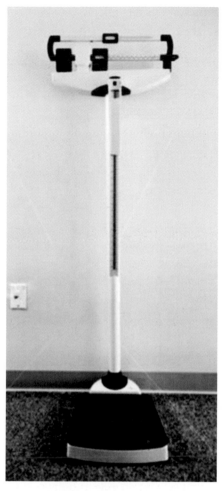

■ **FIGURE 13.4** Weight loss is big business. Hoovers.com reports that the US weight-reduction services industry includes about 1,300 companies with combined annual revenue of about $2 billion. (From: *http://www.hoovers.com/industry/weight-health-management/1220-1.html*)

starvation, vomiting, and/or overexercising to maintain dangerously low body weight.

Bulimia nervosa involves overeating followed by vomiting or laxative abuse. A person with bulimia may appear to be of normal weight or overweight. In addition, overeating or binge eating is also considered an eating disorder. Eating disorders are psychological disorders that require medical treatment. Treatment is provided through a multifactorial team approach that often includes a medical doctor, a therapist, and a RD.

Female athlete triad is common among female athletes (Fig. 13.5). It involves low caloric intake (and low body weight), which leads to cessation of menstruation, which then leads to loss of bone mineral density. It is a serious condition that does require medical intervention as previously noted. If you suspect that someone in your group fitness class may have an eating disorder, let your manager or supervisor know. It is not recommended that you broach the subject with the individual — you may not know how he or she will react.

There are also people who do not fall into a distinct classification for anorexia or bulimia—for whom the term "disordered eating" is the best descriptor.

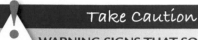

### Take Caution

**⚠ WARNING SIGNS THAT SOMEONE HAS AN EATING DISORDER**

You may come across people in your class that you suspect have an eating disorder. It would not be appropriate for you to confront them, but just be cognizant of how your teaching messages and words may impact them. Some women with eating disorders, wear excessive layers of clothing (even when temperatures are quite warm); you can see their bones and joints rather clearly. Physical signs of anorexia may be more obvious: loss of menstrual periods, lack of energy and weakness, feeling cold all the time, dry yellowish skin, constipation and abdominal pain, restlessness and insomnia, dizziness, fainting and headaches, growth of fine hair all over the face and body. For people who purge, you may see cuts or scars on fingers and swollen cheeks and salivary glands.

## THE DIETARY GUIDELINES FOR AMERICANS

The federal government comes out with new guidelines for nutrient intake and physical activity every 5 years. Science changes every day, and as information from research is collected, the USDA and the Department of Health and Human Services (DHHS) gather groups of scientists (social, academic, research, and so on) together to discuss the latest and greatest ways to improve health. The results are the Dietary Guidelines for Americans. This report contains science-based guidelines for generally healthy Americans over the age of 2. Key components of the most recent (2010) guidelines include

- Consume nutrients and other essential compounds from whole foods and beverages.
- Eat fiber-rich whole grains, fruits, vegetables, fat-free dairy products, and lean "meats."
- Control portion sizes.
- Reduce fat intake, especially saturated fat and trans fat.
- Reduce sodium intake.
- Drink alcoholic beverages in moderation, if at all.
- Maintain appropriate bodyweight, balancing caloric intake with caloric expenditure.
- Engage in regular physical activity for 60 minutes each day and reduce sedentary activities to promote health, psychological well-being, and a healthy bodyweight.

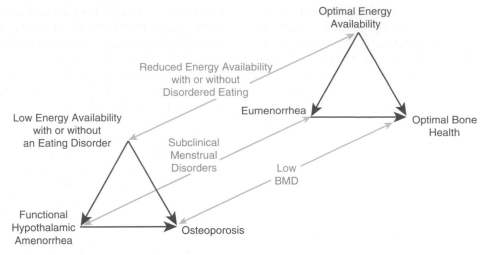

**■ FIGURE 13.5** The female athlete triad. (From - ACSM Position Stand, The Female Athlete Triad. Medicine & Science in Sports & Exercise, October 2007 - Volume 39 - Issue 10 - p. 1868)

- Perform aerobic (cardiovascular), flexibility, strength, and endurance activities.
- Avoid microbial food-borne illness (food safety).

## SPORTS NUTRITION: BEFORE, DURING, AND AFTER

This is a big topic for fitness professionals. Here are a few words of wisdom: Just as practice makes permanent for sports performance, nutritional practices can also affect performance. Eating before (when appropriate) and after a workout or a competition takes practice. In terms of nutrient percentages, the general dietary recommendations that were stated earlier also apply to sports nutrition. What's critical is the timing of food intake in relation to exercise/sport performance. A person who eats dinner at 6 pm, wakes up at 6 am the next day, and shortly thereafter goes running for 30 minutes is running on an "empty" fuel tank. Would you go 12 hours during the day without eating? Generally, full meals can be consumed 3–4 hours before working out or playing sports. As the time gets closer to the activity, the texture of what you eat should go from solid foods to gelatinous foods to liquids.

Some sports have built-in time for eating — such as between games in soccer tournaments — whereas others don't. The important thing to learn about sports nutrition is that establishing good behaviors takes practice. The additional "fuel" should come from wholesome foods, not "junk foods." After you've completed a workout or sport, make sure that you consume plenty of fluids, carbohydrates, protein, and fats.

### HYDRATION

Your class participants' needs vary based on each student's general hydration status. However, experts agree that fluid intake should replace fluid loss. Of course, it's not really practical for everyone to measure their fluid output, but there are some ways to gauge whether or not you're sufficiently hydrated.

For starters, you should urinate multiple times throughout the day. Be sure to assess the color of your urine. Ideally, the desirable color of urine is pale yellow. If it's fluorescent yellow, there's a good chance that you recently had a multivitamin supplement. If your urine is dark yellow, then you may need to drink more fluids (Fig. 13.6).

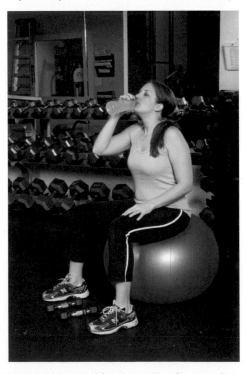

**■ FIGURE 13.6** Thirst is a delayed sensation that your class participants won't feel until they have already lost 1–2 L of water. So it's important to cue your class to drink on a fixed time interval during class rather than letting them rely on thirst to know when to drink.

The best fluid for meeting your hydration needs is water. Electrolytes — especially sodium — and carbohydrates are very important for exercise that lasts more than an hour or is done in extremely hot and humid conditions. Many people are naïve about how many calories they consume from beverages each day. Remember, sodas and other flavored "drinks" can add extra calories with very few other nutritional benefits. That said, electrolytes are found in some sport drinks, and while every athlete does not need sport drinks, if the color and flavor make it more likely for people to drink sport drinks over water, at least they are getting some fluids!

## Hydration Recommendations

- Drink 16 oz of fluid 2 hours before exercise.
- Drink another 8–16 oz 15 minutes before exercise.
- Drink 4–16 oz of fluid every 15–20 minutes during exercise.
- Drink 24 oz of fluid after exercise for every pound lost during exercise to return to full hydration within 6 hours.

## Take Caution

### DEHYDRATION

**You know you're dehydrated when**

- **You are thirsty**
- **Your urine is dark in color**
- **Or you may develop the chills**

**Other symptoms include increased heart rate, increased respiration, decreased sweating, decreased urination, increased body temperature, muscle cramping, extreme fatigue, headaches, and nausea. Having water or a sports drink with electrolytes can be beneficial for restoring serum fluid levels.**

## FOOD LABELS AND NUTRITION FACTS PANEL

Food labels can be an important resource for the individual concerned about the nutrient content of his or her foods (Fig. 13.7). First, there is the list of ingredients; this details, in descending order from greatest to smallest concentration, the actual substances that are in the food. This can be invaluable for people who have food allergies and sensitivities.

Next is the Nutrition Facts Panel. Let's start at the top and work our way down. First you will see the words "serving size," which tells you what the standardized portion for this item is, usually in cups or ounces (it most often adheres to USDA food standardization). After the serving size, you will see the "number of servings" in the package (which means that, for more than one serving, you must multiply the number of servings per package by the Nutrition Information to calculate how much is in the entire package). After serving size and number of servings, the number of "calories" is provided — this is per one serving of the food item.

Then, "calories from fat," which defines fat content by calories with the subgroups "total fat," "saturated fat," and "trans fat." It is challenging to make a recommendation to never eat foods with a certain amount of grams of fat in each serving, because it is about total intake for the day — not just in one food item. For example, nuts have fat — mostly good fats, but they do have fats — so, it would be incorrect to state that if you see a certain quantity of fat on a label, you should not eat that food.

Next on the list of information is "cholesterol" and "sodium." Dietary intake of cholesterol does not increase your serum cholesterol levels, whereas saturated and trans fats can impact those numbers. Foods of plant origin do not contain cholesterol. Foods derived from animals do contain cholesterol. One should consider consuming <300 mg of cholesterol each day. Three ounces of chicken breast meat only has 75 g of cholesterol; 3 oz of steak has 65 g of cholesterol; 3 oz of salmon contains 54 g of cholesterol.

Sodium intake should be <2,400 mg per day for most Americans, and the new Dietary Guidelines suggest 1,500 mg per day. Sodium, as a mineral, is naturally occurring in some foods. However, most sodium in our diets comes from processed and packaged foods. What is the equivalent of 2,400 mg of sodium? Almost one teaspoon of table salt or two tablespoons of soy sauce.

"Carbohydrates" are next; this value can be misleading and, truly, it is best suited for a diabetic who needs to know how many grams of carbohydrates they are eating, so they can moderate their exogenous insulin dosing. Many people avoid carbohydrate-rich foods because they think it has too much "sugar" in the food product. "Fiber" — if by chance, "soluble fiber" or "insoluble fiber" is specified — really doesn't matter for general nutrition and weight loss purposes. "Sugar" is the other word. It is confusing in that it does not represent added "sugars" and it includes naturally occurring "sugars." If you notice, total grams of carbohydrates are often identical to the total grams of sugars.

"Protein" is also listed on the label. You will find a column to the right that reads "% daily values." This represents the percent of nutrients this one food item has relative to the daily caloric intake needs based upon a 2,000-calorie-day diet. The recommended protein requirement is based on bodyweight, and in some cases exercise.

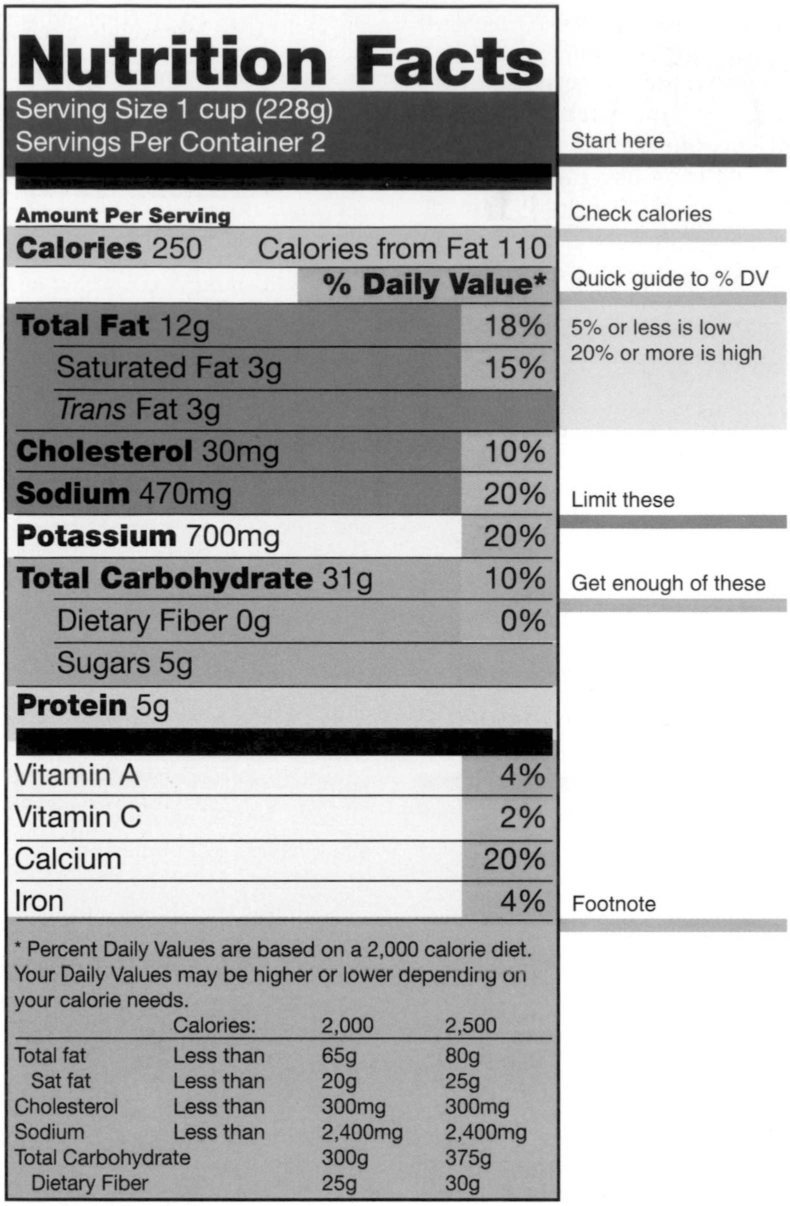

## Nutrition Facts

Serving Size 1 cup (228g)
Servings Per Container 2

| | | Guide |
|---|---|---|
| | | Start here |
| **Amount Per Serving** | | Check calories |
| **Calories** 250 | Calories from Fat 110 | |
| | **% Daily Value*** | Quick guide to % DV |
| **Total Fat** 12g | 18% | 5% or less is low |
| Saturated Fat 3g | 15% | 20% or more is high |
| *Trans* Fat 3g | | |
| **Cholesterol** 30mg | 10% | |
| **Sodium** 470mg | 20% | Limit these |
| **Potassium** 700mg | 20% | |
| **Total Carbohydrate** 31g | 10% | Get enough of these |
| Dietary Fiber 0g | 0% | |
| Sugars 5g | | |
| **Protein** 5g | | |
| Vitamin A | 4% | |
| Vitamin C | 2% | |
| Calcium | 20% | |
| Iron | 4% | Footnote |

* Percent Daily Values are based on a 2,000 calorie diet. Your Daily Values may be higher or lower depending on your calorie needs.

| | Calories: | 2,000 | 2,500 |
|---|---|---|---|
| Total fat | Less than | 65g | 80g |
| Sat fat | Less than | 20g | 25g |
| Cholesterol | Less than | 300mg | 300mg |
| Sodium | Less than | 2,400mg | 2,400mg |
| Total Carbohydrate | | 300g | 375g |
| Dietary Fiber | | 25g | 30g |

■ **FIGURE 13.7** The food label - for more information on how to read a food label, go to: http://www.fda.gov/food/labelingnutrition/consumerinformation/ucm078889.htm (From Thompson W. ACSMs Resources for the Personal Trainer. 3rd ed. Lippincott Williams & Wilkins, Baltimore, MD; 2010. p.181)

## MAGIC PILLS, POTIONS, AND BARS

When asked about ergogenic aids and performance-enhancement products, remember, "There's no such thing in life as a free lunch" (Fig. 13.8). This means that people should assess the risk versus the reward. Is it really worth it? There are no magic substances that are legal. Purported benefits such as increased muscle mass or enhanced sports performance, don't exist without the potential for harm. Understand that the federal government — specifically, the U.S. Food and Drug Administration (FDA) — does not regulate the supplement industry. Contrary to what supplement manufacturers would like you to believe, just because something is "natural" doesn't mean that it's safe to consume. No matter how impressive their "research" may appear to the untrained eye, oftentimes it's contrived and/or manipulated in advertising.

For example, when "energy bars" were first sold, they contained a good percentage of carbohydrates, which truly provides "energy." Now, however, people are gobbling up "protein bars" in lieu of regular food thinking that the products will give them "energy" for their workouts or sports performance. But those products are more likely to quiet hunger pangs than give real "energy." This can be another means of adding extra, unnecessary calories to your daily intake. In short, save your money for buying wholesome foods, and invest in good-quality foods! Protein and energy shakes are expensive replacements for food.

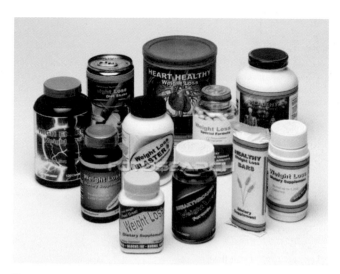

■ **FIGURE 13.8** Magic pills, potions, and bars. Remember there is no "magic" in good, healthy nutrition.

Caffeine is a stimulant that makes one feel alert AND increases heart rate. It not recommended that we encourage our clients to increase their consumption of caffeine before during or after exercise. Every day the FDA sends out advisory sheets about undeclared substances that are in supplements, bars, and shake mixes. For your professional liability protection and to work in your scope of practice, it is best to avoid making recommendations for these products for your clients.

## FAD DIETS

The U.S. Federal Trade Commission estimates that over $30 billion is spent each year on weight loss (1,3). Many of the programs, books, and products can be expensive and offer unrealistic weight-loss goals. Furthermore, most people who use them rarely enjoy long-term success.

Those who do lose weight often gain back most of it — or all of it (Fig. 13.9). And sometimes, they gain back even more than what they had lost. Try to be a savvy shopper of nutritional information. Remember, simply because people have the letters "Dr" in front of their names doesn't make them credible to dispense information about nutrition, diet, exercise, and weight loss. Just because a celebrity looks good in a bathing suit (but has no formal education) doesn't mean that he or she is credible, either. And just because a program worked for your co-worker doesn't mean that it will work for you. Could you imagine what would happen if we tried to self-treat all of our medical conditions through books and Web sites and hired highly unskilled professionals for assistance? Surely, we'd have an enormous medical crisis on our hands.

## SUMMARY: IMPLICATIONS FOR GROUP FITNESS INSTRUCTORS

*Now that you have learned some very basic nutrition information, you can put this into practice for yourself and have the foundation with which to make suggestions and referrals for your students and clients. Below you will find several resources that will help you learn more and assist you in providing the best and most current information available to your clients.*

✔ *RECOMMENDED RESOURCES:*
  *American Cancer Society: www.cancer.org*
  *American College of Sports Medicine: www.acsm.org*
  *American Diabetes Association: www.diabetes.org*
  *American Heart Association: www.americanheart.org*
  *National Heart, Lung and Blood Institute:*
  *www.nhlbi.nih.gov*
  *U. S. Department of Agriculture (USDA):*
  *www.nutrition.gov*

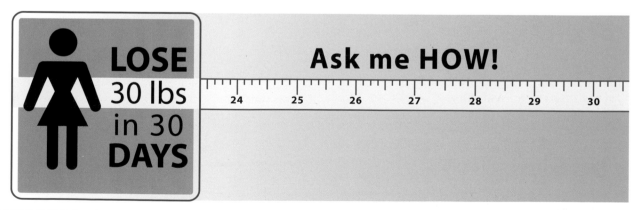

■ **FIGURE 13.9** Promises, promises! If it sounds too good to be true, it probably is. Steer students away from fads and educate them about slow, gradual weight loss for the best result!

# References

1. AHA. "Know Your Fats," Learn and Live. American Heart Association, 2010. Web site: *http://www.heart.org/HEARTORG/Conditions/Cholesterol/PreventionTreatmentofHighCholesterol/Know-Your-Fats_UCM_305628_Article.jsp, accessed on 09/15/2010.*

2. Birch LL. Development of food preferences. *Annu Rev Nutr.* 1999;19:41–62.

3. *http://www.ftc.gov/bcp/reports/weightloss.pdf*

4. *http://www.cancer.org/acs/groups/content/@nho/documents/document/acspc-024113.pdf*

5. Position of the American Dietetic Association, the Canadian Dietetic Association and the American College of Sports Medicine: Nutrition and Athletic Performance. *J Am Diet Assoc.* 2009;109:509–27.

6. US Department of Health and Human Services. *Reducing the Health Consequences of Smoking: 25 Years of Progress. A Report of the SurgeonGeneral.* Rockville, MD: US Department of Health and Human Services, Public Health Service, Centers for Disease Control and Prevention, Center for Chronic Disease Prevention and Health Promotion, Office on Smoking and Health; 1989.

7. Vainio H, Bianchini F. *IARC Handbooks of Cancer Prevention. Volume 6: Weight Control and Physical Activity.* Lyon, (France): IARC Press; 2002.

# Sample Job Descriptions

## GROUP EXERCISE INSTRUCTOR (1)

**POSITION DESCRIPTION**
**GROUP EXERCISE INSTRUCTOR**
**REPORTS TO:   GROUP FITNESS DIRECTOR**

### POSITION SUMMARY

To reflect the enthusiasm and energy required to teach classes safely and effectively while maintaining a professional appearance and attitude that adheres to the Plus One Health Management standards.

### PRINCIPAL DUTES

1. Provide professional, safe, and effective group exercise classes that follow the Plus One Health Management policies and guidelines including the I'm OK policy.
2. Provide ongoing observation and interpersonal feedback around class participation.
3. Actively communicate with the group class coordinator through verbal, written, and scheduled meetings.
4. Attend in house services and group exercise staff meetings.
5. Teach assigned classes on time and take responsibility for covering your class with an appropriate substitute when absent. Arrive 10–15 minutes prior to class start. Prepare studio for the class being given. Restore class to its original state after teaching. Report to class coordinator upon arrival. Have music cued and ready at start of class time. Sign in on all class attendance sheets legibly on the date class is taught.

6. Model health and physical fitness by maintaining a high level of personal fitness.
7. Stay abreast of industry standards. Inform the group exercise coordinator and other fitness staff of any current trends.
8. Maintain current and up-to-date nationally recognized certification in group exercise and CPR/AED.
9. Adhere to the substitution policy. This term is nonnegotiable. All instructors are responsible for obtaining their own class coverage. They must inform the group class coordinator in a timely manner of any substitutions that they must make. No-shows are unacceptable and are grounds for termination.

### KNOWLEDGE

#### REQUIRED

Minimum current nationally recognized Group Exercise Certification and CPR/AED. Three years or more teaching experience.

#### PREFERRED

Degree in Dance, Exercise Science, or similar background. ACSM or ACE certifications. Specialty certifications. Five years or more teaching experience. Prior teaching experience in a corporate setting/background.

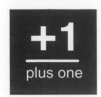

## JOB DESCRIPTION
## EXERCISE SPECIALIST/GROUP FITNESS DIRECTOR
**AREA OF SPECIALIZATION:    GROUP CLASS COORDINATION**
**REPORTS TO:    GENERAL MANAGER, MAY RECEIVE COUNSEL
FROM REGIONAL OR NATIONAL GROUP
FITNESS DIRECTORS**

## POSITION SUMMARY

To develop and implement appropriate exercise routines for members of clubs managed by Plus One Health Management in accordance with established policies, procedures, and protocols. The group fitness director is also responsible for the scheduling and implementing exercise classes and supervising the instructors to ensure member participation and satisfaction. Participate in all center activities with enthusiasm and ensure a safe and effective exercise environment.

## GENERAL RESPONSIBILITIES

1. Follow appropriate fire/emergency protocol to maintain club's safety.
2. Remain aware of potential hazards and unsafe conditions and report them to management.
3. Understand the operational standards for the fitness area.
4. Understand, support, and communicate information on current events/services and programs.
5. Provide inspired and motivational leadership in the training area.
6. Arriving for work at least 10 minutes early and being prepared to begin work on time.
7. Wear club uniform at all times.
8. Attend staff meetings.
9. Make the member the first priority always.
10. Greet all members by name.

11. Perform administrative duties including but not limited to: answering the phones according to Plus One standards, taking phone messages, sending and receiving e-mails, computer entry, faxing, photocopying, creating posters, updating bulletin boards, etc.
12. Routinely inspect training floor, locker areas, and classrooms for neatness and cleanliness including, but not limited to: stacking and restacking weights, classroom equipment, wiping down equipment, keeping areas dust and lint free, vacuuming, operating laundry equipment, folding and stocking towels and uniforms, replenishing locker room amenities, picking up towels, etc.

## PRINCIPAL DUTIES AND FUNCTIONS: EXERCISE SPECIALIST

1. Perform fitness evaluations and orientations in a safe and effective manner.
2. Interpret members' health history; evaluate procedures, and all other pertinent information formulating an appropriate exercise prescription.
3. Communicate information clearly and concisely in a positive manner.
4. Create, safe, effective exercise routines designed to meet individual client needs for apparently healthy and special populations.*
5. *Apply appropriate restrictions or limitations as incited by any physical or medical conditions.

6. Interact with members and prospective members in a friendly, understanding, and professional manner, while providing appropriate supervision at all times.
7. Review members' workouts on a daily basis and adjust accordingly to ensure a safe, effective exercise program.
8. Document incidents, client information, and follow-up as per protocol.
9. Respond immediately to any and all emergency situations in the club.
10. Complete administrative procedures/paperwork required in the fitness area.
11. Inspect all fitness equipment regularly and take corrective action if equipment is unsafe or broken.
12. Perform any job/task in the facility as needed.

## PRINCIPAL DUTIES AND FUNCTIONS: GROUP FITNESS DIRECTOR

1. Provide members with a schedule of classes that meets their needs and a group exercise staff that exceeds members' expectations.
2. Recruit, interview, select, and evaluate qualified instructors in compliance with Plus One Fitness Policy.
3. Ensure that group exercise programming and classes meet with operating standards of the club.
4. Actively participate as an instructor motivating members in classes.
5. Seek member feedback through biannual or annual survey of class participants.
6. Ensure that all classrooms are properly maintained and serviced and that any supplies, including schedules, sign-in sheets, etc. are adequately stocked.
7. Be current on exercise standards and trends in the field. Keep staff up to date on latest research and standards.
8. Maintain administration of classes including schedule changes, promotions, instructor changes, payroll, and substations.
9. Respond to member concerns within 24 hours via phone, email, fax, or personal meeting.
10. Attend Group Fitness Directors meeting via conference call or in person.

## KNOWLEDGE

### REQUIRED

- Minimum current ACE certification
- Current ACSM, ACE, **group exercise certification**

- Current CPR/AED certification
- Knowledge of exercise testing standards and orientations.
- Must secure two current certifications within 1 year of employment
- Willingness to learn or improve computer skills within the first 6 months of employment

### PREFERRED

- Bachelor's degree in Physical Education, Dance, Exercise Science, or related field
- ACSM, NASM, NSCA, indoor cycling, Pilates, yoga, or other specialized certification(s)
- Dance background
- Computer skills

## EXPERIENCE

### REQUIRED

- 3 years experience as personal trainer or fitness floor supervisor
- 1 year teaching group exercise
- Group leadership and motivational skills as demonstrated by audition
- Basic understanding of fitness testing and evaluation concepts, exercise equipment mechanics, and proper body alignment
- Demonstration of communication and service oriented skills

### PREFERRED

- 3+ years experience in the fitness field
- Administering fitness evaluations, orientations, and submaximal fitness tests
- 3+ years leading group exercise
- 1+ year coordinating group exercise programs

Comprehensive understanding of the principles of exercise, cardiovascular, strength, and flexibility training. Thorough understanding of all exercise machines, including proper application and use and correct positioning assuring correct form and technique of all exercises.

## SPECIAL WORK REQUIREMENTS

Flexible hours. Must be willing to work early mornings, evenings, and weekends as required.

# +1

## GROUP FITNESS INSTRUCTOR EVALUATION FORM

EMPLOYEE _____

SITE _____

DATE _____

CLASS _____ TIME _____

EVALUATOR _____

POSITION _____

APPRAISAL PERIOD:

FROM _____ TO _____

ANNUAL _____ OTHER _____

*To the employee,*
*The following evaluation is intended to assist both you and your director/supervisor in the overall assessment of your job. The evaluation will be discussed with you before it is recorded in your personnel record. You are requested to sign the evaluation although it is not necessary.*

*Thank you.*

**Evaluation Scale**

1 = poor  2 = below average  3 = average  4 = above average  5 = excellent
N/A = not applicable          N/O = not observed

## PART 1.  CLASS PREPARATION AND INTRODUCTION

**1.  Cues music before class?**

1            2            3            4            5            N/A            N/O

_____

_____

**2.  Starts class on time?**

1            2            3            4            5            N/A            N/O

_____

_____

**3.  Greets class by introducing self and class type?**

1            2            3            4            5            N/A            N/O

_____

_____

**4.  Asks for newcomers and exercise contraindications?**

1            2            3            4            5            N/A            N/O

_____

_____

**5.  Reminds students to work at their own pace?**

1            2            3            4            5            N/A            N/O

_____

_____

**6. Explains technique guidelines?**

1          2          3          4          5          N/A          N/O

_____

_____

## PART 2.  WARM-UP

**1.  Is appropriately timed?**

1          2          3          4          5          N/A          N/O

_____

_____

**2.  Uses movements designed to increase core temperature?**

1          2          3          4          5          N/A          N/O

_____

_____

**3.  Emphasizes proper muscle groups to type of class?**

1          2          3          4          5          N/A          N/O

_____

_____

**4.  Models new movement patterns?**

1          2          3          4          5          N/A          N/O

_____

_____

**5.  Includes instructional cues (alignment, safety, breathing)?**

1          2          3          4          5          N/A          N/O

_____

_____

# Part 3.  CENTRAL WORKOUT

### 1.  Matches the intensity to the level of the class?

| 1 | 2 | 3 | 4 | 5 | N/A | N/O |
|---|---|---|---|---|-----|-----|

_____

_____

### 2.  Is appropriately timed?

| 1 | 2 | 3 | 4 | 5 | N/A | N/O |
|---|---|---|---|---|-----|-----|

_____

_____

### 3.  Is appropriately paced?

| 1 | 2 | 3 | 4 | 5 | N/A | N/O |
|---|---|---|---|---|-----|-----|

_____

_____

### 4.  Cues in a timely manner?

| 1 | 2 | 3 | 4 | 5 | N/A | N/O |
|---|---|---|---|---|-----|-----|

_____

_____

### 5.  Offers safety, educational, and motivational cues?

| 1 | 2 | 3 | 4 | 5 | N/A | N/O |
|---|---|---|---|---|-----|-----|

_____

_____

### 6.  Interprets the phrasing of the music?

| 1 | 2 | 3 | 4 | 5 | N/A | N/O |
|---|---|---|---|---|-----|-----|

_____

_____

7. **Uses a variety of combinations and movement patterns?**

1                2                3                4                5                N/A                N/O

_____

_____

8. **Balances agonist and antagonist muscle groups?**

1                2                3                4                5                N/A                N/O

_____

_____

9. **Offers modifications and alternatives?**

1                2                3                4                5                N/A                N/O

_____

_____

10. **Is audible?**

1                2                3                4                5                N/A                N/O

_____

_____

11. **Uses RPE or heart rate?**

1                2                3                4                5                N/A                N/O

_____

_____

12. **Keeps the class moving during RPE or heart rate check?**

1                2                3                4                5                N/A                N/O

_____

_____

**13.  Adjusts level, observes students, and makes corrections?**

1                2                3                4                5                N/A                N/O

_____

_____

**14.  Is aware of technical indications and contraindications?**

1                2                3                4                5                N/A                N/O

_____

_____

# Part 4.  COOL-DOWN AND CONCLUSION

**1.  Is appropriately timed?**

1                2                3                4                5                N/A                N/O

_____

_____

**2.  Stretches muscles used during class?**

1                2                3                4                5                N/A                N/O

_____

_____

**3.  Emphasizes breathing?**

1                2                3                4                5                N/A                N/O

_____

_____

**4.  Thanks class for attending?**

1                2                3                4                5                N/A                N/O

_____

_____

**5. Makes necessary announcements?**

1   2   3   4   5   N/A   N/O

_____

_____

**6. Ends the class on time?**

1   2   3   4   5   N/A   N/O

_____

_____

**7. Is available after class for questions and comments?**

1   2   3   4   5   N/A   N/O

_____

_____

## Part 5.  OVERALL WORKOUT

**1. Follows proper BPM guidelines?**

1   2   3   4   5   N/A   N/O

_____

_____

**2. Selects suitable music?**

1   2   3   4   5   N/A   N/O

_____

_____

**3. Uses a variety of cues (auditory, visual, and tactile)?**

1   2   3   4   5   N/A   N/O

_____

**4. Maintains the music volume at an appropriate level?**

1            2            3            4            5          N/A          N/O

_____

_____

**5. Offers smooth transitions between moves?**

1            2            3            4            5          N/A          N/O

_____

_____

**6.  Includes all components as listed in class descriptions?**

1            2            3            4            5          N/A          N/O

_____

_____

**7.  Creates a safe and fun environment for the students?**

1            2            3            4            5          N/A          N/O

_____

_____

# Part 6.  PROFESSIONAL WORK HABITS AND SKILLS

**1.  Is appropriately groomed and attired?**

YES            NO

_____

_____

**2.  Is punctual?**

YES            NO

_____

_____

**3. Relates well to the students?**

YES          NO

_____

_____

**4. Makes eye contact throughout the class?**

YES          NO

_____

_____

**5. Encourages and motivates students?**

YES          NO

_____

_____

**6. Is able to "read" the group?**

YES          NO

_____

_____

**7. Uses proper vocal patterns?**

YES          NO

_____

_____

**8. Is innovative?**

YES          NO

_____

_____

**9.  Displays an appropriate level of personal fitness for the class?**

YES          NO

_____

_____

**10.  Conveys knowledge of fitness to students?**

YES          NO

_____

_____

**ADDITIONAL COMMENTS:**

_____

_____

_____

_____

_____

_____

# EMPLOYEE DEVELOPMENTAL ACTION PLAN

## EMPLOYEE'S MAIN PROFESSIONAL GOALS FOR THE NEXT YEAR

1. _____

_____

2. _____

_____

3. _____

_____

**OTHER:**

_____

_____

_____

**DIRECTOR/SUPERVISOR'S RECOMMENDATIONS:**

_____

_____

_____

**To the employee**:  Do you feel this review was complete, objective and accurate?

_____

_____

Employee's Signature _____    Date _____

*Your signature does not mean that you agree with this review. It is an acknowledgment that you have read and understand the content and have reviewed it with your director/supervisor.*

Director/Supervisor's Signature _____

Date _____

## Reference

1.  Reproduced with permission: Plus One Health management 2010, New York, NY. Reproduced with permission: Grace DeSimone, Plus One Health Management, 75 Maiden Lane, Suite 801 New York, NY 10038; 2010.

# ACSM Certified Group Exercise Instructor Job Task Analysis

The job task analysis (JTA) is intended to serve as a blueprint of the job of an ACSM Certified Group Exercise Instructor. As you prepare for the examination, it is important to remember that all questions are based on this outline.

## JOB DEFINITION

The ACSM Certified Group Exercise Instructor (GEI) (a) possesses a minimum of a high school diploma and (b) works in a group exercise setting with apparently healthy individuals and those with health challenges who are able to exercise independently to enhance quality of life, improve health-related physical fitness, manage health risk, and promote lasting health behavior change. The GEI leads safe and effective exercise programs using a variety of leadership techniques to foster group camaraderie, support, and motivation to enhance muscular strength and endurance, flexibility, cardiovascular fitness, body composition, and any of the motor skills related to the domains of health-related physical fitness.

## PERFORMANCE DOMAINS AND ASSOCIATED JOB TASKS

The JTA for the GEI certification describes what the professional does on a day-to-day basis. The JTA is divided into domains and associated tasks performed on the job. The percentages listed below indicate the number of questions representing each domain on the 100-question GEI examination.

The performance domains are

- Domain I: Participant and Program Assessment — 10%
- Domain II: Class Design — 25%
- Domain III: Leadership and Instruction — 55%
- Domain IV: Legal and Professional Responsibilities — 10%

## DOMAIN I: PARTICIPANT AND PROGRAM ASSESSMENT

### ASSOCIATED JOB TASKS

A. Evaluate and establish participant screening procedures to optimize safety and minimize risk by reviewing assessment protocols based on ACSM standards and guidelines.

1. Knowledge of

   a. appropriate techniques for health history assessment
   b. ACSM standards and guidelines related to preparticipation health history assessment
   c. ACSM preparticipation screening questionnaire related to screening of class participants

2. Skill in

   a. determining the adequacy of a facility's current preparticipation procedures
   b. developing and implementing preparticipation screening procedures

B. Administer and review, as necessary, participants' health risk assessments to determine if medical clearance is needed prior to exercise using PAR-Q, ACSM preparticipation screening, or other appropriate tools.

1. Knowledge of

   a. the use of informed consent and medical clearance prior to exercise participation
   b. ACSM guidelines related to preparticipation screening procedures
   c. ACSM model for classification of risk to aid in preparticipation screening (i.e., low, moderate, high risk)
   d. important health history information (e.g., past and present medical history, orthopedic limitations, prescribed medications, supplements, activity patterns, nutritional habits, stress and anxiety levels, family history of heart disease and other chronic diseases, smoking history, use of alcohol and illicit drugs, etc.)

2. Skill in

   a. determining when to recommend medical clearance
   b. administering preparticipation screening questionnaire
   c. determining classification of risk by evaluating screening questionnaire
   d. making appropriate recommendations based upon the results of screening questionnaire

C. Screen participants, as needed, for known acute or chronic conditions to provide recommendations and/or modifications.

1. **Knowledge of**

   a. common medical conditions and contraindications to group exercise participation
   b. risk factors, signs and symptoms, physical limitations, and medical conditions that may affect or preclude class participation
   c. appropriate criteria for NOT starting or stopping a participant from exercising

2. **Skill in**

   a. determining health status of group exercise class participants prior to each class
   b. determining when to recommend medical clearance
   c. making recommendations based on results of pre-exercise health status determination

## DOMAIN II: CLASS DESIGN

### ASSOCIATED JOB TASKS

A. Establish the purpose and determine the objectives of the class based upon the needs of the participants and facility.

1) **Knowledge of**

   a. methods used to determine the purpose of a group exercise class (e.g., survey, focus group, inquiry, word of mouth, suggestion box)
   b. types of group exercise classes (e.g., land based, water based, equipment based)
   c. types of equipment used in group exercise settings
   d. participant characteristics such as health, fitness, age, gender, ability
   e. health challenges and/or special needs commonly encountered in a group exercise setting
   f. environmental factors as they relate to the safe participation (e.g., outdoor, indoors, flooring, temperature, space, lighting, room size, ventilation)
   g. the types of different environments for group exercise such as outdoor, indoors, flooring, temperature, space, lighting, room size, ventilation and need to potentially adapt that environment

B. Determine class content (i.e., warm-up, stimulus, and cool-down) in order to create an effective workout based upon the objectives of the class.

1. **Knowledge of**

   a. the physiology of warm-up, stimulus, and cool-down
   b. the FITT principle (i.e., frequency, intensity, time, and type) for developing and/or maintaining cardiorespiratory fitness

   c. training principles (e.g., specificity, adaptation, overload)
   d. different training formats (e.g., continuous, circuit, interval, progressive classes such as 4–6-week sessions)
   e. exercise modification to most appropriately meet the needs of the class participants
   f. different teaching styles (e.g., formal, authoritarian, facilitator, nurturer)
   g. different learning styles (e.g., auditory, visual, kinesthetic)
   h. the use of music in group exercise

2. **Skill in**

   a. applying FITT principles (i.e., frequency, intensity, time, type) to class design
   b. organizing the warm-up, stimulus, and cool-down
   c. planning a class for participants with health challenges and special needs
   d. planning a class based on exercise environment and available equipment
   e. applying various styles of learning to most effectively meet the objectives of the class

C. Select and sequence appropriate exercises in order to provide a safe workout based upon the objectives of the class.

1. **Knowledge of**

   a. a variety of exercises used during warm-up, stimulus, and cool-down
   b. a variety of exercises to meet the needs of participants with different skill and fitness levels
   c. cardiovascular training principles and techniques
   d. muscular conditioning principles and techniques
   e. flexibility training principles and techniques
   f. motor fitness components (e.g., balance, agility, speed, coordination)
   g. the principles of muscle balance (e.g., flexion/extension, agonist/antagonist)
   h. exercise progression (e.g., easy/hard, slow/fast)
   i. health challenges and/or special needs commonly encountered in a group exercise setting
   j. risks associated with various exercises
   k. the benefits and use of music in class design

2. **Skill in**

   a. the selection and application of music given class purpose and objectives
   b. selecting and sequencing exercises to maintain muscle balance, minimize risk to the participants, and modify for those with health challenges and special needs
   c. designing transitions between exercises
   D. Rehearse class content, exercise selection, and sequencing, and revise as needed in order to

provide a safe and effective workout based upon the purpose and objectives of the class.

1. **Knowledge of**

   a. the purpose of class rehearsal
   b. proper execution of exercises and movements
   c. verbal and nonverbal cueing techniques for the purpose of providing direction, anticipation, motivation, and safety
   d. a variety of class environments (*e.g.,* outdoor, indoors, flooring, temperature, space, lighting, room size, ventilation) and associated adaptations that may be required

2. **Skill in**

   a. demonstrating exercises and movements
   b. the application of music, if used, given class purpose and objectives
   c. modifying class design based on rehearsal trial and error
   d. applying teaching styles (*e.g.,* formal, authoritarian, facilitator, nurturer)
   e. applying verbal cueing techniques for the purpose of providing direction, anticipation, motivation, and safety
   f. applying nonverbal cueing techniques (visual, directional)
   g. corresponding movements to music phrase and/or counts during selected exercises or segments

# DOMAIN III: LEADERSHIP AND INSTRUCTION

## ASSOCIATED JOB TASKS

A. Prepare to teach by implementing preclass procedures including screening new participants and organizing equipment, music, and room setup.

1. **Knowledge of**

   a. equipment operation (*e.g.,* audio, exercise equipment, facility)
   b. the procedures associated with determining the health status of group exercise class participants prior to each class
   c. class environment (*e.g.,* outdoor, indoors, flooring, temperature, space, lighting, room size, ventilation)

2. **Skill in**

   a. determining health status of group exercise class participants prior to each class
   b. time management
   c. delivering preclass announcements (welcome, instruction, safety, participant accountability)
   d. operating sound equipment
   e. evaluating and adapting, if needed, environment to maximize comfort and safety

B. Create a positive exercise environment in order to optimize participant adherence by incorporating effective motivational skills, communication techniques, and behavioral strategies.

1. **Knowledge of**

   a. motivational techniques
   b. modeling
   c. appropriate verbal and nonverbal behavior
   d. group behavior change strategies
   e. basic behavior change models and theories (*e.g.,* stages of change, self-efficacy, decisional balance, social learning theory)
   f. the types of feedback and appropriate use
   g. verbal (voice tone, inflection) and nonverbal (body language) communication skills

2. **Skill in**

   a. applying behavior change strategies
   b. applying behavior change models and theories
   c. applying communication techniques (verbal and nonverbal/body language)
   d. fostering group cohesion
   e. interacting with class participants
   f. providing positive feedback to class participants
   g. projecting enthusiasm, energy, and passion
   h. applying techniques addressing various styles of learning

C. Demonstrate all exercises using proper form and technique to ensure safe execution in accordance with ACSM standards and guidelines.

1. **Knowledge of**

   a. basic human functional anatomy and biomechanics
   b. basic exercise physiology
   c. basic ergonomic principles
   d. proper alignment, form and technique
   e. high-risk exercises and movements

2. **Skill in**

   a. demonstrating proper alignment, form, and technique
   b. demonstrating exercise modifications
   c. correcting improper form and/or technique
   D. Incorporate verbal and nonverbal instructional cues in order to optimize communication, safety, and motivation based upon industry guidelines

1. **Knowledge of**

   a. anticipatory, directional, educational, motivational, safety, tactile, and visual cueing techniques
   b. proper participant performance

**2. Skill in**

a. applying anticipatory, directional, educational, motivational, safety, tactile, and visual cues
b. monitoring participants' performance
c. instructing participants how to correct their own exercise execution and/or form

E. Monitor participants' performance to ensure safe and effective exercise execution using observation and participant feedback techniques in accordance with ACSM standards and guidelines.

**1. Knowledge of**

a. safe and effective exercise execution
b. the rationale for exercise intensity monitoring
c. exercise intensity monitoring methods and limitations
d. exercise programming (*e.g.,* mode, intensity, frequency, duration)
e. the signs and symptoms of overexertion
f. proper exercise demonstration techniques
g. proper feedback techniques (*i.e.,* visual and auditory)
h. normal and adverse response to exercise
i. appropriate criteria for NOT starting or stopping a participant from exercising

**2. Skill in**

a. safe and effective exercise execution
b. monitoring exercise intensity in class participants
c. recognizing signs and symptoms of overexertion
d. applying the principles of exercise programming (*e.g.,* mode, intensity, frequency, duration)
e. teaching participants how to monitor and modify their own exercise intensity
f. proper exercise demonstration techniques
g. proper feedback techniques (*i.e.,* visual and auditory)

F. Modify exercises based on individual and group needs to ensure safety and effectiveness in accordance with ACSM standards and guidelines.

**1. Knowledge of**

a. cardiovascular response to various environmental conditions
b. how aerobic, strength and flexibility exercise modifications affect intensity and safety
c. various exercise safety and intensity modification techniques (*e.g.,* tempo, range of motion, alternate movements, load)
d. a variety of exercises for any particular muscle group, from easiest to hardest
e. the American Congress of Obstetricians and Gynecologists (ACOG) recommendations for exercise during pregnancy

**2. Skill in**

a. modifying exercise execution and intensity based on environmental conditions
b. modifying aerobic, strength, and flexibility exercise intensity based on environmental condition, individual and/or group needs
c. applying exercise intensity modification techniques (*e.g.,* tempo, range of motion, alternate movements, load)

G. Monitor sound levels of vocal and/or audio equipment following industry guidelines.

**1. Knowledge of**

a. appropriate vocal projection techniques
b. the value of vocal warm-up
c. vocal warm-up techniques
d. safe volume level
e. group exercise sound projection technology (*e.g.,* microphones, amplifiers, speakers)

**2. Skill in**

a. the application of appropriate vocal projection techniques
b. the application of group exercise sound projection equipment (*e.g.,* microphones, amplifiers, speakers)

H. Respond to participants' concerns in order to maintain a professional, equitable, and safe environment by using appropriate conflict management or customer service strategies set forth by facility policy and procedures and industry guidelines.

**1. Knowledge of**

a. conflict prevention
b. basic conflict resolution techniques
c. communication techniques as they relate to conflict resolution (*e.g.,* active listening, mirroring, reflection)
d. specific club policies regarding conflict management and your role in application of policies

**2. Skill in**

a. applying conflict resolution techniques
b. applying empathetic listening skills
c. selecting the appropriate resolution

I. Educate participants in order to enhance knowledge, enjoyment, and adherence by providing health- and fitness-related information and resources.

**1. Knowledge of**

a. basic human functional anatomy and biomechanics
b. basic exercise physiology
c. basic human development and aging

d. the basic principles of weight management and nutrition

e. motivational techniques used to promote behavior change in the initiation, adherence or return to exercise

f. benefits and risks of exercise

g. basic ergonomic principles

h. stress management principles and techniques

i. healthy lifestyle practices and behavior

j. credible, current, and pertinent health-related information

k. risk factors that may require referral to medical or allied health professionals prior to exercise

2. **Skill in**

a. accessing available health- and exercise-related information

b. delivering health- and exercise-related information

c. referring participant to appropriate medical or allied health professional when warranted

# DOMAIN IV: LEGAL AND PROFESSIONAL RESPONSIBILITIES

## ASSOCIATED JOB TASKS

A. Evaluate the class environment (*e.g.,* outdoor, indoor, capacity, flooring, temperature, ventilation, lighting, equipment, acoustics) to minimize risk and optimize safety by following preclass inspection procedures based on established facility and industry standards and guidelines.

1. **Knowledge of**

a. ACSM facility standards and guidelines

b. established regulations and laws (*e.g.,* Americans with Disabilities Act, CDC, OSHA)

c. the procedures associated with determining the health status of group exercise class participants prior to each class

2. **Skill in**

a. evaluating classroom environment

B. Promote participants' awareness and accountability by informing them of classroom safety procedures and exercise and intensity options in order to minimize risk.

1. **Knowledge of**

a. components that contribute to a safe environment

b. safety guidelines as they relates to group exercise

2. **Skill in**

a. communicating safety precautions before and during class

b. observing compliance with instructions provided to participants

c. cueing to reinforce safety precautions during class

C. Follow industry-accepted professional, ethical, and business standards in order to optimize safety and reduce liability.

1. **Knowledge of**

a. appropriate professional behavior and boundaries pertaining to class participants

b. the ACSM code of ethics

c. the scope of practice of an ACSM Certified GEI

d. standards of care for an ACSM Certified GEI

e. informed consent, assumption of risk, and waivers

f. established and applicable laws, regulations, and policies

g. bounds of competence

h. established and applicable laws, regulations, and policies

i. confidentiality, privacy laws, and practice

j. insurance needs (*e.g.,* professional liability, general liability insurance)

k. basic business principles (*e.g.,* contracts, negligence, types of business entities, tax business structure, advertising, marketing)

2. **Skill in**

a. applying professional behavior and in maintaining appropriate boundaries with class participants

b. applying the ACSM code of ethics

c. assuring and maintaining the privacy of all group exercise participants and any pertinent information relating to them or their membership

D. Respond to emergencies in order to minimize untoward events by following procedures consistent with established standards of care and facility policies.

1. **Knowledge of**

a. Adult CPR

b. automated external defibrillator (AED)

c. basic first aid for accidents, environmental and medical emergencies (*e.g.,* heat cramps, heat exhaustion, heat stroke, lacerations, incisions, puncture wounds, abrasions, contusions, simple/compound fractures, bleeding/shock, hypoglycemia, hyperglycemia, sprains, strains, fainting)

d. the standard of care for emergency response (*e.g.,* incident reporting, injury assessment, activating emergency medical services)

e. the Emergency Action Plan, if applicable, for the fitness facility

f. unsafe or controversial exercises

2. **Skill in**

a. activating emergency medical services

b. administering CPR

c. administering an AED

d. administering basic first aid for exercise-related injuries, accidents, environmental and medical emergencies (*e.g.,* assessment, response, management of class or environment)

e. documenting incidents and/or emergencies

f. selecting exercises that are not controversial or high risk

E. Respect copyrights to protect original and creative work, media, etc. by legally securing copyright material and other intellectual property based on national and international copyright laws.

1. **Knowledge of**

a. copyright laws (*e.g.,* BMI, ASCAP)

b. fair use of copyright material

2. **Skill in**

a. acquiring appropriate copyrighted materials and music

F. Engage in healthy lifestyle practices in order to be a positive role model for class participants.

1. **Knowledge of**

a. healthy lifestyle practices

b. lifestyle behavior change strategies (cognitive and behavioral)

c. appropriate modeling behaviors (*e.g.,* nonthreatening, motivating)

d. risks associated with overtraining

e. body image concepts and perceptions

f. risks associated with the female athlete triad

g. referral practices to allied health professionals

2. **Skill in**

a. applying healthy lifestyle practices

b. communicating healthy lifestyle information

c. personalizing behavioral strategies to class participants

d. recognizing the symptoms of overtraining

e. referring participants to appropriate allied health professionals when necessary

f. identifying issues/behavior related to unhealthy body image and making appropriate referrals

G. Select and participate in continuing education programs that enhance knowledge and skills on a continuing basis, maximize effectiveness, and increase professionalism in the field.

1. **Knowledge of**

a. continuing education requirements for ACSM certification

b. continuing education resources (*e.g.,* conferences, workshops, correspondence courses, online, college/university based, journals)

c. credible, current, and pertinent health-related information

2. **Skill in**

a. obtaining relevant continuing education

b. applying credible, current, and pertinent health-related information when leading the class

# Rating of Perceived Exertion (RPE)

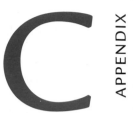

| Table C.1 | CATEGORY (6 TO 20) AND CATEGORY-RATIO (0 – 10) SCALES FOR RATINGS OF PERCEIVED EXERTION | |
|---|---|---|
| **CATEGORY SCALE** | **CATEGORY-RATIO SCALE** | **DESCRIPTOR** |
| 6 No exertion at all | 0 Nothing at all | |
| 7 Extremely light | 0.3 | |
| 8 | 0.5 Extremely weak | Just noticeable |
| 9 Very light | 0.7 | |
| 10 | 1 Very weak | |
| 11 Light | 1.5 | |
| 12 | 2 Weak | Light |
| 13 Somewhat hard | 2.5 | |
| 14 | 3 Moderate | |
| 15 Hard (heavy) | 4 | |
| 16 | 5 Strong | Heavy |
| 17 Very hard | 6 | |
| 18 | 7 Very strong | |
| 19 Extremely hard | 8 | |
| 20 Maximal exertion | 9 | |
| | 10 Extremely strong | "Maximal" |
| | 11 Absolute maximum | Highest possible |

From Resources for the Personal Trainer, 3rd edition, page 180. Copyright Gunnar Borg. Reproduced with permission. For correct use of the Borg scales, it is necessary to follow the administration and instructions given in Borg G. Borg's Perceived Exertion and Pain Scales. Champaign (IL): Human Kinetics; 1998

The RPE scale is a convenient and easy way to monitor how hard you or your students are working during exercise. The RPE scale measures feelings of effort, strain, discomfort, and/or fatigue experienced during both aerobic and resistance exercise. RPE is a guideline to use when setting or determining exercise intensity (1,2).

Two scales are typically used. Table C-1 lists the 6–20 RPE category scale as well as the category ratio scale that rates exercise intensity on a scale of 0 to 10 (1). RPE can be used to rate subjectively overall feelings of exertion and therefore can be helpful in guiding exercise intensity. The threshold level for cardiorespiratory benefits seems to be between 12 and 16 on the original scale and 4 or 5 on the ratio scale (1,2). The verbal descriptors for this range include "somewhat hard" to "hard."

For example, an RPE of "11" should have you breathing a bit quickly but you should be able to continue the activity without too much trouble. An RPE of "19" should be extremely challenging, and you should not be able to continue the activity at that level for a prolonged period of time.

When using RPE, the Group Exercise Instructor should keep in mind that there is variability between individuals. So, the RPE value may not necessarily correspond directly with a particular percentage of maximal heart rate, and the student and the Group Exercise Instructor must then make adjustments as needed (1). RPE is especially helpful for individuals who have difficulty determining exercise heart rate or for those who are taking medications, which influence heart rate (e.g., beta-blockers).

Use RPE to assess how hard students are working after a set or timed interval. Teach the class the range of RPE in which they should be working. This is especially helpful when teaching indoor cycling, strength training, or interval training classes.

## References

1. American College of Sports Medicine. ACSM's Guidelines for Exercise Testing and Prescription, 8th ed. Baltimore: LippincottWilliams & Wilkins, 2010:82–83.

2. Thompson, W (ed.). ACSM's Resources for the Personal Trainer, 3rd ed. Baltimore: Lippincott Williams & Wilkins, 2010:373–374, 380.

# Index

Note: The page numbers in *italics* denote figures; those followed by "t" denote tables; and those followed by "b" denote boxes.